Laboratory/Pathology Words and Phrases

Laboratory Medicine
Anatomic Pathology
Clinical Pathology
Hematology
Dermatopathology

Health Professions Institute • Modesto, California • 1996

Laboratory/Pathology Words and Phrases

Laboratory Medicine, Anatomic Pathology, Clinical Pathology, Hematology, Dermatopathology

Sally Crenshaw Pitman
Editor & Publisher
Health Professions Institute
P. O. Box 801
Modesto, CA 95353-0801
Phone 209-551-2112
Fax 209-551-0404
E-mail: hpi@ainet.com
Web site: http://www.hpisum.com

Printed by
Parks Printing & Lithograph
Modesto, California

ISBN 0-934385-66-1

Last digit is the print number: 9 8 7 6 5 4

To

Leon Sidney Pitman

Contents

Preface

Laboratory/Pathology Words and Phrases is more than an update of the classic *Pathology Words and Phrases* published in 1988. It has been greatly expanded to include over 45,000 entries from laboratory medicine, anatomic and clinical pathology, hematology, and dermatopathology. (In the fall 1996 second printing, the title was changed from *Pathology/Laboratory* to *Laboratory/Pathology* to more accurately reflect the book's emphasis on laboratory terminology, lab values, lab tests, pathogens, and anatomy.)

A special feature includes 80 pages of tables of arteries, bones, muscles, nerves, and veins, listing both English and Latin forms in tabular form for quick reference. The appendix also includes an extensive table of normal laboratory values of blood, urine, and miscellaneous body fluids.

Another useful feature is an extensive list of bacteria, fungi, parasites, and viruses under the broad term *pathogen*. This should make it easier for students and others new to the field of medicine to find the name of a "bug" used in medical reports when it is not known what kind of organism it is.

Much terminology in pathology, laboratory medicine, hematology, and dermatopathology is related to neoplastic disease entities and conditions involving the cellular level, and this book necessarily includes thousands of carcinogen-related terms. A list of over 1200 laboratory tests is provided in the text.

This book is by no means an exhaustive list of words and phrases in the laboratory/pathology specialties, but we are confident that we have gathered the most relevant and useful words and phrases in those specialties. We've culled words and phrases from hundreds of transcripts of medical dictation, as well as laboratory medicine references, anatomy textbooks, scholarly journals in all specialties, and other printed and electronic references.

We hope that this book will be useful for medical transcriptionists in all specialties, not just those who work exclusively in the pathology department or laboratory. Physicians and other healthcare professionals who dictate patient health records refer to laboratory medicine and pathology in almost every report, and use anatomical terms extensively in operative reports, autopsies, and cellular pathology studies. The difficulty in compiling this quick-reference book of laboratory/pathology words and phrases was not in *finding* sufficient terms, but in *limiting* the terms to the ones most likely to be found in dictation of medical reports.

The research, editing, and proofreading of this book were done primarily by Kathy Cameron, Linda Campbell, Catherine Baxter, Dr. John H. Dirckx, and Bron Taylor. My warmest gratitude to all.

Sally Crenshaw Pitman
Editor & Publisher

How to Use This Book

The words and phrases in this book are alphabetized letter by letter of all words in the entry, ignoring punctuation marks and words or letters in parentheses. The possessive form ('s) is omitted from eponyms for ease in alphabetizing. Numbers are alphabetized as if written out, with the exception of subscripts and superscripts which are ignored.

Eponyms may be located alphabetically as well as under the nouns they modify. For example, *acid-fast bacillus (AFB) stain* is found alphabetically under the A's as well as under the main entry *stain*. *Döderlein bacillus* is found in the D's as well as under the broad category *pathogen*, which includes a list of over a thousand organisms. Under *bacillus, bacteria, fungus, organism, parasite,* and *virus,* there is a *see pathogen* reference.

The extensive list of pathogens should be particularly helpful to students and inexperienced medical transcriptionists who find it difficult to determine the correct spelling of "bugs" dictated in medical reports. Physician dictators may not state what kind of organism a term is and thus the student does not know whether to look under *bacillus, bacteria, fungus, organism, parasite,* or *virus* (and usually ends up looking under every possibility before finding the correct term). The physician may dictate the formal name of an organism, such as *Escherichia coli* or *Clostridium difficile,* or part of a name (*Escherichia* or *Clostridium*), or an abbreviated form (such as *E. coli* or "*C. diff*"). All the terms are easily found in this book alphabetically as well as under the broad category *pathogen*.

The main entries *artery, bone, muscle, nerve,* and *vein* include phrases and descriptive terms related to those terms as they are dictated in patient reports, rather than the names of anatomical terms and eponyms which are instead listed in the Appendix in tabular form, with both the English and Latin forms given. The anatomical tables in the Appendix should be helpful to medical transcriptionists trying to find a correct spelling when it may not be clear if the term is in English or Latin, or whether the term is an artery or a muscle.

The fact that many physicians dictate strings of abbreviations and brief forms presents special difficulties for students and less experienced transcriptionists. Laboratory data is particularly difficult to transcribe, yet the accuracy of its transcription is essential to quality patient records. A table of laboratory tests that may be encountered in patient health records is provided in the Appendix, with examples of "normal" laboratory values. Of course, what is determined to be "normal" varies from laboratory to laboratory, and the values presented are intended for reference only.

A, a

A (alpha)
A albumin
AA (amyloid A) protein
AAT (alpha$_1$-antitrypsin)
Ab (antibody)
A band
abapical pole
abarticulation
Abbe-Zeiss counting cell
Abbott VP analyzer
ABC (aspiration biopsy cytology)
ABC peroxidase method of staining
ABC (avidin-biotin complex)
abdomen
   apertures of
   boatlike
   concave
   fascia of
   roof of
   scaphoid
abdominal aorta
abdominal aortic artery
abdominal aortic plexus
abdominal aponeurosis
abdominal apron
abdominal canal
abdominal cavity

abdominal contents
abdominal cramp
abdominal fissure
abdominal fistula
abdominal kidney
abdominal lymph node
abdominal muscle
abdominal ostium
abdominal pad
abdominal panniculus
abdominal pannus
abdominal pregnancy
abdominal pulse
abdominal raphe
abdominal reflex
abdominal region
abdominal ring
abdominal sac
abdominal stoma
abdominal viscera
abdominal wall venous pattern
abdominal zone
abdominis muscle
   rectus
   transversus
abdominocardiac reflex
abdominogenital

1

abdominopelvic cavity
abdominopelvic viscera
abdominoscrotal
abdominothoracic arch
abdominovaginal
abdominovesical
abducens nucleus
abducent nerve
abductor muscle
Abel bacillus
Abell-Kendall method
Abelson murine leukemia virus
Abercrombie degeneration
Abernethy fascia
Abernethy sarcoma
aberrant artery
aberrant bile duct
aberrant bundle
aberrant duct
aberrant ductule
aberrant ganglion
aberrant goiter
aberrant hemoglobin
aberrant tissue
aberration
abetalipoproteinemia, hereditary
ABGs (arterial blood gases)
A bile
abnormal capillary fragility
abnormal formation of connective
   tissue
abnormal hardening of tissue
abnormal increase in circulating
   leukocytes
abnormal mitochondrial protein
abnormal ossification
abnormal test result
abnormal whiteness of skin
abnormalities of development
abnormalities of urine
ABO and Rh blood typing
ABO blood group

ABO blood type
ABO factor
abomasal groove
abomasum
aborted fetus
abortion
   accidental
   ampullar
   artificial
   complete
   complications of
   habitual
   idiopathic
   imminent
   incomplete
   induced
   inevitable
   infected
   missed
   recurrent
   septic
   spontaneous
   therapeutic
   threatened
   tubal
abortion in progress
abortive pneumonia
abortus bacillus
ABP (androgen binding protein)
abraded wound
Abrams needle
abrasion
abruptio placentae
abscess
   acute
   alveolar
   ambolic
   amebic
   apical
   appendiceal
   arthrifluent
   bartholinian

abscess *(continued)*
Bartholin (of vulvovaginal gland)
bartholinitis
Bezold
bicameral
bile duct
biliary
bone
brain
broad ligament
Brodie
bursal
canalicular
caseous
cheesy
cholangitic
chronic
circumtonsillar
cold
collar-button
colonic
crypt
cutaneous
dental
dentoalveolar
diffuse
Douglas
dry
Dubois
encapsulated
epidural
epiploic
extradural
fecal
follicular
frontal
gas
gingival
gravitation
helminthic
hematogenous
hepatic

abscess *(continued)*
hot
hypostatic
iliopsoas muscle
intradural
intramastoid
ischiorectal
kidney
lacrimal
lacunar
luetic
lung
lymphatic
mammary
mastoid
metastatic
metastatic tuberculous
migrating
miliary
Munro
orbital
otic
otogenous
ovarian
palatal
pancreatic
parametrial
parametric
paranephric
parotid
Pautrier
pelvic
pelvirectal
perforating
periapical
periappendiceal
periarticular
pericoronal
perinephric
periodontal
peripleuritic
perirectal

abscess *(continued)*
  peritoneal
  peritonsillar
  periureteral
  phlegmonous
  phoenix
  Pott
  premammary
  prostatic
  psoas
  pulp
  pyemic
  radicular
  renal
  residual
  retrobulbar
  retrocecal
  retroperitoneal
  retropharyngeal
  retrotonsillar
  ring
  root
  satellite
  septicemic
  shirt-stud
  solitary cutaneous
  spermatic
  splenic
  stellate
  stercoral
  sterile
  stitch
  subaponeurotic
  subareolar
  subdiaphragmatic
  subdural
  subepidermal
  subfascial
  subgaleal
  subhepatic
  subpectoral
  subperiosteal

abscess *(continued)*
  subphrenic
  subscapular
  subungual
  sudoriparous
  superficial
  suprahepatic
  syphilitic
  thecal
  thymic
  Tornwaldt
  tropical
  tuberculous
  tubo-ovarian
  tympanitic
  tympanocervical
  tympanomastoid
  urethral
  urinary
  verminous
  vitreous
  wandering
  Welch
  worm
abscess culture
abscess formation
absence of myelin
absence of peripheral pulses
Absidia corymbifera
absolute count
absolute neutrophil count (ANC)
absolute scale
absolute temperature scale
absorption apparatus
absorption band
absorption cell
absorption fever
absorption line
absorption of tissue debris
absorptive cells of intestine
abutting
ACA (anticardiolipin antibody)

acantha
Acanthamoeba
acanthion
acanthocyte (spur cell)
acanthokeratoderma
acantholysis
acanthoma
acanthosis, saw-toothed
acariasis
acarine dermatosis
acarodermatitis
Acarus
Acarus rhyzoglypticus hyacinthi
accelerated hypertension
accelerator factor
accelerator fiber
accelerator globulin (AcG)
accelerator nerve
accelerator urinae muscle
accessioning
accession number
accessory adrenal
accessory atrium
accessory auricle
accessory bone
accessory breast
accessory canal
accessory cartilage
accessory cell
accessory cephalic vein
accessory chromosome
accessory cuneate nucleus
accessory digit
accessory flocculus
accessory gland
accessory hemiazygos vein
accessory hepatic duct
accessory lacrimal gland
accessory ligament
accessory meningeal artery
accessory nasal cartilage
accessory nerve

accessory nerve lymph node
accessory nipple
accessory obturator artery
accessory obturator nerve
accessory olivary nucleus
accessory organ
accessory pancreas
accessory pancreatic duct
accessory parotid gland
accessory phrenic nerve
accessory placenta
accessory plantar ligament
accessory process
accessory pudendal artery
accessory quadrate cartilage
accessory saphenous vein
accessory sinus
accessory spleen
accessory suprarenal gland
accessory thyroid gland
accessory tubercle
accessory vertebral vein
accessory visual apparatus
accessory volar ligament
accidental abortion
accidental proteinuria
accidental termination of pregnancy
accidental tissue
accommodate
accommodation reflex
accompanying vein
accretion line
Accu-Chek glucose monitor
accumulation analysis
accumulation of sphingomyelin in
    marrow histiocytes
accumulation of spinal fluid, abnormal
ACE (angiotensin converting enzyme)
A cell
acellular
acetabular artery
acetabular bone

acetabular fossa
acetabular labrum
acetabular notch
acetabulum
acetaldehyde test
Acetest
acetic acid
acetic acid stain
acetone body
acetone-insoluble antigen
acetone in urine test
acetonitrile
acetowhite epithelium
acetowhite reaction
acetowhite test
acetyl-activating enzyme
acetylcholine receptor antibody
acetylcholinesterase
acetylsalicylic acid
AcG, ac-g (accelerator globulin)
Ac-globulin (accelerator)
ACh (acetylcholine)
A chain
achalasia of esophagus
Achilles bursa
Achilles tendon
achlorhydria, gastric
acholic stool
acholuric jaundice
achondroplasia
achondroplastic dwarfism
AChRab (acetylcholine receptor)
    antibody
achrestic anemia
achromatic apparatus
achromatosis
achromia
achromic nevus
Achromobacter xylosoxidans
acid
    acetic
    acetylsalicylic

acid *(continued)*
    alpha amino
    amino
    aminolevulinic (ALA)
    aromatic amino
    ascorbic
    beta-hydroxybutyric
    bile
    branched chain amino
    carbonic
    choleic
    conjugated bile
    delta-aminolevulinic
    essential fatty
    ethylenediaminetetraacetic (EDTA)
    fatty
    fecal bile
    folic
    glacial acetic
    glucuronic
    homogentisic
    homovanillic (HVA)
    hydrochloric (HCl)
    lactic
    lipid-associated sialic
    medium chain fatty
    nitric
    organic
    osmic
    oxalic
    picric
    propionic
    pyruvic
    salicylic
    short chain fatty
    sialic
    sulfuric
    tartaric
    un-ionized
    uric
    valproic
    vanillylmandelic (VMA)

acid albumin
acid alcohol solution
acid aspiration pneumonitis
acid-base balance
acid-base reaction
acid cell
acid dye
acid elution test for fetal hemoglobin
acidemia
acid environment
acid-fast bacillus (AFB) (pl. bacilli)
acid-fast bacillus (AFB) stain
acid-fastness
acid-fast organism
acid-fast staining
acid fuchsin stain
acid gland
acid hematoxylin stain
acidic metabolite
acidified alcohol
acidified serum test for paroxysmal
 nocturnal hemoglobinuria
acid-lability test
acidophil (also acidophilic)
acidophil adenoma
acidophil body
acidophil cell
acidophil granule
acidophil leukocyte
acidosis
 diabetic
 lactic
 metabolic
 renal tubular
 respiratory
 starvation
 uremic
acid-peptic juice
acid perfusion test
acid phosphatase
 leukocyte
 prostatic

acid phosphatase *(continued)*
 semen
 tartrate resistant acid serum test
acid reflux test
acid serum test
acid-staining cell
acid-wash treatment
acinar architecture
acinar cell
acinar tissue
Acinetobacter calcoaceticus, var.
 anitratus (formerly *Herellea*
 vaginicola)
Acinetobacter calcoaceticus, var. *lwoffi*
 (formerly *Mima polymorpha*)
aciniform
acinitis
acinotubular gland
acinous cell
acinous cell carcinoma
acinous gland
acinus (pl. acini)
 cup-shaped
 flask-shaped
aclasis
acne
acnegenic
acneiform pustule
acne keloid
acne vulgaris
acortical artery
acoustic cell
acoustic crest
acoustic cyst
acoustic immittance test
acoustic meatus
acoustic nerve
acoustic neurilemoma
acoustic neuroma
acousticofacial crest
acousticofacial ganglion
acoustic papilla

acoustic stria
acoustic trauma
acoustic tubercle
acoustic vesicle
acquired aneurysm
acquired cuticle
acquired defect
acquired deficiency
acquired hemolyzing antibodies
acquired immune deficiency
    syndrome (AIDS)
acquired methemoglobinemia
acquired nevus
acquired reflex
acquired tufted angioma
acral-lentiginous melanoma
Acremonium
Acremonium falciforme
Acremonium kiliense
Acremonium recifei
Acremonium restrictum
acrodermatitis
acrodermatitis continua
acrodermatitis enteropathica
acrodermatosis
acrokeratosis
acromegaly
acromial angle
acromial artery
acromial articular facies
acromial articular surface
acromial bone
acromial extremity
acromial process
acromial reflex
acromioclavicular disk
acromioclavicular joint
acromion
acromiothoracic artery
acrosclerosis
acrosomal cap
acrosomal granule

acrosomal vesicle
acrylamide/urea gel
ACTH (adrenocorticotropic hormone)
ACTH antibody
ACTH stimulation test
actin filament
actinic dermatitis
actinic keratitis
actinic keratosis
actinic prurigo
actinium emanation
Actinobacillus actinomycetemcomitans
Actinobacillus equuli
Actinobacillus hominis
Actinobacillus lignieresii
Actinobacillus suis
Actinomadura
Actinomyces
Actinomyces gonidiaformis
Actinomyces in suppurative and
    granulomatous infections
Actinomyces israelii
Actinomyces meyeri
Actinomyces naeslundii
Actinomyces odontolyticus
Actinomyces viscosus
actinomycosis
actinomycotic mycetoma
activated coagulation time (ACT)
activated fatty acid
activated partial thromboplastin
    substitution test
activated partial thromboplastin time
    (APTT)
activated protein C
activation analysis
activator, plasminogen
active congestion
active hyperemia
activity
    enzyme
    mitotic

acuminatum, condyloma
acute abscess
acute arteritis
acute benign pericarditis
acute bronchitis
acute compression triad
acute disseminated myositis
acute eosinophilic pneumonia
acute febrile neutrophilic dermatosis
acute fibrinous pericarditis
acute gastritis
acute glomerulonephritis
acute granulocytic leukemia
acute hemorrhagic cystitis
acute hemorrhagic pancreatitis
acute idiopathic polyneuritis
acute infectious gastroenteritis
acute intermittent porphyria (AIP)
acute interstitial myocarditis
acute interstitial pancreatitis
acute interstitial pneumonitis
acute isolated myocarditis
acute leukemia
acute lymphoblastic leukemia
    B-cell type
    Burkitt-like
    common type
    null cell type
    pre-B-cell type
    T-cell type
acute malaria
acute mastitis
acute mastoiditis
acute megakaryoblastic leukemia
acute monocytic leukemia
acute myelitis
acute myeloblastic leukemia
acute myelogenous leukemia (AML)
acute myelomonocytic leukemia
acute myoendocarditis
acute necrotizing encephalitis
acute nephritis

acute nephrosis
acute osteitis
acute pancreatitis
acute parenchymatous hepatitis
acute phase protein
acute phase reactant
acute pleurisy
acute pneumonia
acute porphyria
acute poststreptococcal glomerulo-
    nephritis
acute progressive myositis
acute promyelocytic leukemia
acute pyelonephritis
acute renal failure
acute rheumatic fever
acute rheumatic myocarditis
acute serum
acute suppurative parotitis
acute thyroiditis
acute tubular necrosis (ATN)
acute undifferentiated leukemia (AUL)
acute vascular purpura
acute yellow atrophy
acyl carrier protein
adamantinoma
Adamkiewicz, spinal artery of
Adam's apple
adaptive enzyme
adaptive hyperplasia
Addis count
Addison disease
addisonian crisis
Addison point
Addis test
adductor canal
adductor muscle
adductor reflex
adductor tubercle
adelomorphous cell
Aden fever
adeno-associated virus

adenocarcinoma
  acinous
  alveolar
  bronchogenic
  cervical
  clear cell
  colon
  cyst
  endometrial
  epithelium
  follicular
  liver
  lung
  moderately differentiated
  mucinous
  ovarian
  papillary
  polypoid
  poorly differentiated
  prostate
  serous
  undifferentiated
  urachal
  vaginal
  well-differentiated
adenocyst
adenocystoma
adenoidal
adenoiditis, follicular
adenoid pattern
adenoids
adenoid tissue
adenoma
  acidophil
  adrenal cortex
  basophil
  chromophobe
  colonic
  epithelial
  Hürthle cell (Huerthle)
  mammary
  parathyroid

adenomatous goiter
adenomatous hyperplasia
adenomatous polyp
adenomatous polyposis coli (APC)
adenomyosis
adenosine deaminase deficiency
adenosine monophosphate (AMP)
adenosine triphosphatase (ATPase)
adenosis
  mammary
  vaginal
adenovirus
adenovirus antibody titer
adenovirus antigen
adenovirus immunofluorescence
adenovirus type 8
adequal cleavage
adermia
adermogenesis
ADH (antidiuretic hormone)
adherent placenta
adhesed
adhesion
  bandlike
  banjo-string
  fibrous
  meningeal
  violin-string
adhesive inflammation
adhesive pericarditis
adhesive pleurisy
adhesive vaginitis
adipocere
adipocyte
adipokinetic hormone
adiponecrosis
adipose capsule of kidney
adipose cell
adipose degeneration
adipose fold
adipose fossa
adipose infiltration

adipose tissue
adiposis dolorosa
adiposity
adiposogenital degeneration
adiposus, panniculus
A disk
adjacent angle
adjuvant
admaxillary gland
admitting diagnosis
admixed
admixture
adnexal
adnexa mastoidea
adnexa oculi
adnexa uteri
adrenal androgen
adrenal antibody
adrenal atrophy
adrenal body
adrenal capsule
adrenal cortex
adrenal cortex adenoma
adrenal cortical deficiency
adrenal failure
adrenal gland
   accessory
   Marchand
adrenal hemorrhage
adrenal hypertension
Adrenalin
adrenaline
adrenaline acid tartrate
adrenal medulla
adrenal mineralocorticoids
adrenal tumor
adrenal weight factor
adrenocortical hyperplasia
adrenocortical steroid therapy
adrenocorticotropic hormone (ACTH)
adrenocorticotropic peptide
adrenocorticotropic releasing factor

adrenogenic tissue
adrenogenital syndrome
adrenotropic hormone
adsorption
adult-onset diabetes
adult-onset diabetes mellitus
adult-onset obesity
adult T-cell lymphoma (ATL)
adult T-cell lymphoma leukemia
adventitial cell
adventitial neuritis
adventitia, tunica
adventitious bursa
adventitious proteinuria
adynamic paralytic ileus
aerate
aeration
Aerobacter (old name for
   Enterobacter)
Aerobacter aerogenes
Aerobacter cloacae
Aerobacter liquefaciens
aerobe microorganism
aerobic bacteria
aerobic culture
Aerococcus
Aeromonas caviae
Aeromonas hydrophila
Aeromonas salmonicida
Aeromonas shigelloides
Aeromonas sobria
aestivoautumnal fever
AFB (acid-fast bacillus)
AFB culture
AFB stain
afferent arteriole
afferent fiber
afferent glomerular arteriole
afferent limb
afferent loop
afferent lymph vessel
afferent nerve

afferent vessel of kidney
affinity column
affinity for acidic stains
affinity for basic stains
affix
A fiber
Afipia felis
AFP (alpha-fetoprotein) test
African hemorrhagic fever
African lymphoma
African sleeping sickness
African tick-borne fever
afterbirth
Ag (antigen)
Ag (silver)
A/G (albumin-globulin) ratio
AGA (appropriate for gestational age)
agammaglobulinemia, congenital
aganglionic bowel
agar
    bile salt
    blood
    Bordet-Gengou
    chocolate
    cornmeal-Tween 80
    egg yolk
    laked blood
    MacConkey
    Nobel
    Sabouraud
agar culture medium
Agaricus
agarose gel
agarose gel electrophoresis
agar plate count
agar slant
age
    bone
    developmental
    gestational (GA)
aged normal serum
agenesis

agent
    antiadrenergic
    antifibrinolytic
    antifoaming
    diuretic
agger nasi cell
agglomeration of cells
agglutinating antibody
agglutination
    heterophile
    latex
    Widal
agglutination of cells
agglutination of latex beads
agglutination test for antibody
agglutination titer for brucellosis
agglutination titer for paratyphoid
agglutination titer for rickettsiae
agglutination titer for tularemia
agglutination titer for typhoid
agglutinin
    blood typing
    brucellosis
    chief
    cold
    cross-reacting
    erythrocyte
    febrile
    production of by immune system
    serum
    Weil-Felix
agglutinin to Rh positive cells in the Rh
    system
agglutinin to type A red blood cells in
    the ABO system
agglutinogen, erythrocyte
agglutinogens in red cells
aggregate dimension
aggregated lymphatic follicle
aggregated lymphatic nodule
aggregate gland
aggregate specimen

aggregations of lymphoid tissue
aging, consequences of
agitans, paralysis
agminated follicles
agminated gland
agnogenic myeloid metaplasia
agonal clot
agonal infection
agonist
agranular lcukocyte
agranular mononuclear cell
agranular reticulum
agranulocytosis
Agrimonia eupatoria
agrypnodal coma
A hemoglobin
A$_{1c}$ hemoglobin
A hemophilia
A hepatitis
AHG (antihemophilic globulin)
AIDS encephalopathy
AIHA (autoimmune hemolytic anemia)
AimV serum-free media
AIP (acute intermittent porphyria)
air-bone gap
airborne infection
air cell
    ethmoidal
    mastoid
air-dried smear
air embolism
airless mass
air sac
airspace-filling pattern
air vesicle
airway pattern
Ajellomyces capsulatus
Ajellomyces dermatitidis
akinesis, anterior wall
Al (aluminum)
AL patch test
AL protein (amyloid light chain)

ala, nasal
alanine aminotransferase (ALT)
    (formerly SGPT)
ala of ethmoid
ala of sacrum
ala of vomer
alar artery
alar bone
alar cartilage
alar fold
alar lamina
alar ligament
alar plate
alar process
alar spine
AlaSTAT latex allergy test
alba, linea
Albarran gland
Albarran test
Albers-Schoenberg disease
Albers-Schoenberg marble bone
albicans, corpus
albinism
albino
Albrecht bone
albuginea, tunica
albumin
    A
    acid
    alkali
    blood
    iodinated I 125 serum (also, ^{125}I)
    iodinated I 131 serum (also, ^{131}I)
    native
    serum
    urine
albumin/globulin (A/G) ratio
albuminocytologic dissociation
albuminoid
albuminous cell
albuminous degeneration
albuminous deposits

albuminous gland
albuminous granule
albumin test
albuminuria
Alcaligenes denitrificans
Alcaligenes faecalis
Alcaligenes odorans
Alcian blue
Alcock canal
alcohol
  acid
  acidified
  blood
  ethyl
  methyl
alcoholic cirrhosis
alcoholic coma
alcoholic formalin
alcoholic hepatitis
alcoholic hyalin
alcoholic pneumonia
alcoholic solution
alcohol intoxication
alcoholism
alcohol poisoning
alcohol-soluble protein
Alder-Reilly granules
aldolase test
aldosterone hormone
aldosterone test
aldosterone, urinary
aldosteronism
  primary
  secondary
aleukemic leukemia
Alexander leukodystrophy disease
algae, red
algid malaria
algid pernicious fever
algoid cell
algor mortis
alimentary apparatus

alimentary canal
alimentary glycosuria
alimentary mucosa
alimentary obesity
alimentary system
alimentary tract smear
aliphatic fatty acids
aliquot
alisphenoid bone
alisphenoids
alizarin stain
alkalemia
alkali albumin
alkali denaturation test
alkaline medium
alkaline phosphatase (ALP)
  leukocyte
  placental (PLAP)
  serum
alkaline phosphatase deficiency
alkaline phosphatase nitroblue
  tetrazolium (NBT)
alkaline phosphatase test
alkaloid test
alkalosis
  hypochloremic
  hypokalemic
  metabolic
  respiratory
alkaptonuria
ALL (acute lymphoblastic leukemia)
allantoic sac
allantoic stalk
allantoic vesicle
allantoid membrane
allantois
allelic gene
Allen-Doisy test
Allen test
allergen
allergic contact dermatitis
allergic dermatitis

allergic eczema
allergic granulomatosis
allergic inflammation
allergic pneumonia
allergic purpura
allergic reaction
allergic stomatitis
allergy
alloantibodies
alloantigen-presenting cell
allocortex
allogeneic disease
Almén test for blood
almond nucleus
alopecia
   androgenic
   cicatricial
   female pattern
   hereditary
   lipedematous
   male pattern
   moth-eaten
   patterned
   postoperative pressure
   postpartum
   pressure
   scarring
   traction
   traumatic
alopecia adnata
alopecia areata
alopecia capitis totalis
alopecia congenitalis
alopecia disseminata
alopecia follicularis
alopecia leprotica
alopecia liminaris frontalis
alopecia marginalis
alopecia medicamentosa
alopecia mucinosa
alopecia pityrodes
alopecia presenilis

alopecia senilis
alopecia symptomatica
alopecia syphilitica
alopecia totalis
alopecia toxica
alopecia triangularis
alopecia triangularis congenitalis
alopecia universalis
Al patch
alpha acid glycoprotein
alpha-adrenergic receptor
alpha amino acid
alpha amino nitrogen
alpha-amylase
alpha-amylose
$alpha_1$-antichymotrypsin (a1AC)
$alpha_1$-antitrypsin (AAT)
$alpha_1$-antitrypsin globulin
alpha-beta variation
alpha-blocker
alpha cell
alpha coma
alpha dinitrophenol
alpha-estradiol
alpha-fetoglobulin
alpha-fetoprotein (AFP)
   amniotic fluid
   fucosylated
   serum
alpha-fetoprotein test
alpha fiber
alpha globulin
alpha globulin antibodies
alpha-glucosidase deficiency
alpha granule
alpha heavy chain disease
alpha hemolysis
alpha-hemolytic streptococcus
alpha-hypophamine
alpha-ketoglutarate dehydrogenase
$alpha_1$-lipoprotein
alpha-naphthol esterase

alpha satellite biotinylated
  chromosome-specific probe
alpha-tocopherol (vitamin E)
alpha-trypsin inhibitor
Alphavirus, alphavirus
alphoid
ALS (amyotrophic lateral sclerosis)
ALT (alanine aminotransferase)
  (formerly SGPT)
Alternaria
Alternaria alternata
Alteromonas putrefaciens
Altmann-Gersh method
Altmann granule
Altmann solution
alum-carmine stain
alum-coated slide
aluminum (Al)
alveolar abscess
alveolar angle
alveolar arch
alveolar artery
alveolar body
alveolar bone
alveolar border of mandible
alveolar canal
alveolar cell
alveolar crest
alveolar dead space
alveolar duct
alveolar foramen
alveolar gland
alveolar hydatids
alveolar macrophage
alveolar mucosa
alveolar necrosis
alveolar nerve
alveolar osteitis
alveolar pattern
alveolar periosteum
alveolar point
alveolar process of maxilla

alveolar ridge
alveolar sac
alveolar septum
alveolar soft part sarcoma
alveolar space
alveolar supporting bone
alveolar wall
alveolar yoke
alveoli (pl. of alveolus)
alveolingual groove
alveolitis, extrinsic allergic
alveolobuccal groove
alveolobuccal sulcus
alveolodental canal
alveolodental ligament
alveolodental membrane
alveololabial groove
alveololabial sulcus
alveololingual groove
alveololingual sulcus
alveolonasal line
alveolus (pl. alveoli)
  dental
  glandular
  pulmonary
Alzheimer cell
Alzheimer disease
Alzheimer neurofibrillary degeneration
Alzheimer stain
AMA (antimitochondrial antibody)
amacrine cells of retina
Amanita
Amanita bisporigera
Amanita muscaria
Amanita ocreata
Amanita phalloides
Amanita verna
Amanita virosa
amastigote
amaurotic familial idiocy
amber streaks in lens
ambiguous external genitalia

ambolic abscess
ambulatory plague
ameba (amoeba)
amebiasis
amebic abscess
amebic dysentery
amebic pneumonia
ameboid astrocyte
ameboid cell
ameboid movement
amelanotic melanoma
amelanotic nevus
ameloblast
ameloblastic odontoma
ameloblastic sarcoma
ameloblastoma
American trypanosomiasis
Ames assay
Ameth index
AMEX method of processing and
   embedding
amino acid
   aromatic
   branched chain
   essential
amino acid cystine
amino acid nitrogen (AAN) test
amino acid screen
aminolevulinate dehydratase test
aminolevulinic acid (ALA) test
aminolevulinic-delta acid
aminopeptidase, serum leucine
aminotransferase, alanine (ALT)
AML (acute myelogenous leukemia)
Ammon horn
ammoniacal silver stain
ammonia dermatitis
ammonia nitrogen test
ammonia, synthesis of
ammonium biurate
ammonium chloride loading test

ammonium magnesium phosphate
   (triple phosphate)
ammonium silver carbonate
amniocentesis, genetic
amnioembryonic junction
amniogenic cell
amnion
amnionic
amnionitis
amnion ring
amniotic band
amniotic cavity
amniotic duct
amniotic fluid, meconium-stained
amniotic fluid embolism
amniotic fold
amniotic raphe
amniotic sac
Amoeba
amorphous debris
amorphous ground substance
amorphous material
amorphous phosphate
amorphous sediment
amorphous sediment in urine
amorphous urate
AMP (adenosine monophosphate)
ampere
amphiarthroses articulation (joint)
amphophil granule
amphophilic matrix
amplicon
ampulla (pl. ampullae)
   duodenal
   ductus deferens
   Henle
   rectal
   semicircular canal
   uterine tube
   Vater
ampullar (also, ampullary)

ampullar abortion
ampullar crest
ampullar limb
ampullar pregnancy
ampullar sulcus
amygdala
amygdaloid body
amygdaloid fossa
amygdaloid nucleus
amygdaloid tubercle
amylaceous corpuscle
amylase
 body fluid
 serum
 urinary
amylase/creatinine
amylase level, serum
amylase test
amyloid A protein
amyloid body
amyloid corpuscle
amyloid degeneration
amyloid kidney
amyloid light chain (AL) protein
amyloidosis
 primary
 renal
 secondary
amyloid precursor protein
amyloid protein
amyloid stain
amyotrophic lateral sclerosis (ALS)
amyotrophy, neuralgic
ANA (antinuclear antibody)
anabiotic cell
anabolic effect
anaerobe
anaerobic bacteria
anaerobic culture of pus or drainage
 from abscess
Anaerobiospirillum succiniciproducens
anal canal, involuntary sphincter of

anal cleft
anal column
anal crypt
anal disk
anal fascia
anal fissure
anal gland
anal intermuscular septum
anal intersphincteric groove
anal membrane
analogous tissue
anal orifice
anal pit
anal plate
anal pruritus
anal reflex
anal region
anal sac
anal sinus
anal sphincter
anal triangle
anal valve
anal vein
anal verge
analysis (pl. analyses)
 activation
 accumulation
 blood gas
 CDK4 amplification
 chemistry
 chromatin
 chromosomal
 DNA
 fetal chromosome
 gastric
 hormone receptor protein
 immunophenotypic
 qualitative
 quantitative
 Northern blot
 segregation
 semen

analysis *(continued)*
  sequence
  sex chromatin
  Southern blot
  stratographic
  volumetric
  Western blot
  zoo blot
analyte
analyzer
  Abbott VP
  ASTRA
  Dade Paramax
  DuPont ACA
  Ektachem
anaphylactic shock
anaphylactoid purpura
anaphylaxis
anaplasia
anaplastic cell
anaplastic epithelial cell
anaplastic tumor
anasarca
anastomoses (pl. of anastomosis)
anastomosing fiber
anastomosing veins
anastomosis (pl. anastomoses)
  arteriolovenular
  arteriovenous
  crucial
  longitudinal
  portacaval
  splenorenal
  supraoptic
anastomosis of arteries
anastomotic area, portal-systemic
anastomotic branch of inferior gluteal
  artery
anastomotic fiber
anastomotic ulcer
anastomotic vein
anatomical dead space

anatomical neck
anatomical neck of humerus
anatomical root
anatomical snuff box
anatomical sphincter
anatomical tooth
anatomical tubercle
anatomic diagnosis
anatomic landmark
anatomic nervous system
anatomic pathology
ANC (absolute neutrophil count)
anchoring villus
"anchovy paste" material in hepatic
  abscess
"anchovy sauce" pus
ancillary
anconeal fossa
anconeus muscle
Ancylostoma americanum
Ancylostoma braziliense
Ancylostoma caninum
Ancylostoma dermatitis
Ancylostoma duodenale
ancylostomatic
ancylostomiasis
Anderson and Goldberger test
Anderson-Collip test
Anderson phenomenon
androgen, adrenal
androgen binding protein (ABP)
androgenic alopecia
androgenic hormone
androgenic zone
androgen level, urine
android pelvis
androstenediol
androstenedione test
anemia
  achrestic
  aplastic
  autoimmune hemolytic (AIHA)

anemia *(continued)*
 chronic disease
 congenital hemolytic
 Cooley
 hemolytic
 hereditary hemolytic
 hypochromic microcytic
 hypoplastic
 iron deficiency
 macrocytic
 Mediterranean
 megaloblastic
 normochromic
 normocytic
 pernicious
 secondary
 sickle cell
 sideroblastic
 spur-cell
anemia, hemolytic, after exposure to
 fava beans
 nitrofurans
 primaquine
 sulfonamides
anemia of chronic disease
anemic infarct
anemic nevus
anencephaly
anergic
anergy
anetoderma
aneuploid
aneuploidy chromosomal abnormality
aneurysm
 abdominal
 abdominal aortic (AAA)
 acquired
 aortic
 aortic sinus
 arterial
 arteriosclerotic
 arteriovenous

aneurysm *(continued)*
 atherosclerotic
 axial
 bacterial
 Bérard
 berry
 brain
 Charcot-Bouchard
 circumscript
 cirsoid
 compound
 congenital
 congenital aortic sinus
 congenital cerebral
 coronary artery
 coronary vessel
 cylindroid
 debulking of
 descending thoracic
 dissecting
 dissecting aortic
 distal aortic arch
 ductal
 ectatic
 embolic
 false
 fusiform
 hernial
 imperforate
 infected
 infraclinoid
 innominate
 intracavernous
 intracranial
 intramural coronary artery
 isthmus
 juxtarenal aortic
 late false
 lateral
 left ventricular
 luetic aortic
 mesh-wrapping of aortic

aneurysm *(continued)*
  miliary
  mixed
  mural
  mycotic
  mycotic suprarenal
  nodular
  orbital
  pararenal aortic
  Park
  pelvic
  peripheral
  phantom
  post infarction ventricular
  Potts
  pulmonary arteriovenous
  pulmonary artery compression
    ascending aorta
  pulmonary artery mycotic
  racemose
  Rasmussen
  renal
  renal artery
  Richet
  Rodriguez
  ruptured
  ruptured aortic
  ruptured cerebral
  ruptured atherosclerotic
  sacciform
  saccular
  sacculated
  serpentine
  Shekelton
  spindle-shaped
  splenic artery
  spontaneous infantile ductal
  spurious
  suprasellar
  syphilitic
  thoracic
  thoracic aorta

aneurysm *(continued)*
  thoracoabdominal
  traumatic
  true
  tubular
  Valsalva sinus
  varicose
  venous
  ventricular
  ventricular septal
  verminous
  windsock
  worm
  wrapping of abdominal aortic
aneurysmal bruit
aneurysmal dilatation
aneurysmal sac
ANF (atrial natriuretic factor)
angiitis
angina pectoris
angioblast
angioblastic cell
angiocentric immunoproliferative
angioedema
angiogenesis factor
angiokeratoma
angiokeratoma corporis diffusum
angiolipoma
angiolithic degeneration
angiolithic sarcoma
angioma (pl. angiomata)
  capillary
  cavernous
  cherry
  hemangioma
  lymphangioma
  petechial
  spider
  telangiectatic
angioma serpiginosum
angiomatosis, bacillary
angioma venosum racemosum

angiomyolipoma
angioneurotic edema
angiotensin converting enzyme (ACE)
angiotensin I test
angiotensin II hormone
angiotensin II test
angle
  acromial
  adjacent
  alveolar
  anopouch
  anorectal
  apical
  axial
  basilar
  beta
  biorbital
  buccal
  bucco-occlusal
  cardiohepatic
  carrying
  cavity line
  cavosurface
  cephalic
  cephalomedullary
  cerebellopontile
  cerebellopontine
  costal
  costophrenic
  costovertebral (CVA)
  craniofacial
  critical
  cusp
  disparity
  duodenojejunal
  epigastric
  ethmoid
  facial
  filtration
  Frankfort-mandibular incisor
  frontal
  gamma

angle *(continued)*
  hepatorenal
  infrasternal
  iridocorneal
  sacrovertebral
  splenorenal (splenic-renal)
  sternal
  subpubic
  subscapular
angle of clitoris
angle of convergence
angle of mandible
angle of refraction
angle of rib
angle of sternum
angle of trigone
angular aperture
angular artery
angular curvature
angular gyrus
angular ligament of wrist
angular movement
angular notch
angular vein
angulated
angulus of stomach
ANH (atrial natriuretic hormone)
anhepatic jaundice
anhidrosis
anhydride-induced immunologic
  respiratory disease
ani (see *levator ani muscle*)
Anichkov cell (also, Anitschkow)
aniline blue
animal bite infection
animal viruses
anion gap test
anisakiasis
Anisakis marina
anisocytosis
anisomorphic
anisonucleosis

anisotropic disk
anisotropic lipoid
Anitschkow cell (also, Anichkov)
ankle articulation
ankle bone
ankle joint
ankle region
ankylosing spondylitis
ankylosis
  bony
  fibrous
annular ligament of ankle
annular ligament of radius
annular ligament of stapes
annular ligament of trachea
annular ligament of wrist
annular pancreas
annulospiral organ
annulus (pl. annuli)
annulus fibrosus of intervertebral
  fibrocartilage
annulus inguinalis
annulus ovalis
annulus tendineus communis
anococcygeal body
anococcygeal ligament
anococcygeal nerve
anococcygeal raphe
anocutaneous line
anogenital band
anogenital raphe
anomalous
anomaly (pl. anomalies)
  Alder
  congenital
  developmental
  May-Hegglin
  Pelger-Huët nuclear
  Undritz
anonychia
anonymous artery
anonymous vein

anopouch angle
anorectal angle
anorectal junction
anorectal line
anorectal lymph node
anorectal ring
anorexia
anospinal center
anovular ovarian follicle
anoxemia test
anoxia
anoxic
ansa
  Haller
  Henle
  lenticular
  peduncular
  Reil
  Vieussens
ansa cervicalis
ansa lenticularis
anserine bursa
anserine bursitis
ansiform lobule
antagonist
antagonistic muscle
antebrachial cutaneous nerve
antebrachial fascia
antebrachial vein
antebrachiocarpal joint
antecubital fossa
antecubital region
antecubital space
anteflexed uterus
antegonial notch
antemortem clot
antemortem thrombus
antenatal diagnosis
anteprostatic gland
anterior abdominal wall
anterior annular ligament of wrist
anterior auricular artery

anterior auricular nerve
anterior band of colon
anterior basis bundle
anterior calcaneoastragaloid ligament
anterior cardiac vein
anterior cell
anterior cerebellar artery
anterior cerebral artery
anterior chamber
anterior choroidal artery
anterior ciliary artery
anterior circumflex artery
anterior clinoid process
anterior communicating artery
anterior condyloid canal of occipital
  bone
anterior condyloid foramen
anterior costotransverse ligament
anterior costovertebral ligament
anterior costoxiphoid ligament
anterior cruciate ligament
anterior crural nerve
anterior curvature
anterior cusp
anterior cutaneous branch
anterior cutaneous nerve
anterior descending artery
anterior ethmoidal nerve
anterior fontanelle
anterior fornix of vagina
anterior horn cells of spinal cord
anterior humeral circumflex artery
anterior inferior cerebellar artery
anterior inferior tibiofibular ligament
anterior intercostal artery
anterior interosseous artery
anterior interosseous nerve
anterior intraoccipital joint
anterior jugular vein
anterior labial commissure
anterior-lateral (anterolateral)
anterior layer of rectus sheath

anterior ligament of head of fibula
anterior ligament of Helmholtz
anterior ligament of knee
anterior ligament of malleus
anterior ligament of wrist
anterior longitudinal ligament
anterior mediastinum
anterior meningeal artery
anterior meningocele
anterior meniscofemoral ligament
anterior muscle, scalenus
anterior nares
anterior nasal aperture
anterior papillary muscle
anterior peroneal artery
anterior pillar of fauces
anterior pituitary-like hormone
anterior pituitary-like substance
anterior pulmonary nerve
anterior radioulnar ligament
anterior recess of ischiorectal fossa
anterior rectus fascia
anterior rectus sheath
anterior sacrococcygeal ligament
anterior sacroiliac ligaments
anterior sacrosciatic ligament
anterior semicircular canal
anterior spinal artery
anterior sternoclavicular ligament
anterior superior dental artery
anterior superior iliac spine
anterior surface of pancreas
anterior surface of prostate
anterior synechiae
anterior talotibial ligament
anterior temporal artery
anterior tibial artery
anterior tympanic artery
anterior uveitis of iris
anterior vagal trunk
anterior wall akinesis
anteroinferiorly

anterolateral (anterior-lateral)
anterolateral central artery
anterolateral column
anterolateral fontanelle
anterolateral groove
anterolateral striate artery
anterolateral sulcus
anterolateral surface
anteromedial central artery
anteromedial surface
anteromedial thalamostriate artery
anteromedian gap
anteromedian groove
anteroposterior (AP) diameter
anteverted uterus
anthracene laxative
anthracosis
anthracotic
anthrax bacillus
anthrax, inhalational
anthrax pneumonia
anthropoid pelvis
anti-A agglutinins in serum
anti-ACh receptor antibody
anti-AChR (antiacetylcholine receptor)
   antibody
antiacrodynia factor
antiadrenergic agent
antialopecia factor
antianemic factor
anti-antibody
anti-B agglutinins in serum
antiberiberi factor
antibiotic-containing disks
antibiotic sensitivity test(ing)
anti-black-tongue factor
antibody (Ab) (pl. antibodies)
   acetylcholine receptor (AChR)
   acquired hemolyzing
   ACTH (adrenocorticotropic
     hormone)
   adrenal

antibody *(continued)*
   AE1
   AE3
   agglutinating
   alpha-globulin
   anti-ACh receptor
   anti-AChR (antiacetylcholine
     receptor)
   anti-B
   anticardiolipin (aCA)
   anticentromere (ACA)
   anticolonic
   anticytoplasmic (ACPA)
   antidelta IgM
   antidermatitis factor
   anti-DNA
   anti-EA (early antigen) of
     Epstein Barr virus
   anti-ENA
   antifibrin
   anti-GBM
   antigliodin
   antiglioma monoclonal antibody
     kinase C
   anti-HA (hepatitis A)
   anti-HAV (hepatitis A virus)
   anti-HB (hepatitis B)
   anti-HB$_c$ (hepatitis B core)
   anti-HB$_e$ (hepatitis B "e")
   anti-HB$_s$ (hepatitis B surface)
   anti-HEV (hepatitis E virus)
   antihuman globulin
   antihyaluronidase
   anti-idiotype
   anti-idiotypic
   anti-IL-2 receptor monoclonal
   anti-kidney
   anti-La
   antimitochondrial (AMA)
   anti-MPO
   anti-nRNP
   antinuclear (ANA)

antibody *(continued)*
  antiphospholipid
  anti-PR3
  anti-receptor
  anti-Rh
  anti-Ro
  anti-Scl-70
  anti-Sm
  anti-SS-A
  anti-SS-B
  anti-TBM
  antithyroglobulin
  anti-VCA (viral capsid antigen)
  A33 monoclonal
  biotinylated secondary
  CAM 5.2
  CC49 monoclonal
  CD5+ monoclonal
  cell-bound
  centromere
  CF (complement fixation)
  C-58 monoclonal
  complement fixation (CF)
  C100-3 hepatitis C virus (anti-HIV)
  cross-reacting
  cryptosporidiosis
  cytotrophic
  disease caused by
  Donath-Landsteiner
  Duffy blood antibody type
  eastern equine encephalitis
  E5 monoclonal
  EMA (epithelial membrane antigen)
  endomysial
  extractable nuclear (ENA)
  fluorescent
  fluorescently tagged
  fluorescent treponemal
  fungal
  GFAP (glial fibrillary acidic
    protein)
  glomerular basement membrane

antibody *(continued)*
  HA-1A monoclonal
  HAMA (human antimurine)
  HBe
  HIV
  HLA-DR monoclonal
  HLe-1 monoclonal
  idiotypic
  IgG
  IgM
  IgM anti-HAV
  IgM anti-HBc
  Ig2b kappa monoclonal
  inhibiting
  insulin
  intrinsic factor
  kinase C antiglioma monoclonal
  La (SS-B)
  Leu2a monoclonal
  Leu3a+3b monoclonal
  Leu4 monoclonal
  Leu5b monoclonal
  Leu17 monoclonal
  Leu23 monoclonal
  luteinizing hormone
  lym-1 monoclonal
  lymphocytotoxic
  milk protein
  mitochondrial
  monoclonal (MOAB, MoAb, MAB)
  MB1 monoclonal
  MSL-109 monoclonal
  MT2 monoclonal
  MT3 monoclonal
  Muromonab-CD3 monoclonal
  mycobacterial
  NCL-Arp monoclonal
  NCL-ER-LHZ monoclonal
  NCL-PGR monoclonal
  NSE (neuron-specific enolase)
  OKT3 monoclonal
  OKT4 monoclonal

antibody *(continued)*
  OKT8 monoclonal
  OPD4 monoclonal
  parietal cell
  PBC-associated
  pemphigus
  platelet
  PM-81 monoclonal
  production
  prolactin hormone
  Proteus OX-2
  Proteus OX-19
  Proteus OX-K
  Rh
  Ro (SS-A)
  scleroderma
  17-1A monoclonal SFHb
    (pyridoxilated stroma-free
    hemoglobin)
  6B6 monoclonal
  65-2A6 monoclonal
  Sjögren
  smooth muscle
  S-100 protein
  sperm
  staining
  teichoic acid
  testing
  3F8 monoclonal
  thyroglobulin
  thyroid microsomal
  thyrotropin hormone
  thyrotropin receptor
  TI-23 (CMV monoclonal a.)
  2A11 monoclonal
  UCHL1 monoclonal
  western equine encephalitis
antibody labeled with radioisotope
antibody technique, fluorescent
antibody titer
anticardiolipin antibody (aCA)
antichymotrypsin, alpha$_1$–

antichymotrypsin test
anticoagulant
  circulating
  coumarin
  Coumadin
  heparin
  lupus
anticoagulant heparin solution
anticoagulant-treated blood
anticolonic antibody
anticomplementary factor
anticytoplasmic antibody (ACPA) test
antidelta IgM antibody
anti-deoxyribonuclease-B titer
  (anti-DNAse titer)
anti-D immunoglobulin
antidiuretic hormone (ADH) test
antidiuretic hormone–water deprivation
  stimulation test
anti-DNA antibody
  Farr
  Ginsberg/Keiser
  indirect fluorescence
anti-DNA test
anti-double-stranded DNA test
anti-EA (Epstein-Barr) antibody
anti-ENA antibody
antifibrinolytic agent
antifoaming agent
anti-GBM antibody
antigen (Ag)
  acetone-insoluble
  adenovirus
  alpha-fetoprotein (AFP)
  antiproliferating cell nuclear
  Au (gold)
  Australian
  bile
  CA (cancer)
  C carbohydrate
  CA 15-3 antigenic tumor marker
  CA 19-9 carbohydrate

antigen *(continued)*
  CA 72-4 antigenic tumor marker
  CALLA (common acute lympho-
    blastic leukemia antigen)
  cancer (CA)
  capsular
  carcinoembryonic (CEA)
  CDE
  CD3
  CD45 leukocyte common
  Chr a
  common acute lymphoblastic
    leukemia (CALLA)
  conjugated
  delta (delta-Ag)
  Di
  ECA (enterobacterial common)
  EMA (epithelial membrane)
  ENA (extractable nuclear)
  enterobacterial common (ECA)
  epithelial membrane (EMA)
  erythrocyte
  extractable nuclear (ENA)
  febrile
  Forssman
  Goa (Gonzales blood)
  HBAg (hepatitis B antigen)
  hepatitis associated (HAA)
  hepatitis B
  hepatitis B core (HB$_c$Ag)
  hepatitis B e (HB$_e$Ag)
  hepatitis B surface (HB$_s$Ag)
  hepatitis D virus
  HLA (human lymphocytic)
  HPA (*Histoplasma capsulatum*)
  inhalant
  latex particles coated with
  Ly
  Lyb
  membrane
  nonspecific
  p24

antigen *(continued)*
  pancreatic oncofetal (POA)
  PHA (phytohemagglutinin)
  polypeptide
  prostate specific (PSA)
  Rh (Rhesus factor)
  rheumatoid-associated nuclear
    (RANA)
  rotavirus
  serum hepatitis (SH)
  Sm
  streptococcal
  streptococcus M
  T-dependent
  T-independent
  Thy-1
  tissue
  tissue polypeptide (TPA)
  tumor
  VDRL
  von Willebrand factor (vWF)
antigen-antibody complex
antigen-antibody reaction
antigenically stable
antigenic change
antigenic complex
antigenic drift
antigenic profile
antigenic properties of blood
antigen labeled with radioisotope
antigen-presenting cell (APC)
antigen-reactive cell
antigen-responsive cell
antigen-sensitive cell
antigliodin antibody
antiglioma monoclonal antibody
    kinase C
antiglobulin
antiglobulin consumption test
antiglobulin test (AGT)
anti-glomerular basement membrane
    (anti-GBM) antibody disease

antigonadotropic hormone
antigravity muscle
anti-HA antibody
anti-HAV (hepatitis A virus) antibody
anti-HB antibody
anti-HB$_c$ antibody (antibody to core
    antigen of hepatitis B virus)
anti-HB$_e$ antibody (antibody to e
    antigen of hepatitis B virus)
anti-HB$_s$ antibody (antibody to surface
    antigen of hepatitis B virus)
antihelix (also, anhelix)
antihemophilic factor
antihemophilic globulin (AHG)
antihemophilic plasma
antihemorrhagic factor
anti-HEV (hepatitis E virus) antibody
antihuman globulin antibody
antihyaluronidase antibody
antihyaluronidase titer (AH titer)
anti-idiotype antibody
anti-idiotype autoantibody
anti-IL-2 receptor monoclonal antibody
antiketogenesis
anti-kidney antibody
anti-LA/SS-B test
antimesenteric border of the distal
    ileum
antimesenteric fat pad
antimesenteric surface
antimesocolic side of cecum
antimicrobial removal device
antimitochondrial antibody (AMA)
anti-Monson curve
anti-MPO antibody
antineuritic factor
antineuritic vitamin
anti-nRNP autoantibody
antinuclear antibody (ANA)
antinuclear factor
antioncogene (see *tumor suppressor
    gene*)

antipellagra factor
antiphospholipid antibody
antiphospholipid syndrome
antiplasmin, alpha
antipodal cell
anti-Pr cold autoagglutinin
anti-PR3 antibody
antipyretic
antireceptor antibody
anti-Rh antibody
anti-Rh antiglobulins
anti-Ro/SS-A test
anti-Scl-70 autoantibody
antiseptic
antiserum (pl. antisera)
anti-Sm test
anti-SS-A antibody
anti-SS-B antibody
antisterility factor
antistreptolysin O titer (ASO titer)
anti-TBM antibody
antithrombin III (ATIII)
antithyroglobulin antibody
antitoxin
antitragicus muscle
antitragohelicine fissure
antitragus
antitrypsin
    alpha$_1$-
    PiZZ
antitrypsin globulin, alpha
antitrypsin test
anti-VCA (viral capsid antigen)
    antibody
antivenin of animal origin
antivenom (also, antivenin)
antivenomous serum
antiviral interferon
antiviral protein
Antoni type A neurilemoma
Antoni type B neurilemoma
antral gastric cell

antral gastritis
antral mucosa
antral pouch
antral sphincter
antrum
   aditus ad
   cardiac
   ethmoid
   gastric
   mastoid
   maxillary
   prepyloric
   pyloric
   stomach
   Willis
   Highmore
   pyloric
   tympanic
   Valsalva
antrum cardiacum
anuli fibrosi
anus
   imperforate
   preternatural
AoBP (aortic blood pressure)
aorta (pl. aortae)
   abdominal
   arch of
   ascending
   buckled
   calcified
   coarctation
   descending
   descending thoracic
   dynamic
   esophageal artery of
   kinked
   overriding
   shaggy
   supraceliac
   thoracic
   tortuous

aorta *(continued)*
   transverse
   primitive
   ventral
aortic aneurysm
aortic arch
aortic arch syndrome
aortic area
aortic artery
aortic blood pressure (AoBP)
aortic body
aortic bulb
aortic cusp
aortic foramen
aortic glands
aortic hiatus
aortic isthmus
aortic knob
aortic knuckle
aortic lymph node
aortic nerve
aortic notch
aortic opening
aorticorenal disease
aorticorenal ganglia
aortic orifice
aortic ostium
aortic plexus
aortic receptor
aortic sac
aortic semilunar valve
aortic septal defect
aortic septum
aortic sinus
aortic sinus aneurysm
aortic spindle
aortic sulcus
aortic valve
aortic valve stenosis
aortic valvular leaflet
aortic vestibule
aortitis, syphilitic

aortopulmonary septum
Apathy mounting medium
apatite
APC (adenomatous polyposis coli)
APC antioncogene
APC tumor suppressor gene
aperistalsis
aperture
   angular
   anterior nasal
   inferior pelvic
   inferior thoracic
   superior pelvic
   superior thoracic
apertures of abdomen
apex (pl. apices)
   bladder
   cordis
   duodenal bulb
   external ring
   fibrous
   fibula
   heart
   ischiorectal fossa
   lingual
   lung
   nose
   prostate
   pulmonis
apex of femur
apex pneumonia
aphakic eye
aphtha (pl. aphthae)
aphthoid
aphthosis
aphthous stomatitis
aphthous ulcer
apical abscess
apical angle
apical area
apical canaliculus
apical complex

apical dendrite
apical ectodermal ridge
apical foramen
apical gland
apical infection
apical ligament
apical lymph node
apical periodontal abscess
apical pneumonia
apical process
apical recess
apical segment
apical space
apical zone
apicoposterior segment
aplasia
aplastic anemia
aplastic anemia due to marrow
   suppression
aplastic anemia syndrome
aplastic lymph
apocrine adenosis
apocrine cell
apocrine gland
apocrine metaplasia of breast
apolar cell
aponeurosis (pl. aponeuroses)
   abdominal
   bicipital
   epicranial
   extensor
   external oblique muscle
   gluteal
   internal oblique muscle
   lingual
   lumbar
   lumbocostal
   palatine
   palmar
   palmaris
   pharyngeal
   plantar

aponeurosis *(continued)*
    plantaris
    suprahyoid
aponeurotic portion of diaphragm
apophyseal point
ApopTag molecular biological-
   histochemical system
apoptosis
apoptotic oligodendrocyte
aporic gland
apparatus
    absorption
    accessory visual
    achromatic
    alimentary
    Barcroft-Warburg
    Benedict-Roth
    central
    chromatic
    chromidial
    digestive
    Golgi
    Haldane
    juxtaglomerular
    lacrimal
    respiratory
    Tiselius
    urogenital
    vasomotor
    vestibular
appearance
    beefy
    cobblestone
    dewy
    granular
    ground-glass
    hobnailed (of liver)
    honeycomb(ed)
    meaty
    mottled
    nutmeg
    onionskin

appearance *(continued)*
    speckled
    steamy
    tigroid
appearance infarct
appendage
    auricular
    cecal
    epiploic
appendages of testis
appendectomy
appendiceal abscess
appendiceal lumen
appendiceal mass
appendiceal stump
appendicitis
appendicular artery
appendicular colic
appendicular lymph node
appendicular muscle
appendicular skeleton
appendicular vein
appendix (pl. appendices)
    auricular
    cecal
    ensiform
    epiploic
    inflammation
    mesentery of
    Morgagni
    orifice of
    paracecal
    preileal
    retrocecal
    retrocolic
    retroileal
    right auricular
    serpentine
    subcecal
    testis
    ventricle of larynx
    vermiform

appendix *(continued)*
  vesicular
  xiphoid
appendix of epididymis
appendix of testis
apperceptive mass
appetite juice
apple, Adam's
apple-green fluorescence
apple jelly nodules
apple-peel bowel
appose
apposed
apposition
appropriateness of treatment
apron
  abdominal
  vascular
Apt test for differentiating fetal from
  adult hemoglobin
APTT (activated partial thromboplastin
  substitution test)
APUD cell (amine precursor uptake
  and decarboxylation)
apyrexia
aquagenic pruritus
Aqua-Mount
aqueduct
  cerebral
  cochlear
  fallopian
  sylvian
  ventricular
aqueduct of cochlea
aqueduct of Sylvius
aqueduct of vestibule
aqueous humor
aqueous-influx phenomenon
aqueous solution
aqueous vein
arachidonic acid metabolites
Arachnia

Arachnia propionica
arachnodactyly
arachnoidal foramen
arachnoidal membrane
arachnoid granulation
arachnoiditis, chronic adhesive
arachnoid matter
arachnoid membrane
arachnoid space
arachnoid villi
Aran-Duchenne muscular atrophy
Arantius body
Arantius canal
Arantius duct
Arantius ligament
Arantius nodule
Arantius ventricle
arbitrary unit
arborescence
arborescent
arborization of blood vessels
  (collateral circulation)
arbovirus
arc
  auricular
  binauricular
  bregmatolambdoid
  crater
  interauricular
  longitudinal
  nasobregmatic
  naso-occipital
  neural
  reflex
arcade
  gastroepiploic
  mitral
arcade of jejunum, arterial
arcade of Struthers
arch
  abdominothoracic
  alveolar

arch *(continued)*
  aortic
  arterial
  axillary
  branchial
  carotid
  carpal
  coracoacromial
  cortical
  costal
  crural
  dental
  diaphragmatic
  expansion
  fallopian
  femoral
  fibrous
  glossopalatine
  hyoid
  inguinal ligament
  jugular
  lateral lumbosacral
  lumbocostal
  mandibular
  medial lumbosacral
  nasal
  neural
  palatal
  palatoglossal
  palatopharyngeal
  palpebral
  pharyngeal
  pharyngopalatine
  plantar
  pubic
  Riolan
  superciliary
  tarsal
  tendinous
  Treitz
  venous dorsal
  visceral

arch *(continued)*
  Zimmermann
  zygomatic
arched crest
archenteric canal
arch formation, Gothic
architecture
  hepatic
  lobular
archival tissue
arch of aorta
arch of aortic artery
arch of atlas
arch of bone
arch of fauces
arch of foot
arch of pelvic fascia
arciform vein
arcuate artery
arcuate crest
arcuate eminence
arcuate fiber
arcuate ligament
arcuate line
arcuate nucleus
arcuate popliteal ligament
arcuate pubic ligament
arcuate vein
arcuate vessel
arcuate zone
arcus aortae (arch of aorta)
arcus senilis
ardent fever
area (see also *region*)
  aortic
  apical
  association
  auditory
  basal seat
  cochlear
  cribriform
  denture-bearing

area *(continued)*
   denture foundation
   denture-supporting
   dermatomic
   embryonic
   entorhinal
   excitable
   frontal
   fronto-orbital
   gastric
   gastrohepatic bare
   germinal
   pubo-obturator
   subhepatic
area of cardiac dullness
areatus
arenavirus
areola of bone
areolar connective tissue
areolar gland
areolar membrane
areolar sheet
areolar tissue
argentaffin cells of Kultschitzky
argentaffin granule
argentaffinoma
argentaffin stain
Argentinian hemorrhagic fever
Argentinian hemorrhagic fever virus
arginine 358 alpha$_1$-antitrypsin
   (Pittsburgh mutation)
arginine vasopressin (AVP)
arginosuccinicaciduria
ARGUS flow cytometer
argyrophil cell
argyrophil fiber
argyrophilic fibrillary tangle
argyrophil plaque
Arias-Stella cell
Arias-Stella reaction
A ring of esophagus
Arizona hinshawii

Armanni-Ebstein cell
Armanni-Ebstein disease
Armanni-Ebstein kidney
Armanni-Ebstein lesion
armed macrophage
Arneth classification of polymorphonuclear neutrophils
Arnold canal
Arnold-Chiari deformity
Arnold-Chiari malformation
Arnold ganglion
Arnold nerve
aromatic amino acid (AAA)
array, organoid
arrector pili muscle
arrest, cardiac
arrested growth lines
arrhenoblastoma
arsenic (As)
   blood
   hair analysis for
   nail analysis for
   urinary
arsenic poisoning
ART (automated reagin test)
arteria (see Table of Arteries)
arterial arcades of the jejunum
arterial arch
arterial blood
arterial blood gases (ABGs)
arterial bulb
arterial canal
arterial capillary
arterial carbon dioxide
arterial circle
arterial cone
arterial duct
arterial gases (blood)
arterial gland
arterial groove
arterial ligament
arterial line culture

arterial mesocardium
arterial nephrosclerosis
arterial obstruction
arterial oxygen
arterial oxygen saturation
arterial puncture
arterial stenosis
arterial stenosis from embolism
arterial stenosis without thrombosis
arterial transfusion
arterial vein
arteries (see Table of Arteries)
arteriococcygeal gland
arteriolar necrosis
arteriolar nephrosclerosis
arteriole
    afferent
    afferent glomerular
    capillary
    efferent
    efferent glomerular
arteriolitis in kidneys, necrotizing
arteriolovenular anastomosis
arteriolovenular bridge
arteriosclerosis
    cerebral
    coronary
    hyaline
    hypertensive
    infantile
    intimal
    medial
    Mönckeberg (Moenckeberg)
    peripheral
    presenile
    senile
arteriosclerosis obliterans
arteriosclerotic aneurysm
arteriosclerotic kidney
arteriosclerotic nephritis
arteriosclerotic plaque
arteriostenosis

arteriosus
    conus
    ductus
    embryonic truncus
    remnant of the ductus
arteriovenous anastomoses
arteriovenous fistula
arteriovenous shunt
arteritis
    acute
    giant cell
    infantile
    necrotizing
    syphilitic
    temporal
arterivirus
artery (pl. arteries)—descriptive terms.
    (See Table of Arteries for
    anatomical terms.)
    aberrant
    Abbott
    accessory
    accompanying
    Adamkiewicz
    adipose
    afferent
    anastomosis of
    anastomotic
    angular
    anonymous
    anterior
    anterolateral
    arcuate
    articular
    ascending
    atrial
    auricular
    axillary
    azygos
    calcaneal
    carotid
    central

artery *(continued)*
   Charcot
   chief
   circumflex
   Cohnheim
   coiled
   collateral
   common
   communicating
   companion
   conducting
   copper-wire
   corduroy
   corkscrew
   deferential
   degeneration of
   descending
   dorsal
   Drummond
   efferent
   elastic
   end
   external
   great
   hardening of
   Heubner
   highest (superior)
   inferior
   inflammation of
   innominate
   intercostal
   interlobular
   intermediate
   internal
   interosseous
   intersegmental
   interventricular
   Kugel anastomotic
   labial
   labyrinthine
   lateral
   left

artery *(continued)*
   lesser
   long
   Louis
   lowest
   medial
   middle
   Müller (Mueller)
   Neubauer
   nutrient
   parietal
   perforating
   pipestem
   postcentral
   posterior
   posterolateral
   posteromedial
   precentral
   pre-Rolandic
   principal
   proper
   radial
   recurrent
   right coronary (RCA)
   Rolandic
   segmental
   short
   spinal
   screw
   sheath of
   sheathed
   straight
   superficial
   superior
   superior articular
   transverse
   vidian
   Wilkie
   Willis
   Zinn
arthralgia
arthrifluent abscess

Arthrinium
arthritic atrophy
arthritis
  gouty
  infectious
  juvenile rheumatoid
  rheumatoid
  septic
  tuberculous
arthritis panel including
  antinuclear antibody
  antistreptolysin O titer
  C-reactive protein
  erythrocyte sedimentation rate
  rheumatoid factor by latex
    agglutination
  serum uric acid
Arthroderma
arthrodial articulation
arthrodial cartilage
arthrodial joint
Arthropoda
arthropod-borne relapsing fever
arthropod-borne viruses
arthropod vectors
arthroscope
articular artery
articular capsule
articular cartilage, hyaline
articular chondritis
articular corpuscle
articular crescent
articular crest
articular disk
articular eminence
articular facet
articular fluid
articular fossa
articular labrum
articular lamella of bone
articular lip
articular margin

articular meniscus
articular muscle
articular nerve
articular network
articular pit
articular process of vertebrae
articular surface
articular system
articular tubercle of temporal bone
articular vascular circle
articulated skeleton
articulating surface
articulatio (pl. articulationes)
  (see *articulation*)
articulation (also, joint)
  acromioclavicular
  amphiarthroses
  ankle
  arthrodial
  atlantoaxial
  atlanto-occipital
  balanced
  ball-and-socket
  bicondylar
  brachiocarpal
  brachioradial
  brachioulnar
  calcaneocuboid
  capitular
  carpal
  carpometacarpal
  cartilaginous
  chondrosternal
  Chopart
  composite
  compound
  condylar
  condyloid
  confluent
  costocentral
  costochondral
  costosternal

articulation *(continued)*
   costotransverse
   costovertebral
   coxal
   coxofemoral
   craniovertebral
   cricoarytenoid
   cricothyroid
   crurotalar
   cubital
   cubitoradial
   cuboideonavicular
   cuneocuboid
   cuneometatarsal
   cuneonavicular
   dental
   dentoalveolar
   diarthroses
   digit
   distal radioulnar
   elbow
   ellipsoidal
   femoral
   fibrous
   glenohumeral
   gliding
   gomphosis
   hip
   humeral
   humeroradial
   humeroulnar
   iliofemoral
   iliosacral
   immovable
   incudomalleolar
   incudostapedial
   intercarpal
   interchondral
   intercostal
   intercuneiform
   intermetacarpal
   intermetatarsal

articulation *(continued)*
   interphalangeal
   intertarsal
   intervertebral
   knee
   laryngeal
   lower extremity
   lumbosacral
   mandible
   manubriosternal
   maxillary
   metacarpophalangeal
   metatarsophalangeal
   movable
   multiaxial
   occipitoatloid
   ovoid
   patellofemoral
   peg-and-socket
   petrobasilar
   petro-occipital
   phalangeal
   pisiform bone
   pisocuneiform
   pivot
   plane
   proximal radioulnar
   pubis
   radiocarpal
   radiohumeral
   radioulnar
   sacrococcygeal
   sacroiliac
   sacrum and coccyx
   saddle
   scapuloclavicular
   schindylesis (wedge-and-groove
     joint)
   shoulder
   simple
   spheroid (ball-and-socket joint)
   sternal

articulation *(continued)*
  sternoclavicular
  sternocostal
  sternum
  subtalar
  superior tibial
  sutura
  synarthrosis
  synchondrosis
  syndesmosis
  synovial
  talocalcaneal
  talocalcaneonavicular
  talocrural
  talonavicular
  tarsometatarsal
  tarsus
  temporomandibular
  temporomaxillary
  tibiofibular
  tibiotarsal
  transverse tarsal
  trochoid (pivot joint)
  xiphisternal
  zygapophyseal
articulation by reciprocal reception
articulation of atlas with axis or
  epistropheus
articulation of atlas with occipital bone
articulation of auditory ossicles
articulation of Buisson
articulation of calcaneus and
  astragalus
articulation of digits of foot
articulation of digits of hand
articulation of hand
articulation of head of humerus
articulation of head of rib
articulation of hip
articulation of metacarpal bones
articulation of metatarsal bones
articulation of phalanges of foot

articulation of phalanges of hand
articulation of trunk
articulation of vertebral arches
articulator
artifact, suction
artifacts of resuscitation
artificial abortion
artificial eye
artificial heart
artificial kidney
aryepiglottic fold
aryepiglottic muscle
arylsulfatase test for differentiating
  species of rapid-growing
  mycobacteria
arytenoepiglottic
arytenoidal articular surface
arytenoid cartilage
arytenoid gland
arytenoid muscle
arytenoid swelling
As (arsenic)
asbestosis
ascariasis
Ascaris lumbricoides
ascending aorta
ascending aortic artery
ascending artery
ascending branch of uterine artery
ascending cervical artery
ascending colon
ascending degeneration
ascending frontal convolution
ascending lumbar vein
ascending lymphangitis
ascending myelitis
ascending nerve tracts
ascending neuritis
ascending oblique muscle
ascending palatine artery
ascending parietal convolution
ascending part

ascending pharyngeal artery
ascending process
ascending pyelonephritis
ascending ramus of ischium
ascending ramus of os pubis
Aschoff body
Aschoff cell
Aschoff-Rokitansky sinus
ascites
ascitic fluid
Ascoli precipitin test for anthrax
ascorbate-cyanide test
ascorbic acid
Aselli gland
Aselli pancreas
aseptate hyphae
aseptic fever
aseptic myocarditis of newborn
aseptic necrosis
aseptic wound
Ashby method
ashen tubercle
ashen wing
ashy dermatitis
ashy dermatosis
Asiatic cholera
Askanazy cell
Askin tumor
Ask-Upmark kidney
ASO (antistreptolysin O) titer
aspartate aminotransferase (AST)
   (formerly SGOT)
aspergillosis
Aspergillus
Aspergillus flavus
Aspergillus fumigatus
Aspergillus glaucus
Aspergillus niger
Aspergillus terreus
aspiration
  bronchial
  fine-needle (FNA)

aspiration *(continued)*
  lymph node
  marrow
  percutaneous epididymal sperm
  Vabra
aspirating needle
aspiration biopsy
aspiration biopsy cytology (ABC)
aspiration pneumonia
aspiration pneumonitis
aspiration trocar
aspirin tolerance test
asplenia
assay (see also *test*)
  biological activity
  CA-125
  Cardiac T Rapid
  competitive binding
  Clostridium difficile toxin
  1,25-dihydroxycholecalciferol
    (1,25-OH-D$_3$)
  enzyme
  enzyme-linked immunosorbent
    (ELISA)
  estrogen receptor
  fluorescent cytoprint
  Guthrie bacterial inhibitor (GBIA)
  hamster egg penetration
  histoculture drug response (HDRA)
  hormone
  25-hydroxyvitamin D (25-OH-D)
  immune complex
  Limulus amebocyte lysate
  lipoprotein
  microcytotoxicity
  PHA (phytohemagglutinin)
  plasma
  plasminogen activator inhibition
  progesterone receptor
  radioallergosorbent (RAST)
  radioceptor
  Raji cell

assay *(continued)*
   rapid flow cytometry
   Rio-rad protein
   sperm penetration
   stem cell
   T and B lymphocyte subset
   Vitamin D
assimilation pelvis
assimilation sacrum
association area
association cortex
association fiber
association tract
AST (aspartate aminotransferase)
   (formerly SGOT)
asteatosis
asterion
asteroid body
asthma
asthmaticus, status
Astler-Coller modification of Dukes
   classification of carcinoma
ASTRA analyzer
astragaloid bone
astragaloscaphoid bone
astragalus
astringent solution
astroblastoma
astrocyte
   ameboid
   proliferating
astrocytoma, gemistocytic
astroglia
astroglial cell
astroglial scarring
astrovirus
asymmetrical
asymmetry
asymptomatic gluten-sensitive
   enteropathy
asynchronism
asynchronous

asynchrony
asynergic
asynergy
atavistic epiphyses
ataxia, Friedreich
ataxic lymphopathy
atelectasis
atelectatic lung
atherogenic
atheroma
atheroma embolism
atheromatous degeneration
atheromatous plaque
atheromatous streaking
atherosclerosis
atherosclerotic
athlete's foot (tinea pedis)
athlete's heart
ATIII (antithrombin III)
atlantoaxial articulation
atlantoaxial joint
atlanto-occipital articulation
atlanto-occipital joint
atlanto-occipital membrane
atlas, arch of
atlas bone
atlas with axis, articulation of
atlas with epistropheus, articulation of
atlas with occipital bone, articulation of
atmospheric oxygen
ATN (acute tubular necrosis)
atopic dermatitis
atopic eczema
atopy
ATPase (adenosine triphosphatase)
atraumatic injury
atresia
   cardiac
   esophageal
atresia of ovarian follicle
atretic follicles
atretic ovarian follicle

atria (pl. of atrium)
atrial artery
atrial auricle
atrial auricula
atrial canal
atrial complex
atrial myxoma
atrial natriuretic factor (ANF)
atrial natriuretic hormone (ANH)
atrial septal defect
atrioventricular (AV or A/V)
atrioventricular band
atrioventricular block
atrioventricular bundle of His
atrioventricular canal
atrioventricular conduction
atrioventricular gradient
atrioventricular groove
atrioventricular nodal artery
atrioventricular nodal branch
atrioventricular node
atrioventricular node of His
atrioventricular opening of His
atrioventricular orifice
atrioventricular sulcus
atrioventricular trunk
atrioventricular valve
atrium (pl. atria)
   accessory
   left
   right
atrium dextrum of left heart
atrium dextrum of nasal fossa
atrium dextrum of primitive heart
atrium dextrum of right heart
atrophic change
atrophic gastritis
atrophic inflammation
atrophic kidney
atrophic pulp degeneration
atrophic vaginitis

atrophy
   acute yellow
   adrenal
   Aran-Duchenne muscular
   arthritic
   basal cell
   black
   blue
   bone
   breast
   brown
   cerebral
   cervical
   Charcot-Marie
   Charcot-Marie-Tooth
   circumscribed cerebral
   compensatory
   compression
   concentric
   correlated
   cortical
   Cruveilhier
   cutaneous
   degenerative
   Dejerine-Sottas
   Dejerine-Thomas
   denervated muscle
   disuse
   Duchenne-Aran muscular
   eccentric
   Eichhorst
   endocrine
   endometrial
   epidermal
   Erb
   exhaustion
   facial
   fatty
   Fazio-Londe
   gastric
   gastric mucosa

atrophy *(continued)*
  granular
  hepatic
  Hoffmann
  inflammatory
  interstitial
  ischemic muscular
  juvenile muscular
  lacrimal gland
  Landouzy-Dejerine
  laryngeal
  leaping
  Leber optic
  lingual
  lobar
  macular
  mammary
  multiple system
  muscular
  myelopathic muscular
  myopathic
  neural
  neuritic muscular
  neuromuscular
  neuropathic
  neurotrophic
  numeric
  optic
  otic
  pancreatic acini
  pathologic
  penile
  peroneal
  physiologic
  pigmentary
  post-traumatic
  postmenopausal
  pressure
  progressive choroidal
  progressive muscular
  progressive neuromuscular
  progressive spinal muscular

atrophy *(continued)*
  progressive subcortical
  progressive unilateral facial
  pseudohypertrophic muscular
  red
  renal
  rheumatic
  salivary gland
  senile
  serous
  simple
  spinal muscular
  splenic
  subacute
  subchronic
  Sudeck
  testicular
  thymic
  thyroid
  Tooth (Charcot-Marie-Tooth)
  toxic
  transneuronal
  unilateral facial
  vaginal
  vascular
  villous
  Vulpian
  Werdnig-Hoffmann spinal muscular
  white
  yellow
  Zimmerlin
atrophy of breast
atrophy of hair cells
atrophy of ovary
atrophy of pancreatic acini
atrophy of parenchyma of lacrimal and
  salivary glands
atrophy of skin, diffuse idiopathic
atrophy of tubular cells
atropine test
attenuation
attic recess

attolens aurem muscle
attrahens aurem muscle
atypia
    architectural
    cytologic
    koilocytotic
atypical bronchial pneumonia
atypical change
atypical interstitial pneumonia
atypical lymphocyte
atypical phenylketonuria
atypical pneumonia
atypical verrucous endocarditis
Au (gold) antigen
Auberger blood group
auditory area
auditory artery
auditory canal
auditory capsule
auditory cartilage
auditory cell
auditory cortex
auditory field
auditory ganglion
auditory meatus
auditory mucosa
auditory nerve
auditory nucleus
auditory ossicle
auditory pit
auditory plate
auditory process
auditory radiation
auditory receptor cell
auditory stria
auditory teeth of Huschke
auditory tooth
auditory tract
    cartilaginous portion of
    cushion of
    isthmus of
    pharyngeal orifice of

auditory tract *(continued)*
    pharyngeal ostium of
    tonsil of
    torus tubarius
auditory vein
auditory vesicle
Auerbach ganglia
Auerbach mesenteric plexus
Auerbach myenteric plexus
Auer body
Auer rod
augmented histamine test of gastric
    function
augmenting factor
augmentor fiber
augmentor nerve
AUL (acute undifferentiated leukemia)
auramine O dye
auramine–rhodamine fluorescent stain
auramine–rhodamine fluorochrome
    stain
auramine–rhodamine stain
aurantiasis
aurem muscle
    attolens
    attrahens
Aureobasidium pullulans
auricle
    accessory
    atrial
    cervical
auricle of left atrium
auricle of right atrium
auricula dextra
    cartilage of
    ligaments of
    muscles of
    nerves of
    vessels of
auricular appendage
auricular appendix
auricular arc

auricular artery
auricular canaliculus
auricular cartilage
auricular complex
auricular ganglion
auricular ligament
auricular lymph nodes
auricular nerve
auricular notch
auricular point
auricular reflex
auricular surface
auricular surface of ilium
auricular surface of sacrum
auricular triangle
auricular tubercle of Darwin
auricular vein
auriculo-infraorbital plane
auriculotemporal nerve
auriculoventricular groove
auscultation
auscultatory gap
Australian antigen
Australian Q fever
autemesia
autoagglutinin, anti-Pr cold
autoantibody, anti-idiotype
autoantigen
autochthonous malaria
autoclasis
autoclave
autoerythrocyte sensitivity test
autoerythrocyte sensitization syndrome
autograft
autohemolysis test
autoimmune disease
autoimmune hemolytic anemia (AIHA)
autoimmune hepatitis
autoimmune mechanism
autoimmune thyroiditis
autoimmunity
autoinfection

autoinoculation
autointerference
Autolet blood glucose test
autologous blood
autologous protein
autologous transfusion
autolysis, postmortem
autolytic enzyme
autolyze
automated reagin test (ART)
automatic cell
autonomic ganglion
autonomic motor neuron
autonomic nerve
autonomic nervous system
autonomic plexus
autoparenchymatous metaplasia
AutoPap 300 QC automatic PAP
   screener system
Autopath QC test
autophagic vacuole
autophagosome
autoprothrombin
autopsy (also called postmortem,
    postmortem examination,
   or "the post")
  consent for
  coroner
  medicolegal
autopsy room
autopsy specimen
autopsy subject, names for
  the body
  the cadaver
  the deceased
  the decedent
  the patient
  the name of the late patient
  the remains
  the subject
autopsy surgeon
auxiliary ventricle of heart

avascular necrosis
avian excreta
avian leukosis viruses
avian malaria
avian tuberculosis
aviator's ear
avidin-biotin complex (ABC)
avidin-biotin peroxidase complex
avidin-biotinylated peroxidase complex
Avipoxvirus
A vitamin

AV (atrioventricular) node
AV (arteriovenous) shunt
avulsed wound
A wave
axial aneurysm
Ayala index
Ayre spatula
azoospermia
azotemia
Aztec ear
azurophilic granule

B, b

Babesia bigemina
Babesia microti
babesiosis
Bachman-Pettit test
Bachman test
bacillary angiomatosis
bacillary dysentery
bacillary embolism
bacillary hemoglobinuria
bacillary necrosis
bacille Calmette-Guérin
bacilli in urine
bacilluria
bacillus (pl. bacilli) (see *pathogen*
    for names of organisms)
bacitracin
backbone
back-flow of blood
back-to-back configuration
back tooth
backward curvature
BACTEC bottle
bacteremia
bacteria (pl. of bacterium) (see *patho-*
    gen for names of organisms)
    acid-fast
    aerobic

bacteria *(continued)*
    anaerobic
    corkscrew-shaped
    defense against
    fibrillary
    funguslike
    gram-negative
    gram-positive
    helical
    intracellular
    pathogenic
    pus-forming
    pyogenic
    spiral-shaped
bacteria in stool
bacteria in urine
bacterial cellular protein
bacterial colonies
bacterial culture
bacterial culture media
bacterial dissociation
bacterial flora
bacterial gastroenteritis
bacterial infection
bacterial lipopolysaccharide
bacterial meningitis
bacterial myocarditis

bacterial nephritis
bacterial pericarditis
bacterial pneumonia
bacterial pneumonitis
bacterial protein
bacterial toxemia
bacterial toxins
bacterial vaginosis
bacterial virus
bactericidal concentration, minimum
   (MBC)
bacteriologic smear
bacteriological
bacteriology
bacteriolytic test
bacteriophage
bacteriophage plaque
bacterium (pl. bacteria) (see *bacteria*)
bacteriuria
Bacteroides (see *pathogen*)
Baehr-Lohlein lesion
Baerensprung erythrasma
Baermann concentration
bag, body
bagassosis
Bagros space
Baker cyst
baker's eczema
BAL (bronchoalveolar lavage)
balance
  acid-base
  electrolyte
balanced articulation
balanitis
balanitis xerotica obliterans
balanoposthitis
Balantidium coli
baldness (see *alopecia*)
  congenital
  female pattern
  male pattern
Balkan nephritis

ball-and-socket articulation
ball-and-socket joint
ballerina-foot pattern
balloon cell
balloon cell nevus
ballooning degeneration
ball valve
balsam mounting medium
Balser fatty necrosis
bamboo hair
band
  A
  absorption
  amniotic
  anogenital
  atrioventricular
  BB
  Bechterew
  Broca
  Bungner
  chromosome
  Clado
  contraction
  coronary
  Crooke-Russell
  delta
  diagonal
  Essick cell
  fibroelastic
  fibromuscular
  fibrous
  Gennari
  H
  Harris
  His
  Hunter-Schreger
  I
  iliotibial
  Ladd
  Lane
  longitudinal
  M

band *(continued)*
  Mach
  Maissiat
  matrix
  MB
  Meckel
  mesocolic
  MM
  moderator
  N-b
  oligoclonal
  omental
  pecten
  perioplic
  peritoneal
  pseudokeloidal
  Q
  R
  Reil
  septomarginal
  Silastic
  Simonart
  Soret
  Streeter
  tendinous
  transverse
  Z
band cell
bandlike adhesion
band neutrophil
band of Broca
band of colon
  anterior
  free
band of Giacomini
band of Gosset, spiral
band of Kaes-Bechterew
band-pass filter
band-shaped nucleus
band visualization
Bang bacillus
banjo-string adhesions

Bankart lesion
bank
  blood
  bone
  eye
  human milk
  skin
  tissue
Banti syndrome
Bárány caloric test
barber's pilonidal sinus
barbiturates, blood
Barcroft-Warburg apparatus
Bardinet ligament
Bard-Parker blade
bare area for colon
bare area of liver
barium meal
barium sulfate-absorbed plasma
Barkow ligaments
baroreceptor nerve
Barr body
Barr-Epstein virus
Barré-Guillain syndrome
barrel-shaped stone
Barrett epithelium
Bart abnormal hemoglobin
Bartholin abscess of vulvovaginal
  gland
Bartholin cyst
Bartholin duct
Bartholin gland
bartholinian abscess
Bartonella bacilliformis
basal body temperature (BBT)
basal bone
basal cell atrophy
basal cell carcinoma
basal cell epithelioma
basal cell layer
basal cell nevus
basal cell of skin

basal cell of vagina
basal cell papilloma
basal cell, swollen
basal corpuscle
basal epithelial hyperplasia
basal ganglia
basal granular cells
basal granule
basal lamina
basal layer
basal metabolism
basal nucleus
basal pigmentation
basal plate
basal plate cotyledon
basal ridge
basal rod
basal seat area
basal sphincter
basal squamous (basosquamous)
basal striation
basal surface
basal vein
basale, stratum
basalis decidua
basaloid cell
basaloma
base
   cement
   cranial
Basedow goiter
base excess test
base finger
baseline
baseline test
base material
basement lamina
basement membrane
basement tissue
base of bladder
base of ischiorectal fossa
base of lung

base plate or baseplate
basibregmatic axis
basic fuchsin
basic function
Basidiobolus ranarum
basihyal bone
basilar angle
basilar artery
basilar bone
basilar cartilage
basilar cell
basilar crest
basilar lamina
basilar membrane
basilar meningitis
basilar part
basilar plexus
basilar process
basilar sinus
basilar sulcus
basilar vertebra
basilic vein
basinasal line
basioccipital bone
basiotic bone
basipharyngeal canal
basis bundle, anterior
basisphenoid bone
basisphenoid vein
basket cell
basketweave pattern
baso (slang for basophil)
basopenia
basophil adenoma
basophil, beta
basophil cell
basophil degranulation test
basophil granule
basophil substance
basophilia
basophilic cell
basophilic cytoplasmic granules

basophilic leukemia
basophilic leukocyte
basophilic nuclear remnants in
  erythrocytes
basophilic stippling of erythrocytes
basosquamous (basal squamous)
basosquamous cell carcinoma
bath, flotation
bathing trunk nevus
bath itch
bath pruritus
battery of tests
Battey bacillus
battledore placenta
Bauhin gland
Bauhin valve
Baumé scale
BB bands
B bile
BB isoenzyme
BBT (basal body temperature)
BCAA (branched chain amino acid)
B (beta)
B cell
B-cell differentiating factor
B-cell lymphoma
B-cell monocytoid lymphoma
B-cell stimulatory factor
B chain
BCIP (5-bromo-4-chloro-3-indolyl
  phosphate)
bcl-2 gene (oncogene)
beach ear
beaded hepatic duct
beaked pelvis
beaker cell
beaklike projections of cartilage
Beale cell
Beale ganglion cells
Beau line
Bechterew band
Becker nevus

bed
  bladder
  capillary
  gallbladder
  hepatic
  liver
  nail
  portal vascular
  stomach
beef heart cardiolipin
beef heart infusion
beefy appearance
beefy red appearance of tongue
beefy texture
Behçet syndrome
BEI (butanol-extractable iodine)
bejel
bell clapper deformity
Bellini ligament
belly button
belly of muscle
B-emission counter
Bence Jones body
Bence Jones protein in urine
Bence Jones proteinemia
Bence Jones proteinuria
Bence Jones reaction
bench test
Benedict-Roth apparatus
Benedict test for glucose
benign epidermal tumor
benign false positive
benign familial chronic pemphigus
benign fibrous histiocytoma
benign hypertension
benign juvenile melanoma
benign lymphocytic meningitis
benign lymphoepithelial lesion
benign lymphoreticulosis
benign mucosal pemphigoid
benign neoplasm
benign nephrosclerosis

benign pigmented nevus
benign polyp
benign prostatic hyperplasia
benign recurrent hematuria
benign squamous papilloma
benign tertian malaria
bentiromide test
bentonite flocculation test
benzene nucleus
benzene poisoning
benzene ring
benzidine test for occult blood in urine
  or feces
Bérard aneurysm
Berger cells
Berger space
Bergmann cells
beriberi
berlock dermatitis
Bernard canal
Bernstein esophageal acid infusion test
berry aneurysm
berry cell
Berry ligaments
Berson test
Bertin bone
Bertin, columns of
Bertin ligament
berylliosis
beryllium dust
beryllium granuloma
Besnier-Boeck disease
Besnier-Boeck-Schaumann disease
Besnier prurigo
Bessey-Lowry unit
Best carmine stain
beta-adrenergic receptor
beta angle
beta basophil
beta blocker
beta-carotene cleavage enzyme
beta-cell

beta-endorphin
beta factor
beta fiber
beta fraction
beta globulin
beta granule
beta-HCG (human chorionic
  gonadotropin)
beta hemolysin
beta-hemolytic streptococcus
beta-hydroxybutyric acid
beta-lactamase
beta leukocyte
$beta_1$-lipoprotein
beta lipoprotein fraction
$beta_2$-microglobulin
beta particle
beta phage
Betascope 630 Biot Analyzer
beta substance
beta-thromboglobulin
Bethesda PAP smear classification
Bethesda system
Betke-Kleihauer stain
Bettendorff test for arsenic
Betz cell
Bevan-Lewis cell
bevel, cavosurface
Bezold abscess
B_T factor
B fiber
B5 fixative
BFP (biological false positive)
BGM cell
B hemophilia
B hepatitis
BHI (brain-heart infusion)
BHS-RFC A3 fluorescence microscope
Bial test
Bi antigen
biauricular axis
biaxial joint

bicameral abscess
bicameral uterus
bicanalicular sphincter
bicarbonate ion
bicarbonate, plasma
bicarbonate test
biceps brachii muscle
biceps tendon
Bichat canal
Bichat ligament
bicipital aponeurosis
bicipital bursitis
bicipital fascia
bicipital groove
bicipital rib
bicipital ridge
bicipital tuberosity
bicipitoradial bursa
bicondylar articulation
bicondylar joint
bicornuate uterus
bicuspid tissue
bicuspid tooth
bicuspid valve
Biebrich scarlet stain
Bielschowsky method
Bielschowsky stain
bifid rib
bifida, spina
Bifidobacterium
bifurcated ligament
bifurcation of lymph node
bifurcation of pulmonary trunk
Bigelow ligament
bigeminal body
bigeminal pregnancy
bilateral cortical necrosis
bilaterally
bilayer, outer lipoprotein
bile
  A
  B

bile *(continued)*
  C
  canaliculus
  extrahepatic
  gallbladder
  liver
  viscid
  viscous
  white
bile acid
  conjugated
  fecal
  total
bile acid pool
bile acid tolerance test
bile antigen
bile capillary
bile concretion
bile duct
  common (CBD)
  infundibulum
  interlobular
  preampullary portion of
  sphincter of
bile duct abscess
bile duct carcinoma
bile duct lumen
bile duct stone
bile esculin test
bile lake
bile papilla
bile pigment in basal ganglia
bile salts
bile sludge
bile solubility test for differentiation
  of pneumococci from other
  streptococci
bilharziasis
"bili" (slang for bilirubin)
biliary abscess
biliary apparatus
biliary calculus

biliary cirrhosis
biliary duct
biliary ductule
biliary fistula
biliary gland
biliary obstruction
biliary passage
biliary plexus
biliary radicle
biliary sludge
biliary structure
biliary tract
biliary tract stone
biliary tree
bilious diarrhea
bilious pneumonia
bilious remittent malaria
bilious vomiting
bilirubin
   conjugated
   deposition of unconjugated
   direct-reacting
   indirect-reacting
   serum
   total
   unconjugated
   urine
bilirubinate
bilirubin glucuronyltransferase
bilirubin infarct
bilirubin in urine
bilirubinuria (choluria)
Billheimer assay method
bilobate
bilobate placenta
bilobed (bi-lobed)
bilobed gallbladder
bilobular
bilobulate
bilocular joint
bilocular stomach
binary fission

binauricular arc
binding protein
Binz test for quinine in urine
biochemical profile
biochemical reaction
biochemistry
biological activity assay
biological false positive (BFP)
biological vector
biopsy (bx)
   aspiration
   bone marrow
   brain
   brush
   chorionic villus
   cold cup
   cone
   cytological
   dermis
   excisional
   exploratory
   fine-needle aspiration
   incisional
   Keyes punch
   mirror image breast
   needle
   needle core
   open
   punch
   shave
   skin
   stereotactic
   surface
   thin-needle
   Vabra aspirate
biopsy of myocardium via transvenous
   catheter
biopsy specimen
bioptome, Caves-Schutz-Stanford
Biopty cut needle
Biorad MRC 600 scanning system
Bio-rad protein assay

biorbital angle
biotin-dependent carboxylase
  deficiency
biotinylated secondary antibody
biparietal diameter (BPD)
bipartite patella
bipartite uterus
bipennate muscle
bipolar cell
bipolar retinal cell
Bipolaris australiensis
Bipolaris hawaiiensis
Bipolaris spicifera
Birbeck granule
bird's nest lesion
birefringence
birefringent crystal
birth canal
birth defect
birthmark, vascular
birth trauma
bisect
bisected
bisection
bismuth stomatitis
bite cell
bite plane
biuret test for serum proteins
biventral lobule
biventricular configuration
biventricular dilatation
biventricular hypertrophy
bizarre cell
bizarre mitotic figures
bizarre nuclei
Bizzozero red cell
BK DNA virus
black atrophy
black degeneration of brain
black eye
black fever
black induration

black light
black liver
black lung
black plague
black, Sudan
black tarry stool
black vomit
blackwater fever
bladder
  apex of
  base of
  exstrophy of
  hypertrophy
  hypotonic
  inflammation of
  neck of
  neurogenic
  papilloma of
  trigone of
  urinary
  uvula of
bladder bed
bladder capacity
bladder carcinoma
bladder cell
bladder diverticulum
bladder fundus
bladder tumor
bladder washing
blade bone
bland embolism
bland endometrium
Blandin and Nuhn gland
Blandin gland
blast cell
blast form
blastic lesion
blast injury
blastocyst
blastoderm
blastodermic disk
blastodermic layer

blastodermic vesicle
Blastomyces dermatitidis
blastomycetic dermatitis
blastomycosis
    European
    North American
    South American
blastoporic canal
Blastoschizomyces pseudotrichosporon
bleb
    cutaneous
    emphysematous
bleeding
    dysfunctional uterine (DUB)
    excessive
    postcoital
    postmenopausal
    purpuric
    recurrent
    widespread
bleeding from wounds, prolonged
bleeding gums
bleeding into a joint
bleeding polyp
bleeding time (BT)
    Duke
    Ivy
    Mielke
    Simplate
blennoid
blennorrhagia
blennorrhea, inclusion
blepharitis
blepharoplast
Blessig cyst
blighted ovum
blind foramen
blind gut
blindness
blind pouch
blind spot
blister cell

blistering
bloc (see *en bloc*)
Bloch scale
block
    atrioventricular
    cell
    occult
    paraffin
    tissue
    wax
blockade, ganglionic
blocked pleurisy
blocking and sectioning
blood
    anticoagulant-treated
    antigenic properties of
    arterial
    capillary
    circulating
    defibrinated
    degenerated
    donor
    extravasated
    hemolyzed
    iron-binding capacity of
    laky
    mass of congealed
    mixed venous
    nonoxygenated
    occult
    oxygen-carrying capacity of
    oxygenated
    peripheral
    platelet-poor (PPB)
    stagnation of
    sludged
    transfusion of incompatible
    typing and crossmatching of
    venous
    whole
blood agar, Bordet-Gengou
blood albumin

blood alcohol level
blood arsenic
blood barbiturate
blood-borne infection
blood-borne organism
blood-borne parasite
blood-brain barrier
blood cell
blood-clot lysis time (BLT)
blood clotting
blood coagulation
blood corpuscle
blood count
   complete
   differential
blood crystal
blood culture
blood ethanol
blood factor
blood fluke
blood-forming organ
blood-forming tissue
blood gas analysis
blood gases, arterial
blood gland
blood glucose
blood group (also, blood type)
   ABO
   Auberger
   autologous
   Cartwright
   Diego
   Dombrock
   Duffy
   high frequency
   I
   Kell
   Kidd
   Lewis
   low frequency
   Lutheran
   MNS

blood group *(continued)*
   P
   Rh
   Rh negative
   Rh positive
   Sutter
blood grouping
blood-influx phenomenon
blood lactic acid
blood lead level
bloodless field
blood loss
blood mole
blood pigment
blood plasma
blood plasma fraction
blood platelet
blood pool
blood pressure
blood serum
blood sludge
blood smear
blood specimen
bloodstained effusion
blood stream (also, bloodstream)
bloodsucking intestinal parasite
blood sugar test, fasting
blood tests (see Table, pp. 576-590)
blood-tinged fluid
blood-tinged sputum
blood transfusion, mismatched
blood type (see *blood group*)
blood typing
blood typing agglutinin
blood urea nitrogen (BUN)
blood vessel gland
blood volume
blood work
bloody diarrhea
bloody fluid
bloody spinal fluid
bloody stools

Bloom syndrome
blot, blotting
  Northern
  Southern
  Western
blotchy clumping of pigment
blotchy facial hyperpigmentation
blot-dot hybridization
Blount disease
blowing wound
blue aniline dye
blue aniline stain
blue atrophy
blue-black pigmentation (ochronosis)
    of cartilage, tendons, arterial intima
blue dome cyst
blue fever
blue-green pus
blue liver
blue nevus
blue ocular sclera
blue pus
blue pus bacillus
blue rubber bleb nevus
bluetongue virus
bluish macule
Blumenthal lesion
blunt trauma
B lymphocyte
Boas-Oppler bacillus
Boas point
boatlike abdomen
Bochdalek foramen
Bochdalek gap
Bockhart impetigo
Bodansky unit
Bodian method of staining
body (pl. bodies)
  acetone
  acidophilic
  adrenal
  alveolar

body *(continued)*
  Amato
  amyloid
  angularis
  anococcygeal
  aortic
  Arantius
  Arnold
  asbestos
  Aschoff
  asteroid
  Auer
  Barr
  Bence Jones
  bigeminal
  Bracht-Wachter
  Cabot ring
  Call-Exner
  carotid
  cavernous
  cell
  central
  chromaffin
  chromatin
  ciliary
  coccygeal
  colloid
  compressible cavernous
  conchoidal
  Councilman
  crystalloid
  cytoid
  Deetjen
  demilune
  dense
  Döhle (Doehl) inclusion
  Donovan
  Dutcher
  Ehrlich hemoglobinemic
  elementary
  epithelial
  esophageal

body *(continued)*
  Exner-Call
  fat
  fibrin
  foreign
  fuchsin
  fungal
  geniculate
  glomus
  Guarnieri
  Heinz
  Heinz-Ehrlich
  Herring
  Hirano
  Howell-Jolly
  immune
  inclusion
  inner
  Jolly
  Jolly-Howell
  ketone
  Lafora
  Leishman-Donovan
  Lewy
  Lewy inclusion
  Lipschütz
  lymphoglandular
  lyssa inclusion
  Mallory
  Mallory malpighian
  malpighian
  Masson
  Molluscum
  Negri
  Nissl
  Pappenheimer
  paravertebral
  Pick
  Pick inclusion
  psammoma
  Russell
  Schaumann

body *(continued)*
  Schmorl
  Stieda
  Toxoplasma
  vermiform
  vertebral
  Weibel-Palade
  Y
  zebra
body bag
body cavity
body cell mass
body fluid
body fluid amylase
body fluid glucose
body louse
body of epididymis
body of femur
body of gallbladder
body of Retzius
body of sternum
body of vertebra
body stalk
body wall
Boeck disease
Boeck sarcoid
Boehmer hematoxylin
Boerhaave gland
Boettcher (see *Böttcher*)
boggy uterus
Bogros space
boil
Bolivian hemorrhagic fever
Bolivian hemorrhagic fever virus
Boll cell
Bollinger granule
bolster fingers
bone (see Table of Bones)
  acetabular
  acromial
  alar
  Albers-Schoenberg marble

bone *(continued)*
   Albrecht
   alveolar
   alveolar supporting
   ankle
   arch of
   areolae of
   articular lamella of
   articular tubercle of temporal
   basal
   basihyal
   basilar
   basioccipital
   basisphenoid
   Bertin
   blade
   breast
   Breschet
   brittle
   bundle
   calcaneal
   calf
   cancellous
   cannon
   capitate
   carpal
   cartilage
   cavalry
   central
   chalky
   cheek
   coccygeal
   coffin
   collar
   compact
   convoluted
   coronary
   cortical
   costal
   coxal
   cranial
   cribriform

bone *(continued)*
   cubital
   cuboid
   cuneiform
   dead
   dense
   dermal
   destruction of
   devitalized portion of
   dorsal talonavicular
   ear
   eburnated
   elbow
   endochondral
   enetral
   epactal
   epihyal
   epiphysis of
   epipteric
   episternal
   erosion of epiphyseal
   eburnated
   ethmoid
   exercise
   exoccipital
   facial
   femoral
   fibular
   first cuneiform
   flank
   flat
   Flower
   fourth turbinated
   fragile
   freeze-dried
   frontal
   funny
   Goethe
   greater multangular
   hamate
   haunch
   heel

bone *(continued)*
  highest turbinated
  hip
  hollow
  hooked
  hyoid
  hyperplastic
  iliac
  immature
  incarial
  incisive
  inferior turbinated
  inflammation of
  innominate
  intermaxillary
  intermediate cuneiform
  interparietal
  intracartilaginous
  intrachondral
  intramembranous
  irregular
  ischial
  ivory
  ivorylike
  jaw
  jugal (zygomatic)
  Krause
  lacrimal
  lamellar
  lamellated
  lateral cuneiform
  lenticular
  lentiform
  lesser multangular
  lingual
  long
  lunate
  malar
  marble
  mastoid
  maxillary
  maxilloturbinal

bone *(continued)*
  medial cuneiform
  medullary
  metacarpal
  metastasis to
  metatarsal
  middle cuneiform
  middle turbinated
  multangular
  nasal
  navicular
  necrotic
  neoplasm of
  new
  newly woven
  nonlamellar
  nonlamellated
  occipital
  odontoid
  orbicular
  orbitosphenoidal
  osteoporosis of
  osteoporotic
  palate
  palatine
  parietal
  pedal
  pelvic
  penis
  perichondral
  periosteal
  periotic
  peroneal
  petrosal
  petrous
  phalangeal
  ping-pong
  pipe
  Pirie
  pisiform
  pneumatic
  postsphenoid

bone *(continued)*
- preinterparietal
- premaxillary
- presphenoid
- pterygoid
- pubic
- pyramidal
- quadrilateral
- radial
- redness of
- replacement
- resurrection
- reticulated
- rider's
- Riolan
- rudimentary
- sacral
- sacred
- scaphoid
- scapular
- sclerotic
- scroll
- second cuneiform
- semilunar
- septal
- sesamoid
- shank
- shin
- short
- sieve
- skull
- sphenoid
- sphenoidal turbinated
- sphenoturbinal
- splint
- spoke
- spongy
- squamo-occipital
- squamous
- squamous-type
- stifle
- stirrup

bone *(continued)*
- substitution
- superior turbinated
- supernumerary
- suprainterparietal
- supraoccipital
- suprapharyngeal
- suprasternal
- supreme turbinated
- sutural
- tail
- tarsal
- temporal
- thigh
- thoracic
- three-cornered
- trabecular
- trapezium
- trapezoid
- triangular
- tuberculosis of
- turbinate
- turbinated
- tympanic
- tympanohyal
- ulnar
- unciform
- upper jaw
- vascular
- vesalian
- Vesalius
- vomer
- wedge
- weightbearing
- whettle
- woven
- xiphoid
- yoke
- zygomatic

bone abscess
bone age
bone architecture

bone atrophy
bone bank
bone calcification
bone canaliculus
bone cell
bone corpuscle
bone cortex
bone cyst
bone deformity
bone degeneration
bone dysplasia
bone erosion
bone fracture
bone fragment, jagged
bone infarct
bone lacuna
bonelet
bone marrow
bone marrow biopsy
bone marrow degeneration
bone marrow, differential count:
  lymphocytes
  metamyelocytes
  monocytes
  myeloblasts
  myelocytes: neutrophilic,
    eosinophilic, basophilic
  plasma cells
  polymorphonuclear basophils,
    eosinophils, neutrophils
  promyelocytes
  reticulum cells
bone marrow embolism
bone marrow failure
bone marrow study
bone marrow transplantation
bone matrix
bone medulla
bone mineral density
bone morphogenetic protein
bone pain
bone plate

bone resorption
bone salts
bone softening
bone splitting
bone spur
bone tissue, normal
bone tumor
bone wax
Bonnot gland
bony ankylosis
bony callus
bony eburnation
bony fossa
bony labyrinth
bony landmarks
bony palate
bony pelvis
bony proliferation
bony semicircular canal
bony thoracic cage
bony tissue
booster phenomenon on TB test
border
  alveolar
  brush
  crescentic
  interosseous
border cell
border disease virus
borderline diabetes
borderline hypertension
borderline leprosy
borderline malignancy
borderline normal
borderline test result
border of distal ileum, antimesenteric
border of heart
  inferior
  left
  right
  superior
border of mandible, alveolar

border zone
Bordet-Gengou agar
Bordet-Gengou bacillus
Bordet-Gengou blood agar
Bordet-Gengou phenomenon
Bordetella bronchiseptica
Bordetella parapertussis
Bordetella pertussis
Bornholm disease
Borrelia burgdorferi
Borrelia hermsii
Borrelia kochii
Borrelia mazzottii
Borrelia parkeri
Borrelia recurrentis
Borrelia turicatae
boss
bosselated
Boston exanthem
Botallo ligament
Botryodiplodia theobromae
botryoides sarcoma
botryomycosis
borderline normal
Böttcher (Boettcher)
Böttcher canal
Böttcher cell
Böttcher space
bottle, BACTEC
bottle-shaped hair cells
botulism
Bouin fixative
Bouin fluid
Bouin picroformol-acetic fixative
Bouin solution
boundary membrane
Bourgery ligament
bouquet fever
boutonneuse fever
boutonnière deformity
bowed tendon

bowel
  aganglionic
  apple-peel
  dead
  infarcted
  intussuscepted
  ischemic
  kink in
  large
  small
  strangulated
bowel axis
bowel contents
bowel disease with protein loss
bowel gases
bowel gas pattern
bowel loop
bowel lumen
bowel sounds
bowel stenosis
bowel stoma
bowel tones
bowel wall
Bowen disease
bowenoid cell
bowenoid papulosis
Bowen precancerous dermatosis
Bowie stain
bowing of long bones
bowleg, nonrachitic
Bowman capsule
Bowman disease
Bowman gland
Bowman membrane
Bowman space
boxer's encephalopathy
box, snuff
Boyden sphincter
Bozicevich test
BPD (biparietal diameter)
Br (bromine)

brachial artery
brachial fascia
brachial gland
brachial lymph node
brachial muscle
brachial neuritis
brachial plexus
brachial vein
brachii, biceps
brachii muscle
brachiocarpal articulation
brachiocephalic artery
brachiocephalic trunk
brachiocephalic vein
brachioradial articulation
brachioradial muscle
brachioradial tendon
brachioulnar articulation
Bracht-Wachter lesion
brachypellic pelvis
bradycardia
brain
   edematous
   inflammation of
   metastasis to
   respirator
   sand
   split
   wet
brain abscess
brain artery
brain biopsy
brain damage, irreversible
brain dead
brain death
brain degeneration
brain disease, demyelinating
brain fissure
brain-heart infusion (BHI)
brain heart infusion agar
brain laceration
brain mantle

brain stem
brain substance
brain sugar
brain swelling
brain tissue
brain tumor
brain wave
branch
   anterior cutaneous
   circumflex
   cutaneous lateral
   inferior cardiac
   perforating
   pudendal
branched chain alpha-ketoacids,
   block in decarboxylation of
branched chain amino acid (BCAA)
branched tubular glands of Littré
brancher (also, branching)
brancher enzyme
brancher enzyme deficiency
brancher factor
branches
   paired parietal
   paired visceral
   unpaired parietal
   unpaired visceral
branchial arch
branchial cartilage
branchial cell
branchial cleft
branchial cleft cyst
branchial cyst
branchial duct
branchial efferent column
branchial fistula
branchial groove
branchial pouch
branching enzyme
branching factor
branching filaments
branching pattern

branchiomeric muscle
branchiomotor nucleus
Branhamella catarrhalis (formerly
   Neisseria catarrhalis)
brass founder's fever
Braune canal
Brazilian spotted fever
bread-and-butter heart
bread-and-butter pericardium
breakbone fever
breakdown hemoglobin
breakdown of muscle tissue
breakdown of red blood cells
breast
   accessory
   biopsy of
   fibroadenoma of
   fibrocystic
   proemial
   shotty
breast atrophy
breast biopsy
breast bone (also, breastbone)
breast carcinoma
breast degeneration
breast inflammation
breast milk jaundice
breast neoplasm
breast tumor
breath analysis test
breath-holding test
bregmatic bone
bregmatic fontanel
bregmatolambdoid arc
Brenner tumor
Breschet bone
Breschet canal
Breslow classification of malignant
   melanoma
Breus mole
breviradiate cells
Brewer infarct

bridge
   arteriolovenular
   cell
   cytoplasmic
   intercellular
   mucosal
bridge corpuscle
bridge of nose
bridging epithelium
bridging necrosis
Brill-Zinsser disease
brim, pelvic
B ring of esophagus
Brinton disease
bristle cell
brittle bone
brittle diabetes
brittle mass
broadest muscle
broad fascia
broad flat nose
broad ligament abscess
broad ligament of uterus
broad ligament pregnancy
Broca area
Broca band
Broca center
Broca diagonal band
Broca pudendal pouch
Brockenbrough needle
Brodel white line
Broder criteria
Broders index of tumor malignancy
Brodie abscess
Brodie joint
Brodie knee
Brodie ligament
broken-down erythrocytes
Brolacin agar
bromine (Br)
bromosulfophthalein (also, sulfo-
   bromophthalein sodium) (BSP)

bromphenol test
bronchial artery
bronchial aspirate
bronchial asthma
bronchial brushing
bronchial fremitus
bronchial gland
bronchial mucosa
bronchial pneumonia
bronchial polyp
bronchial stenosis
bronchial tube
bronchial vein
bronchial washing
bronchic cell
bronchiectasis
bronchiolar edema
bronchiolar exocrine cell
bronchiolar spasm and edema
bronchiole
   conducting
   respiratory
   terminal
bronchiolitis obliterans organizing
   pneumonia
bronchiolitis, obliterative
bronchitis
   acute
   chronic
bronchoalveolar lavage (BAL)
bronchoalveolar lavage fluid
bronchobiliary fistula
bronchocavitary fistula
bronchoesophageal fistula
bronchoesophageal muscle
bronchogenic adenocarcinoma
bronchogenic carcinoma
bronchogenic cyst
bronchomediastinal lymph trunk
bronchomediastinal trunk
bronchopleural fistula
bronchopneumonia, hypostatic

bronchopulmonary dysplasia
bronchopulmonary lymph node
bronchopulmonary segment
bronchoscopic smear
bronchus (pl. bronchi)
   branch
   eparterial
   hyparterial
   inferior lobe
   inflammation of
   intermediate
   left main
   lobar
   main stem
   major
   middle lobe
   mucoid impaction of
   primary
   principal
   right lobe
   right main
   segmental
   superior
   superior lobe
bronchus intermedius
bronchus principalis sinister
bronchus principalis dexter
bronchus segmentalis
bronze diabetes
bronze edema
bronze pigmentation of skin
brood capsule
brood cell
Brooker periarticular heterotopic
   ossification (PHO)
broth, nutrient
brown adipose tissue
brown atrophy
Brown-Brenn Gram stain
brown fat
brown fat tissue
Brown-Hopp tissue Gram stain

brown induration
brown reaction product
brown stool
brown stria
brown-tail moth dermatitis
brown tissue
brown tumor
Brucella abortus
Brucella canis
Brucella melitensis
Brucella suis
brucellosis agglutinins
Bruch gland
Bruch membrane
Brücke line
Brunner gland
Brunn nest
Bruns glucose medium
brush biopsy
brush border
brushing, bronchial
Bruton disease
B_T factor
bubble gum dermatitis
bubonic plague
bucca (pl. buccae)
buccal angle
buccal artery
buccal cavity
buccal curve
buccal fat pad
buccal flange
buccal gingiva
buccal gland
buccal lymph node
buccal mucosa
buccal nerve
buccal occlusion
buccal region
buccal shelf
buccal smear
buccal surface

buccal ulcer
buccal vestibule
buccinator artery
buccinator crest
buccinator lymph node
buccinator nerve
buccocervical ridge
buccogingival ridge
bucconasal membrane
bucconeural duct
bucco-occlusal angle
buccopharyngeal fascia
buccopharyngeal membrane
buccopharyngeal part
buckled aorta
Bucky diaphragm
bud
    dorsal pancreatic
    end
    ventral pancreatic
budding platelet
Budin obstetrical joint
Buerger disease
buffalo hump
buffer capacity
buffered formalin
buffered neutral formalin
buffered solution
buffer, plasma
buffy coat
buffy coated cells
buffy coat smear
buffy coat smear test
Buhl desquamative pneumonia
Buisson, coxofemoral articulation of
bulb
    aortic
    arterial
    carotid
    dental
    duodenal
    end

bulb *(continued)*
  hair
  olfactory
bulbar conjunctiva
bulbar myelitis
bulbar ridge
bulbar septum
bulb artery, urethral
bulbi, phthisis
bulbi urethrae, arteria
bulbocavernosus muscle
bulbocavernous gland
bulb of penis
bulb of urethra
bulboid corpuscle
bulbosacral system
bulbospongiosus muscle of penis
bulbourethral artery
bulbourethral gland
bulb vestibule
bulging of bleb
bulging of mucosa between trabeculae
bulging of sac
bulging of sclera
bulky stool
bulla (pl. bullae)
Bullard hematoxylin
bullous emphysema
bullous fever
bullous impetigo of newborn
bullous pemphigoid
bull's-eye lesion
bumpy texture
BUN (blood urea nitrogen)
BUN/creatinine ratio
bundle
  aberrant
  atrioventricular (AV)
  collagen
  comma
  neurovascular
bundle bone

bundle of His, atrioventricular
Bungner band
Bunyamwera viruses
Bunyavirus encephalitis
Burdwan fever
buret (burette)
Burkitt lymphoma
Burkitt tumor
burned skin
burn infection
burn, powder
burns classification
Burns ligament
Burns space
Burow solution
burr cell
burrow
burrowing pus
bursa
  Achilles
  adventitious
  anserine
  bicipitoradial
  omental
bursal abscess
bursal equivalent tissue
bursitis
  anserine
  bicipital
  calcaneal
  chronic
  intertubercular
  olecranon
  prepatellar
  severe
  subacromial
  subdeltoid
  trochanteric
bursting of cells
bursting of red blood cells
Butchart staging classification
butter bacillus

butterfly rash
buttery texture
button, cell
buttonlike necrotic lesion at inoculation
　site
B virus hepatitis
B_1 vitamin

B_6 vitamin
B_{12} vitamin
Bwamba fever
B wave
bx (biopsy)
bypass graft
Byzantine arch palate

C, c

C (carbon)
C (Celsius)
C (cervical)
cablelike connection
Cabot ring body
cachectic fever
cachexia, malarial
cadaver
cadaveric
CAE (carcinoembryonic) antigen
caecum (cecum)
CA (cancer antigen)
CA 15-2 RIA test
CA 15-3 antigen
CA 15-3 antigenic tumor marker
CA 15-3 breast cancer tumor marker
CA 15-3 RIA test
CA 19-9 antigenic tumor marker
CA 19-9 carbohydrate antigen
CA 27.29 tumor marker
CA 50 tumor marker
CA 72-4 antigen
CA 72-4 antigenic tumor marker
CA 125 antigen
CA 125 assay
CA 125 cross-reactivity
CA 125 ovarian tumor marker

CA 125-11 tumor marker
CA 195 tumor marker
CA 549 breast cancer tumor marker
CA M26 tumor marker
CA M29 tumor marker
CA virus
caddy (dark, sandy mud) stool
café au lait spots on skin
cage
    bony thoracic
    osseocartilaginous thoracic
Cajal gold sublimate
Cajal, interstitial cells of
Cajal trichrome
cake kidney
Calabar swelling
calcaneal artery
calcaneal articular surface
calcaneal bone
calcaneal bursitis
calcaneal process
calcaneal region
calcaneal spur
calcaneal sulcus
calcaneal tendon
calcaneal tubercle
calcaneal tuberosity

calcaneoastragaloid ligament
calcaneocuboid articulation (or joint)
calcaneocuboid ligament
calcaneofibular ligament
calcaneonavicular ligament
calcaneotibial ligament
calcaneus and astragalus, articulation of
calcaneus bone
calcaneus, tendo
calcareous degeneration
calcareous infarct
calcareous infiltration
calcareous material
calcareous metastasis
calcareous pancreatitis
calcarine artery
calcarine fasciculus
calcarine fissure
calcarine sulcus
calciferous canal
calcification
   dystrophic
   metastatic
   Mönckeberg (Moenckeberg)
   normal
calcification line
calcification of bone
calcification of cysts
calcification of osseous matrix
calcific plaque
calcified aorta
calcified cartilage
calcified pericardium
calcified thrombus inside a vein
calcinosis
calcinosis cutis
calcinuric diabetes
calcitonin
calcitonin–calcium infusion stimulation
   test
calcitonin hormone
calcitonin test

calcium
   ionized
   total
calcium crystals
calcium deposition in osteoid tissue
calcium deposits
calcium infiltration
calcium oxalate
calcium oxalate calculus
calcium oxalate crystals in urine
calcium phosphate salt in bones and
   teeth
calcium pyrophosphate crystals in
   pseudogout
calcium resorption
calcium salts
   crystals of
   deposition of in kidney tissue
calculus (pl. calculi)
   alternating
   alvine
   articular
   biliary
   calcium oxalate
   cholesterol
   combination
   cystine
   decubitus
   encysted
   fibrin
   fusible
   gastric
   gallbladder
   gonecystic
   hemic
   hemp seed
   hepatic
   indigo
   intestinal
   joint
   lacrimal
   lacteal

calculus *(continued)*
   lung
   mammary
   matrix
   metabolic
   mulberry
   nasal
   nephritic
   oxalate
   pancreatic
   phosphate
   pocketed
   preputial
   prostatic
   renal
   salivary
   serumal
   shellac
   spermatic
   staghorn
   stomach
   stonelike
   struvite
   subgingival
   submorphous
   supragingival
   tonsillar
   urate
   urethral
   uric acid
   urinary
   urostealith
   uterine
   vesical
   vesicoprostatic
   xanthic
Caldani ligament
Caldwell-Moloy classification
calf bone
calf muscle
caliber of stool
calibration of testing instrument

calibration of testing method
calibration, standard
Calicivirus, calicivirus
California encephalitis virus
calix (pl. calices) (see *calyx*)
CALLA (common acute lymphoblastic
   leukemia antigen)
Call-Exner body
callosal convolution
callosal gyrus
callosal sulcus
callosity
callosomarginal artery
callosomarginal fissure
callous (adj.)
callus (noun)
   bony
   ensheathing
callus formation (*not* callous)
Calmette-Guérin bacillus
caloric deficiency in children
calorics
   cold water
   ice water
caloric test
Calot triangle
Calmette test
calvaria
calvaria dura mater
calvarium
Calvé-Perthes-Legg disease
calvities (baldness)
calyceal
calyces (pl. of calyx)
Calymmatobacterium granulomatis
   (formerly *Donovania granulomatis*)
calyx (pl. calyces) (also, calix)
   major
   minor
   renal
cameloid cell
CAM 5.2 antibody

Campbell ligament
Camper fascia
Camper ligament
camp fever
CAMP (Christie, Atkins, and Munch-
  Petersen) factor
CAMP test for Group B beta-hemo-
  lytic streptococci
Campylobacter cinaedi
Campylobacter coli
Campylobacter fennelliae
Campylobacter fetus (formerly *Vibrio
  fetus*)
Campylobacter gastroenteritis
Campylobacter jejuni
Campylobacter laridis
Campylobacter parahemolyticus
Campylobacter pylori
Campylobacter vulnificus
canal
  abdominal
  accessory
  adductor
  Alcock
  alimentary
  alveolar
  alveolodental
  ampulla of semicircular
  anal
  anterior condyloid
  anterior semicircular
  archenteric
  Arnold
  arterial
  artery of pterygoid
  atrial
  atrioventricular (AV)
  auditory
  basipharyngeal
  Bernard
  Bichat
  biliary (interlobular)

canal *(continued)*
  biliary (intralobular)
  birth
  blastoporic
  bony semicircular
  Böttcher
  Braune
  Breschet
  calciferous
  caroticotympanic
  carotid
  carpal
  caudal
  central
  cerebrospinal
  cervical (of uterus)
  cervical axillary
  cervicoaxillary
  ciliary
  Civinini
  Cloquet
  cochlear
  common atrioventricular
  condylar
  condyloid
  connecting
  Corti
  Cotunnius
  craniopharyngeal
  crural
  deferent
  dental
  dental root
  dentinal
  diploic
  Dorello
  Dupuytren
  ear
  endocervical
  endodermal
  ethmoid
  eustachian

canal *(continued)*
- external auditory
- facial
- fallopian
- femoral
- Ferrein
- flexor
- Fontana
- galactophorous
- ganglionic
- Gartner
- gastric
- genital
- greater palatine
- gubernacular
- Guyon
- gynecophoric
- hair
- Hannover
- haversian
- hemal
- Henle
- Hensen
- hernial
- Hirschfeld
- His
- Holmgren-Golgi
- Hoyer
- Huguier
- Hunter
- Huschke
- hyaloid
- hypoglossal
- iliac
- incisive
- incisor
- inferior dental
- infraorbital
- inguinal
- interdental
- interfacial
- intersacral

canal *(continued)*
- intestinal
- intracytoplasmic
- Jacobson
- Kovalevsky
- Kuersteiner
- lacrimal
- lateral
- lateral semicircular
- Lauth
- Leeuwenhoek
- Löwenberg (Loewenberg)
- mandibular
- marrow
- maxillary
- medullary
- mental
- Müller (Mueller)
- musculotubal
- nasal
- nasolacrimal
- nasopalatine
- neural
- neurenteric
- notochordal
- nutrient
- obstetric
- obturator
- olfactory
- optic
- orbital
- palatine
- palatomaxillary
- palatovaginal
- paraurethral
- parturient
- pelvic
- pericardioperitoneal
- perivascular
- persistent atrioventricular
- persistent common atrioventricular
- Petit

canal *(continued)*
   pharyngeal
   pleural
   pleuropericardial
   pleuroperitoneal
   portal
   posterior semicircular
   principal artery of pterygoid
   pterygoid
   pterygopalatine
   pudendal
   pulmoaortic
   pulp
   pyloric
   recurrent
   Reichert
   rigid
   Rivinus
   root (of tooth)
   Rosenthal
   sacculocochlear
   sacculoutricular
   sacral
   Santorini
   Schlemm
   scleral
   semicircular
   sheathing
   small (of chorda tympani)
   Sondermann
   sphenopalatine
   sphenopharyngeal
   spinal
   Stensen
   Stilling
   subsartorial
   Sucquet-Hoyer
   supraciliary
   supraoptic
   supraorbital
   tarsal
   temporal

canal *(continued)*
   Theile
   Tourtual
   tubal
   tubotympanic
   tympanic
   umbilical
   uniting
   urogenital
   uterine
   uterocervical
   uterovaginal
   utriculosaccular
   vaginal
   van Horne
   Velpeau
   ventricular
   Verneuil
   vertebral
   vesicourethral
   vestibular
   vidian
   Volkmann
   vomerine
   vomerobasilar
   vomerorostral
   vomerovaginal
   vulvar
   vulvouterine
   Walther
   Wirsung
   zygomaticofacial
   zygomaticotemporal
canal for tensor tympani muscle
canalicular abscess
canalicular duct
canalicular sphincter
canaliculus (pl. canaliculi)
   apical
   auricular
   bile
   bone

canaliculus *(continued)*
  cochlear
  haversian
  innominate
  intercellular
canalization
canal of Cuvier
canal of Guidi
canal of Guyon
canal of Hering
canal of Nuck
canal of Oken
canal of Recklinghausen
canal of Scarpa
canal of Schlemm
canal of Steno
canal of Stilling
canal of stomach
Canavan disease
Canavan–van Bogaert–Bertrand disease
cancellated bone
cancellous bone
cancellous tissue
cancer (see *carcinoma, sarcoma, tumor*)
  aniline
  betel
  chimney-sweep's
  clay pipe
  colloid
  contact
  cystic
  dendritic
  dye worker's
  hereditary
  latent
  melanotic
  mule-spinner's
  non-small cell lung
  occult
  paraffin
  pitch worker's
  scirrhous

cancer *(continued)*
  small-cell lung
  swamp
  tar
  tubular
cancer antigen (CA)
cancer cell
cancer embolism
cancer-inducing virus
cancerization
candela (cd)
Candida
Candida albicans
Candida guilliermondii
Candida krusei
Candida lusitaniae
Candida parapsilosis
Candida pseudotropicalis
Candida pulcherrima
Candida ravautii
Candida rugosa
Candida stellatoidea
Candida tropicalis
Candida viswanathii
candidal granuloma
candidal infection
candidiasis
candidosis
C&S (culture and sensitivity)
canicola fever
canine tissue
canine tooth
canis
canities
cannabinoids
cannon bone
CA 125 glycoprotein
caoutchouc pelvis
cap, cervical
capacity
  bladder
  buffer

capacity *(continued)*
  cranial
  forced vital (FVC)
  functional residual (FRC)
  heat
  hemoglobin-binding
  inspiratory
  iron-binding (IBC)
  lung
  maximum breathing
  oxygen
  residual
  respiratory
  thermal
  total iron-binding (TIBC)
  total lung (TLC)
  vital (VC)
capillary
  arterial
  bile
  continuous
  lymph
  sinusoidal
  venous
capillary angioma
capillary bed
capillary blood
capillary dilatation and proliferation
capillary embolism
capillary endothelial cell
capillary fenestrated
capillary fragility, abnormal
capillary fragility test
capillary gap method
capillary hemangioma
capillary hereditary fragility
capillary lake
capillary loops of glomerulus
capillary microaneurysms of retina
capillary nevus
capillary permeability factor
capillary pneumonia

capillary resistance test
capillary thrombosis
capillary tube
capillary valve
capillary vein
capillary vessel
capillary zone electrophoresis (CZE)
capitate bone
capitate facet
capitate hamate
capitate-hamate joint
capitate soft spot
capitate, volar
capitis, tinea
capitolunate joint
capitular articulation
capitular joint
capitulum bone
Capnocytophaga canimorsus
Capnocytophaga ochracea
Capripoxvirus
capsid
capsid formation
capsular antigen
capsular artery
capsular ligament
capsular nephritis
capsular polysaccharide
capsular space
capsular swelling
capsulatum
capsule
  adrenal
  articular
  auditory
  Bowman
  brood
  cartilage
  cricoarytenoid articular
  cricothyroid articular
  fatty renal
  fibrous

capsule *(continued)*
  fibrous renal
  Gerota
  Glisson
  hepatic
  joint
  organ
  splenic
  thyroid
  tough
  tough fibrous
  tumor
capsule cell
capsule of connective tissue
capsule of joint
capsule of liver
capture ELISA
caput medusae
caput succedaneum
carate
carbohydrate metabolism
carbohydrates, test on venous blood for
carbohydrate utilization test
carbolfuchsin stain
carbon (C)
carbon-containing fuels, combustion of
carbon dioxide (CO_2)
  arterial
  metabolism
  partial pressure of (PCO_2)
  pulmonary excretion of
  pulmonary retention of
  tests for
  total (TCO_2)
carbon dioxide gases
carbon dioxide tension
carbonic acid in blood
carbonization
carbon monoxide (CO)
carbon monoxide poisoning
carbon 13-labeled ketoisocaproate
  breath test

Carbowax embedding medium
carboxyhemoglobin in blood
carbuncle
carbunculosis
Carcassonne ligament
carcinoembryonic antigen (CEA) test
carcinoid syndrome
carcinoid tumor
carcinoma (see also *cancer, sarcoma,*
   tumor)
  acinous cell
  adenocystic
  adenoid cystic
  adenoid squamous cell
  adenosquamous
  adnexal
  adrenocortical
  aldosterone-producing
  aldosterone-secreting
  alveolar
  alveolar cell
  ameloblastic
  anaplastic c. of thyroid gland
  apocrine
  basal cell
    alveolar
    comedo
    cystic
    morphea-like
    multicentric
    nodulo-ulcerative
    pigmented
    sclerosing
    superficial
  basaloid
  basosquamous cell
  bile duct
  bilharzial
  bladder
  breast
  bronchioalveolar
  bronchioloalveolar

carcinoma *(continued)*
 bronchogenic
 cerebriform
 cholangiocarcinoma
 cholangiocellular
 chorionic
 choroid plexus
 clear cell
 colloid
 comedo
 corpus
 cortisol-producing
 cribriform
 cylindrical
 ductal
 ductal carcinoma in situ (DCIS)
 ductal carcinoma of prostate
 duct cell
 eccrine
 embryonal
 embryonal cell
 endometrial
 epidermal, epidermoid
 exophytic
 extrahepatic bile duct
 fibrolamellar
 follicular
 gastric
 gelatinous
 genital
 giant cell
 giant cell c. of thyroid gland
 glandular
 glans, intraepidermal
 granulosa cell
 hepatic
 hepatocellular
 hereditary
 Hürthle cell
 hypernephroid
 infantile embryonal
 infiltrating ductal

carcinoma *(continued)*
 infiltrating lobular
 inflammatory c. of breast
 intraductal
 intraepidermal
 intraepithelial
 invasive
 invasive lobular
 juvenile embryonal
 Kulchitzky cell
 large cell
 lenticular
 leptomeningeal
 lobular
 lobular c. in situ (LCIS)
 Lucké
 medullary
 melanotic
 meningeal
 Merkel cell
 metastatic
 metatypical
 microinvasive
 micropapillary
 moderately well-differentiated
 mucinous
 mucoepidermoid
 mucous
 nasopharyngeal
 neuroendocrine c. of skin
 noninfiltrating lobular
 oat cell
 osteoid
 Paget
 pancreatic
 papillary
 papillary c. of thyroid gland
 poorly differentiated
 preinvasive
 prickle cell
 primary
 primary intraosseous

carcinoma *(continued)*
  rectosigmoid
  renal cell
  residual
  retinoblastoma hereditary human
  scar
  schistosomal bladder
  schneiderian
  scirrhous
  sebaceous
  signet ring
  small cell
  small cell lung c. (SCLC)
  small round cell
  spindle cell
  squamous
  squamous cell (SCC)
  staging of cervical
  string cell
  systemic effects
  terminal duct
  thyroid
  trabecular c. of skin
  transitional cell
  tubular
  undifferentiated
  undifferentiated c. of thyroid gland
  undifferentiated squamous cell
  uterine cervix
  uterine corpus
  verrucous
  villous
  well-differentiated
carcinoma in situ
  ductal (DCIS)
  lobular (LCIS)
carcinoma en cuirasse
carcinoma ex mixed tumor
carcinoma ex pleomorphic adenoma
carcinomatosis
carcinomatous pericarditis
carcinosarcoma

cardia
  crescent of
  gastric
cardia of stomach
cardiac aneurysm
cardiac anomaly
cardiac antrum
cardiac area of stomach
cardiac arrest
cardiac atresia
cardiac branch
cardiac cirrhosis
cardiac congestion
cardiac dilatation
cardiac dullness
cardiac edema
cardiac failure
cardiac ganglion
cardiac gland
cardiac histiocyte
cardiac hormone
cardiac hypertrophy
cardiac impression on liver
cardiac index
cardiac isoenzymes (see *isoenzymes*)
cardiac liver
cardiac lung
cardiac mucosa
cardiac muscle fiber
cardiac muscle, striated
cardiac muscle tissue
cardiac nerve, parasympathetic
cardiac notch
cardiac obstruction
cardiac opening
cardiac orifice
cardiac output
cardiac part
cardiac plexus
cardiac polyp
cardiac prominence
cardiac reflex

cardiac segment
cardiac shadow
cardiac skeleton
cardiac stomach
cardiac tamponade
Cardiac T Rapid Assay
cardiac troponin T marker in blood
cardiac valve, vegetations of
cardiac valvular abnormality
cardiac valvular defect
cardiac valvular lesion
cardiac valvular stenosis
cardiac vein
cardinal ligament of uterus
cardinal point
cardinal vein
Cardiobacterium hominis
cardioesophageal (CE) junction
cardiogenic embolism
cardiogenic plate
cardiogenic shock
cardiohepatic angle
cardiohepatic triangle
cardiomegaly
cardiomyopathy, hypertrophic
cardiorrhexis
cardiovascular silhouette
caries, dental
carinal lymph node
carina of the trachea
carinatum, pectus
cariniform cartilage
carmine
carnassial tooth
carneous degeneration
Carney complex
Carnoy fixative
Carnoy solution
carotene absorption test
carotene-containing vegetables and
    fruits
carotene test

carotenoderma
carotenoids
caroticoclinoid ligament
caroticotympanic artery
caroticotympanic canal
caroticotympanic nerve
carotid arch
carotid artery
carotid gland
carotid sheath
carotid sinus
carotid sinus nerve
carpal arch
carpal artery
carpal articular surface
carpal articulation
carpal bone
carpal canal
carpal groove
carpal joint
carpal tunnel
carpometacarpal articulation
carpometacarpal joint
carpometacarpal ligament
carpus bone
carrier cell
carrier electrophoresis
carrier protein
Carr-Price test
carrying angle
Carter fever
cartilage
    accessory
    accessory nasal
    alar
    arthrodial
    articular
    arytenoid
    auditory
    auricular
    basilar
    branchial

cartilage *(continued)*
  calcified
  cariniform
  cells of
  cellular
  ciliary
  circumferential
  conchal
  connecting
  corniculate
  costal
  cricoid
  cuneiform
  diarthrodial
  elastic
  ensiform
  epiglottic
  epiphyseal
  falciform
  fibroelastic
  fibrous
  floating
  hyaline
  hyaline articular
  loss of elasticity of
  pitted
  roughened
  scored
  thinned
  yellow
cartilage bone
cartilage capsule
cartilage cell
cartilage corpuscle
cartilage lacuna
cartilage matrix
cartilage model
cartilaginous articulation
cartilaginous joint
  primary
  secondary
  symphysis

cartilaginous part
cartilage plate, epiphyseal
cartilage space
cartilaginous portion of auditory tube
cartilaginous septum
cartilaginous tissue
cartilaginous viscerocranium
cartilago (pl. cartilagines)
cartwheel pattern
Cartwright blood group
caruncle, hymenal
cascade, diagnostic
cascara
caseating
caseation
caseous abscess
caseous necrosis
caseous nephritis
caseous pneumonia
Casoni intradermal test for hydatid
  disease
Casoni skin test
Caspersson type B cell
casserian ligament
Casser ligament
cast (pl. casts)
  abnormal c. in urine
  epithelial
  granular c. in urine
  homogeneous c. in urine
  hyaline
  RTE (renal tubular epithelial)
  waxy c. in urine
casting
Castle intrinsic factor
castrate cell
castration cell
catabolic
catabolism of fatty acids
catacrotic pulse
catadicrotic pulse
catagen phase of hair growth

catalase test
cataract
   congenital
   senile
cataract needle
catarrh
catarrhal fever
catarrhal inflammation
catarrhal pneumonia
catarrhal stomatitis
cat-bite fever
catecholamines
   fractionated
   free
   plasma
   total
   urinary
caterpillar cell
"cath" (slang for catheter, catheterized)
cathepsin D
catheter
   central venous pressure (CVP)
   Foley
   indwelling
   fluid-filled
   intracranial pressure (ICP)
   urinary bladder
catheter fever
catheter-induced embolism
catheterized specimen
cation
cationic protein
cat-scratch disease
cat-scratch fever
CA II flow cytometer
cauda equina
caudal
caudal canal
caudal flexure
caudal ligament
caudal neuropore
caudal neurosecretory system

caudal pancreatic artery
caudal pharyngeal complex
caudal retinaculum
caudal sheath
caudal vertebra
caudate lobe of liver
caudate nucleus
caudate process
cauliflower ear
cauliflower-like polyp
caval cuff, suprahepatic
caval fold
cavalry bone
cavalryman osteoma
caval valve
caveolated cell
cavernosa penis, corpora
cavernosum, corpus
cavernous angioma
cavernous artery
cavernous body
cavernous groove
cavernous hemangioma
cavernous nerve
cavernous part
cavernous plexus
cavernous sinus
cavernous tissue
cavernous vein
Caves-Schutz-Stanford bioptome
caviar lesion
cavitary dilatation of central canal
   of spinal cord
cavitary fluid
cavitary myelitis
cavitation
cavity
   abdominal
   abdominopelvic
   amniotic
   axillary
   body

cavity *(continued)*
  buccal
  chest
  cleavage
  cotyloid
  cranial
  crown
  endometrial
  epamniotic
  epidural
  funnel-shaped
  glenoid
  joint
  medullary
  oral
  pericardial
  peritoneal
  pleural
  retroperitoneal
  thoracic
  tubular
  uterine
cavity line angle
cavity margin
cavity of tunica vaginalis
cavity wall
cavosurface angle
cavosurface bevel
cavum (pl. cava)
CBC (complete blood count)
  hematocrit
  hemoglobin
  MCH (mean corpuscular
    hemoglobin)
  MCHC (mean corpuscular
    hemoglobin concentration)
  MCV (mean corpuscular volume)
  RBC (red blood cell) count
  WBC (white blood cell) count
CBD (common bile duct)
C bile

C_4 binding protein
cc (cubic centimeter)
C carbohydrate antigen
CCAT (conglutinating complement
  absorption test)
C cell
CCK (cholecystokinin)
CCK-PZ (cholecystokinin-
  pancreozymin)
C_3 complement
C_4 complement
CD (cluster of differentiation)
CDC (Centers for Disease Control)
CDC classification of HIV infection
CD4 count
CD4 lymphocyte count (T4)
CD4+ lymphocyte
CD14 membrane protein
CD45 leukocyte common antigen
CDE antigen
"C. diff" (slang for *Clostridium
  difficile*) toxin assay
CDK4 amplification analysis
CDLHb (diaspirin-cross-linked
  hemoglobin)
CE (cardioesophageal) junction
CEA (carcinoembryonic antigen)
cecal appendage
cecal appendix
cecal artery, ileocolic
cecal fold
cecal foramen
cecal recess
cecal volvulus
cecum (also, caecum)
  antimesocolic side of
  subhepatic
Cedecea
Cedecea davisae
Cedecea lapagei
Cedecea neteri
Celani method

celiac artery
celiac axis
celiac disease
celiac ganglion
celiac gland
celiac lymph node
celiac plexus
celiac sprue
celiac trunk
celite-absorbed plasma
cell
    A (alpha)
    absorption
    absorptive
    accessory
    acid
    acidophil
    acidophilic
    acid-staining
    acinar
    acinous
    acoustic
    adenomorphous
    adipose
    adventitial
    agger nasi
    agglomeration of
    agglutination of
    air
    albuminous
    algoid
    alloantigen-presenting
    alpha
    alveolar
    Alzheimer
    amacrine
    ameboid
    amniogenic
    anabiotic
    anaplastic
    anaplastic epithelial
    aneuploid

cell *(continued)*
    angioblastic
    anterior
    anterior ethmoidal air
    anterior horn
    antigen-presenting (APC)
    antigen-reactive
    antigen-responsive
    antigen-sensitive
    antral gastric
    apocrine
    apolar
    APUD (amine precursor uptake
        and decarboxylation)
    argentaffin
    argyrophil
    argyrophilic
    Arias-Stella
    Armanni-Ebstein
    Aschoff
    Askanazy
    astroglia
    atrophy of hair
    atypical
    auditory
    auditory receptor
    automatic
    B (beta)
    balloon
    band
    basal granular
    basaloid
    basilar
    basket
    basophil
    basophilic
    beaker
    Beale
    Beale ganglion
    Berger
    Bergmann
    berry

cell *(continued)*
   beta
   Betz
   Bevan-Lewis
   BGM
   bipolar
   bipolar retinal
   bite
   bizarre
   Bizzozero red
   bladder
   blast
   blister
   blood
   Boll
   bone
   border
   Böttcher (Boettcher)
   bottle-shaped hair
   bowenoid
   branchial
   breakdown of red blood
   breviradiate
   bristle
   bronchial mucosal
   bronchic
   bronchiolar exocrine
   brood
   burr
   bursting of
   C
   Cajal
   Cajal interstitial
   cameloid
   cancer
   capillary endothelial
   capsule
   carrier
   cartilage
   Caspersson type B
   castration
   caterpillar

cell *(continued)*
   caveolated
   CD45RO+
   cement
   central
   centroacinar
   chalice
   chief
   chromaffin
   chromophobe
   chromophobic
   chromosomal structure of
   ciliated
   Clara
   Clarke
   Claudius
   clear
   cleavage
   cleaved
   clonogenic
   clue
   clump
   clumping of
   cochlear hair
   collenchyma
   column
   columnar
   columnar epithelial
   columnar sustentacular
   commissural
   compound granule
   cone
   connective-tissue
   contractile fiber
   contrasuppressor
   cordlike arrangement of
   corneal
   Corti
   corticotroph-lipotroph
   cover
   crescent
   cribrate

cell *(continued)*
 Crooke
 cuboid
 cuboidal
 cuboidal epithelial
 cuboidal glandular
 cultured
 Custer
 cylindrical
 cytomegalic
 cytotoxic
 cytotoxic T
 cytotrophoblastic
 D (delta)
 damaged nerve
 dark
 Daudi
 daughter
 Davidoff
 dead nerve
 decidual
 decoy
 deep
 deficient production of red blood
 definition
 degenerating nerve
 Deiters
 delomorphous
 delta
 demilune
 dendritic
 dendritic reticular
 denture
 devitalized nerve
 Dogiel
 dome
 donor
 Dorothy Reed
 Downey
 duct
 ductal
 dust

cell *(continued)*
 dyskeratotic
 ECL (enterochromaffin-like)
 effector
 egg
 electrolytic
 elementary
 embryonic
 embryonic mesenchymal
 enamel
 enamel-forming
 encasing (also incasing)
 endocervical
 endodermal
 endometrial
 endothelial
 enterochromaffin
 enteroendocrine
 entodermal
 ependymal
 epidermic
 epithelial
 epithelial reticular
 epithelioid
 erythrocyte progenitor
 erythroid
 ethmoid air
 ethmoidal
 excitable
 external pillar
 exudation
 Fananás
 fasciculata
 fat
 fat-storing
 fatty granule
 Ferrata
 fiber
 Finkeldey-Warthin
 flagellate
 flat
 floor

cell *(continued)*
   foam
   follicular
   follicular epithelial
   follicular ovarian
   foreign
   foreign body giant
   formative
   foveolar
   fuchsinophil
   fusiform
   G
   galvanic
   gametoid
   gamma
   ganglion
   gastrin-secreting
   Gaucher
   Gegenbaur
   gemistocytic
   germ
   germinal
   ghost
   giant
   giant Betz
   Gierke
   gitter
   Gley
   glia
   glial
   glitter
   globoid
   glomerular
   glomus
   goblet
   Golgi epithelial
   Goormaghtigh
   granular
   granule
   granulocytic white
   granulosa
   granulosa lutein

cell *(continued)*
   grape
   great alveolar
   ground-glass
   guanine
   gustatory
   gyrochrome
   hair
   hairy
   Haller
   heart-disease
   heart-failure
   heart-lesion
   heckle
   Heidenhain
   HeLa
   helmet
   helper (inducer)
   helper/inducer T cell
   helper T
   hemolymphatic
   hemolyzed red blood
   HEMPAS
   Hensen
   hepatic parenchymal
   heteromeric
   hexagonal
   hilar
   hilus
   hobnail
   Hodgkin
   Hofbauer
   homozygous typing (HTC)
   horizontal
   horn
   horny
   Hortega
   host
   Hürthle
   hyperchromatic
   I (inclusion)
   immature

cell *(continued)*
    immature red blood
    immature white blood
    immunologically activated
    immunologically competent
    incasing (also encasing)
    inclusion
    indifferent
    inflammatory
    inflammatory response
    initial
    injured nerve
    innocent bystander
    intercalary
    intercapillary
    interdigitating
    interfollicular
    intermediate
    internal pillar
    interstitial
    irritability of nerve
    irritation
    islet
    Ito
    juvenile
    juxtaglomerular
    K (killer)
    karyochrome
    keratinized
    keratinized epithelial
    killer T
    koilocytotic
    Kulchitsky
    Kupffer
    L
    lacis (meshwork)
    lacrimoethmoid
    lacunar
    LAK
    Langerhans
    Langhans
    Langhans giant

cell *(continued)*
    large
    large cleaved
    large granule
    large noncleaved
    lattice
    LE (lupus erythematosus)
    Leishman chrome
    lepra
    Leydig
    light (of thyroid)
    lining
    Lipschütz
    littoral
    liver
    Loevit
    lupus erythematosus (LE)
    luteal
    lutein
    luteinizing theca
    lymph
    lymphadenoma
    lymphoid
    lymphokine-activated killer (LAK)
    lymphoreticular
    lysis of
    macroglia
    male sex
    malignant
    malpighian
    Marchand wandering
    marrow
    Martinotti
    mast
    mastoid
    mastoid air
    matrix
    Mauthner
    McCoy
    megakaryocyte progenitor
    megaspore mother
    melanin-containing

cell *(continued)*
    memory
    meningothelial
    Merkel
    Merkel-Ranvier
    Merkel tactile
    mesangial
    mesenchymal
    mesoglial
    mesothelial
    metaplastic squamous
    Mexican hat
    Meynert
    microglia
    microglial
    middle
    middle ethmoidal air
    midget bipolar
    migratory
    Mikulicz
    mirror-image
    mitral
    monocytoid
    monomorphous oval
    mononuclear
    Mooser
    mossy
    mother
    motor
    Mott
    mucin-secreting columnar
    mucoalbuminous
    mucoserous
    mucous
    mucous neck
    mucus-secreting
    mulberry
    Müller radial (Mueller)
    multinucleated giant
    multinucleate globoid
    multipolar
    mural

cell *(continued)*
    muscle
    mycosis
    myeloid
    myeloma
    myoepithelial
    myoepithelioid
    myoid
    myointimal
    Nageotte
    natural killer (NK)
    neoplastic
    nerve
    nerve sheath
    Neumann
    neurilemma
    neuroendocrine
    neuroendocrine transducer
    neuroepithelial
    neuroglia
    neuroglial
    neuromuscular
    neurosecretory
    nevus
    nevus-type giant
    Niemann-Pick
    NK (natural killer)
    non-alpha, non-beta pancreatic islet
    non-beta
    nonclonogenic
    nonglandular
    nonmalignant
    non-nerve
    nonspecialized
    nucleated
    nucleated red blood
    null
    nurse
    oat
    OKT
    olfactory
    olfactory receptor

cell *(continued)*
  oligodendroglia
  Onodi
  Opalski
  osseous
  osteochondrogenic
  osteogenic
  osteoprogenitor
  oval
  oxygen-carrying material
    of red blood
  oxyntic
  oxyphil
  P
  pacemaker
  packed human blood
  packed red blood
  pagetoid
  Paget
  palisade
  pancreatic islet
  panel
  Paneth granular
  papillary
  parafollicular
  paraganglionic
  paraluteal
  paralutein
  parenchymal
  parent
  parietal
  Pelger-Huët
  peptic
  pericapillary
  peripolar
  perithelial
  peritubular contractile
  permissive
  pessary
  phagocytic stellate
  phalangeal
  pheochrome

cell *(continued)*
  photo
  photoreceptor
  physaliphorous
  Pick
  pigment
  pillar
  pineal
  plasma
  platelike
  pleomorphic
  pluripotent
  pluripotential
  pneumatic
  PNH (paroxysmal nocturnal
    hemoglobinuria)
  polar
  polychromatic
  polychromatophil
  polygonal
  polyhedral
  polymorphic pigment-producing
  polyplastic
  posterior
  posterior ethmoidal air
  PP (pancreatic polypeptide)
  pre-B
  precursor
  prefollicle
  pregnancy
  pregranulosa
  pre-T
  prickle
  primary embryonic
  primitive
  primitive granulosa
  primitive reticular
  primitive wandering
  primordial
  primordial germ
  principal
  prokaryotic

cell *(continued)*
   prolactin
   proliferating
   pseudo-Gaucher
   pseudounipolar
   pseudoxanthoma
   ptyocrinous
   pulmonary endothelial
   pulmonary epithelial
   pulpar
   Purkinje
   pus
   pyramidal
   pyrrol
   quiescent
   RA (ragocyte)
   radial
   Raji
   reactive
   reactive mesothelial
   recipient
   red blood
   Reed
   Reed-Sternberg
   Renshaw
   reserve
   residential
   resting
   retina (amacrine)
   resting wandering
   restructured
   reticular
   reticularis
   reticuloendothelial
   reticulum
   rhagiocrine
   Rieder
   Rindfleisch
   rod
   rod nuclear
   Rohon-Beard
   Rolando

cell *(continued)*
   root
   rosette-forming
   Rouget
   round
   S
   Sala
   sarcogenic
   satellite
   scalelike
   scavenger
   Schilling band
   Schultze
   Schwann
   sclerenchyma
   secretory
   segmented
   seminal
   sensitized
   sensory
   sentinel
   septal
   seromucous
   serous
   Sertoli
   sex
   Sézary
   shadow
   sheep red blood (sRBC)
   shrinking of
   sickle
   signet ring
   silver
   skein
   skeletogenous
   slender elongated
   small
   small cleaved
   small granule
   smooth-muscle
   smudge
   solitary

cell *(continued)*
    somatic
    somatostatin
    specialized
    sperm
    spermatogenic
    sphenoid
    spider
    spindle
    spindle-shaped
    splenic
    spur
    squamous
    squamous alveolar
    squamous epithelial
    stab
    staff
    standard
    star
    star-shaped
    stellate
    stem
    Sternberg
    Sternberg-Reed
    strap
    structure of
    superficial
    supporting
    suppressor
    suppressor T
    surface mucous
    sustentacular
    swelling of
    swollen basal
    sympathetic formative
    sympathicotropic
    sympathochromaffin
    syncytial
    synovial
    T (thymus, thymus-dependent, or
      thymus-derived lymphocytes)
    T cytotoxic

cell *(continued)*
    T effector
    T helper
    T lymphocyte
    T4 helper
    T8 suppressor
    tactile
    tanned red (TRC)
    target
    tart
    taste
    TDTH
    teardrop
    tendon
    Tg
    theca
    theca lutein
    thymus-dependent (T cells)
    thymus-independent (B cells)
    tightly packed round
    Tiselius electrophoresis
    Tm
    totipotent
    touch
    Touton giant
    transducer
    transepithelial migration of
      chronic inflammatory
    transitional
    transitional epithelial
    TRC (tanned red cell)
    tufted
    tunnel
    Türk
    tympanic
    tympanic air
    type I alveolar
    type II alveolar
    Tzanck
    umbrella
    undegenerated nerve
    undifferentiated

cell *(continued)*
  undifferentiated columnar epithelial
  undifferentiated mesenchymal
  unipolar
  urothelial
  vacuolated
  vacuolation of
  vasoformative
  veil
  veiled
  Vero
  vestibular hair
  veto
  Virchow
  virus-transformed
  visual receptor
  vitreous
  volume of packed
  von Kupffer
  wandering
  Warthin
  Warthin-Finkeldey giant
  wasserhelle
  water-clear
  white blood (WBC)
  WI-38 (Wistar Institute)
  wing
  xanthoma
  yolk
  zymogen
  zymogenic
cell aggregations, normal
cell assay test, Raji
cell block of paraffin
cell block, opening
cell bodies, chromatolysis
cell body of motor neuron
cell-bound antibody
cell bridge
cell button
cell center
cell cluster

cell count
cell count of cerebrospinal fluid
cell count of urine
cell culture
cell death
cell layer
cell line
cell-mediated immunity
cell membrane
cell nest
celloidin
Cellosolve dehydrating agent
cell plate
cell polarity
cell prep, LE (lupus erythematosus)
cell sac
cell-serum mixture in saline
cell sheet
cell strand
cell tubule
cellular blue nevus
cellular bone marrow
cellular debris
cellular embolism
cellular immunity
cellular infiltrate
cellularity, scant
cellular organelle
cellular polyp
cellular repair
cellular tissue
cellulitis of scalp, dissecting
cellulitis, periurethral
cellulocutaneous
cellulose
cellulosity
cell wall
celom, extraembryonic
celomic bay
celomic pouch
Celsius scale (C)
cement base

cement cell
cement corpuscle
cement line
cement substance
cementodentinal junction
cementum
center
    anospinal
    Broca
    ciliospinal
    diaphyseal
    epiotic
    germinal
    ossification
    swallowing
center cell
centigrade scale
centigram (cg)
centigray (cGy)
centiliter (cL)
centimeter (cm)
centimole (cmol)
central apparatus
central artery of retina
central bone of ankle
central canal of spinal cord
central canal of vitreous
central canal of cochlea
central cell
Central European tick-borne fever
central gray substance
central groove
central incisor
central lesion
central lobule
central lymph node
central myelitis
central necrosis
central nervous system
central perineal tendon
central pit
central pneumonia

central sulcus
central tegmental fasciculus
central tegmental tract
central tendon of diaphragm
central tendon of perineum
central vein of liver lobule
central venous pressure (CVP) catheter
central zone of amyloid
centralis retinae, arteria
centrifugation
centrifuge
centrilobar pancreatitis
centrilobular congestion
centrilobular emphysema
centrilobular necrosis of liver
centrilobular region of liver
centripetal nerve
Centri-Sep spin column
centroacinar cell
centrocyte
centrodistal joint
centromedian nucleus
centromere antibody
centromere, chromosomal
centromeric index
centrosome
centrum
CEP (congenital erythropoietic
    porphyria)
cephalic angle
cephalic flexure
cephalic pole
cephalic triangle
cephalic vein
cephalic ventricle
cephalocaudal axis
cephalomedullary angle
ceramide trihexosidase
ceramide trihexosidase deficiency
ceratocricoid ligament
ceratopharyngeal part
c-erb protein

cercariae of avian schistosomes in skin
cercarial dermatitis
cerebellar artery
cerebellar cortex
cerebellar fissure
cerebellar fossa
cerebellar notch
cerebellar pyramid
cerebellar sulcus
cerebellomedullary cistern
cerebellopontine angle
cerebellopontine angle meningioma
cerebellopontine recess
cerebellorubral tract
cerebellothalamic tract
cerebellum
cerebral aqueduct
cerebral arteriosclerosis
cerebral artery
cerebral atrophy
cerebral concussion
cerebral congestion
cerebral contusion
cerebral cortex
cerebral cranium
cerebral cyst
cerebral death
cerebral edema
cerebral embolism
cerebral fissure
cerebral flexure
cerebral hemisphere
cerebral infarction
cerebral malaria
cerebral meningitis
cerebral parenchyma
cerebral part
cerebral petechiae
cerebral pneumonia
cerebral sulcus
cerebral surface
cerebral vein

cerebral ventricle
cerebral vesicle
cerebromacular degeneration (CMD)
cerebroretinal degeneration
cerebrospinal axis
cerebrospinal canal
cerebrospinal fluid (CSF)
cerebrospinal fluid glucose
cerebrospinal fluid glutamine
cerebrospinal fluid lactic acid
cerebrospinal fluid otorrhea
cerebrospinal fluid pressure
cerebrospinal fluid protein
cerebrospinal fluid volume
cerebrospinal meningitis
cerebrospinal system
cerebrovascular accident (CVA)
cerebrum
    first ventricle of
    lateral ventricle of
    second ventricle of
    third ventricle of
ceroid-laden macrophage
ceruloplasmin
ceruminous gland
cervical adenocarcinoma
cervical aortic knuckle
cervical artery
cervical atrophy
cervical auricle
cervical axillary canal
cervical canal
cervical cap
cervical chain
cervical condyloma
cervical cone biopsy
cervical cytology
cervical disk
cervical dysplasia
cervical erosion
cervical eversion
cervical fascia

cervical flexure
cervical ganglion, uterine
cervical gland
cervical incompetence
cervical interspinal muscle
cervical intraepithelial neoplasia (CIN)
cervical ligament
cervical line
cervical loop
cervical margin
cervical motion tenderness (CMT)
cervical mucus
cervical nerve
cervical os
cervical paratracheal lymph node
cervical part
cervical pleura
cervical plexus
cervical polyp
cervical pregnancy
cervical rib
cervical rotator muscle
cervical sinus
cervical smear
cervical spine
cervical stenosis
cervical stump
cervical transformation zone
cervical triangle
cervical ulcer
cervical vein
cervical vertebra
cervical vesicle
cervical zone
cervicalis, ansa
cervicitis
cervicoaxillary canal
cervicothoracic ganglion
cervicovaginal artery
cervix (pl. cervixes, cervices)
  biopsy of
  cone biopsy of

cervix *(continued)*
  conization of
  fish-mouth
  incompetent
  uterine
C_1 esterase
C_1 esterase inhibitor
C factor
CF (complement fixation)
CF antibody
C fiber
C-14 cholate breath
cg (centigram)
cGMP (cyclic guanosine-3-5'-
  monophosphate)
cGy (centigray)
Chaetoconidium
Chagas disease
chain (pl. chains)
  A
  B
  branched
  heavy
  kappa
  light
  long
  monoclonal light
  polypeptide
  short
chain amino acid, branched
chain disease, heavy alpha
chain fatty acid (see also *fatty acid*)
  medium
  short
chain reaction, polymerase
chalazion
chalice cell
chalky bone
chamber
  anterior
  pulp
Champy fixative

chancre, syphilitic
chancriform pyoderma
chancroid
change
   antigenic
   atrophic
   koilocytotic cellular
   malignant
   post-radiation
   pregangrenous
   radiation cell
   reparative
   solar degenerative
channel
   gastric
   pancreaticobiliary common
   pyloric
Charcot-Bouchard aneurysm
Charcot cirrhosis
Charcot intermittent fever
Charcot joint
Charcot-Leyden crystals
Charcot-Marie atrophy
Charcot-Marie-Tooth atrophy
Charcot triad
charring
Chassaignac space
Chauffard point
Chaussier line
check ligaments
Chédiak-Higashi granules
Chédiak-Steinbrinck-Higashi syndrome
cheek
   gluteal
   infraorbital
cheek bone
cheek gland
cheek muscle
cheek tooth
cheesy abscess
cheesy discharge
cheesy necrosis

cheesy nephritis
cheesy pneumonia
cheesy pus
cheilitis
cheiloschisis
cheilosis
"chem 6" (SMA-6)
"chem 12" (SMA-12)
"chem 20" (SMA-20)
chemical cleavage
chemical debris
chemical dermatitis
chemical diabetes
chemical irritant
chemical pneumonitis
chemical poisoning
chemical poison
chemical test
chemistry, blood
chemistry panel
chemistry profile
C hemoglobin
chemotactic response
chemotactic sexual hormone
chemotaxis
chemotherapy code
Chemstrip bG dipstick
Chemstrip urine dipstick
chenodeoxycholic acid, total
chenodeoxycholylglycine, conjugated
C hepatitis
cherry angioma
chest tube
chest wall
chevron bone
Chiari-Arnold malformation
Chiari reticulum
chiasm, optic
chiasmatic cistern
chiasmatic sulcus
Chiba aspiration biopsy needle
chicken fat clot

chickenpox (varicella)
chickenpox immunoglobulin
Chick-Martin test
chiclero ulcer
chief agglutinin
chief artery
chief cell
chief complaint
chikungunya virus
chilblain
Child classification of hepatic risk
   criteria
Child-Pugh A, B, C, classification
Child-Turcotte classification
chills
chip, prostate (prostatic)
chisel
   Councilman
   Virchow bone-splitting
chlamydia
Chlamydia pneumoniae
Chlamydia psittaci
Chlamydia trachomatis
Chlamydiazyme test
chloasma
chloracne
chloride
   mercuric
   serum
   sweat
   urine
chloride test
chloroazotemic nephritis
chloroform poisoning
chlorpalladium
choana (pl. choanae)
choanal polyp
cholangiole
chocolate agar
chocolate cyst
Chodosh macroscopic appearance
choked disk disease

cholangiocarcinoma
cholangiogram
cholangitic abscess
cholangitis
cholecystectomy
cholecystitis
cholecystoduodenal fistula
cholecystoduodenal ligament
cholecystoduodenocolic fold
cholecystokinin (CCK)
cholecystokinin-pancreozymin
   (CCK-PZ)
choledochous duct
choledochal sphincter
choledochoduodenal junction
choledocholithiasis
choledochopancreatic ductal junction
choleic acid
cholelithiasis
cholemic nephrosis
cholera
cholestasis
cholestatic jaundice
cholesteatoma
Cholestec L-D-X system to measure
   total cholesterol and glucose
cholesterol
   serum
   total
cholesterol cleft
cholesterol crystals
cholesterol deposition
cholesterol embolism
cholesterol gallstone
cholesterol granuloma
cholesterol pleurisy
cholesterol pneumonitis
cholesterolosis
cholic acid, total
cholinergic fiber
cholinergic receptor
cholinesterase II test

choluria (bilirubinuria)
choluric jaundice
chondritis, articular
chondrocyte
chondroid tissue
chondroma
chondropharyngeal part
chondrosarcoma
chondrosternal articulation
chondroxiphoid ligament
Chopart articulation
Chopart joint
chorda (pl. chordae)
chorda saliva
chorda tendinea (pl. chordae tendineae)
chorda tympani nerve
chordal tissue
chordoma
chorea, Huntington
chorioallantoic graft
chorioallantoic membrane
chorioallantoic placenta
chorioamnionitis
choriocapillary layer
choriocarcinoma
chorioepithelioma
choriomeningitis, lymphocytic
chorionic disk
chorionic gonadotropic hormone
chorionic gonadotropin in urine
chorionic growth hormone
chorionic plate
chorionic sac
chorionic tissue
chorionic villi biopsy
chorionic villus (pl. villi)
chorioretinitis
choristoma
choroidal nevus
choroidal ring
choroid artery
choroid coat

choroiditis
choroid layer
choroid plexus
choroid plexus papilloma
choroid vein
Chr a antigen
Christchurch (Ch[1]) chromosome
Christian-Hand-Schüller disease
Christmas disease
Christmas factor
chromaffin body
chromaffin cell
chromaffinoma
chromaffin reaction
chromaffin tissue
chromate
chromatic apparatus
chromatic fiber
chromatic granule
chromatin analysis, sex
chromatin body
chromatin, clumped
chromatin nucleolus
chromatin particle
chromatin pattern
chromatin reservoir
chromatin test for genetic sex
    determination
chromatography
    gas
    high-performance liquid
    high-pressure liquid
    ion-exchange
    liquid
    paper
    thin-layer
chromaffinoma
chromatolysis of cell bodies
chromatophore
chromatophorotropic hormone
chromatosis
chromic acid

chromidial apparatus
chromium, radioactive
chromium red blood cell survival test
Chromobacterium violaceum
chromoblastomycosis
chromocenter
chromogenic enzyme substrate test
chromogranin A
chromomycosis
chromophil (also chromophilic)
chromophil granule
chromophil substance
chromophobic adenoma
chromophobic cell
chromophobic granule
chromophytosis
chromoprobe
chromosomal abnormality
   aneuploidy
   deletion
   inversion
   reduplication
   translocation
chromosomal analysis
chromosomal centromere
chromosomal disorder
chromosomal gap
chromosomal structure of cell
chromosome
   accessory
   Christchurch (Ch 1)
   fragile X
   giant
   Philadelphia
   ring
chromosome analysis
chromosome band(ing)
chromosome in situ hybridization
chromosome satellite
chronic abscess
chronic acholuric jaundice
chronic active hepatitis

chronic adhesive arachnoiditis
chronic bacillary diarrhea
chronic bone marrow failure
chronic bowel disease with protein loss
chronic bronchitis
chronic bullous dermatosis
   of childhood
chronic constrictive pericarditis
chronic diffuse sclerosing osteomyelitis
chronic eczema
chronic eosinophilic pneumonia
chronic Epstein-Barr virus infection
chronic exposure to loud noise
chronic familial jaundice
chronic fibrous thyroiditis
chronic fissure
chronic focal sclerosing osteomyelitis
chronic gastritis
chronic glomerulonephritis
chronic granulocytic leukemia
chronic hypertrophic myocarditis
chronic idiopathic
chronic inflammation
chronic interstitial myocarditis
chronic interstitial salpingitis
chronic leukemia
chronic lymphocytic leukemia (CLL)
chronic meningitis
chronic myelitis
chronic myelomonocytic leukemia
chronic myocarditis
chronic nephritis
chronic nutritional deficiency
chronic obstructive pulmonary disease
   (COPD)
chronic osteitis
chronic pancreatitis
chronic passive congestion
chronic pernicious myocarditis
chronic persistent hepatitis
chronic pleurisy
chronic pneumonia

chronic pneumonitis
chronic pyelonephritis
chronic ulcer
chronicity
chronicum migrans, erythema
Chrysosporium
Chrysosporium parvum
Churg-Strauss syndrome
chyle
chyle cistern
chyle corpuscle
chyle lymph
chyle vessel
chyliferous vessel
chyliform pleurisy
chylomicron
chylous pleurisy
chyme, fat-containing
Ciaccio gland
cicatricial alopecia
cicatricial horn
cicatricial kidney
cicatricial pemphigoid
cicatricial tissue
cicatrix
cicatrization
CIE (counterimmunoelectrophoresis)
cilia
ciliary artery
ciliary body
ciliary canal
ciliary cartilage
ciliary crown
ciliary disk
ciliary fold
ciliary ganglion
ciliary ganglionic plexus
ciliary gland
ciliary ligament
ciliary margin
ciliary muscle
ciliary process

ciliary ring
ciliary vein
ciliary zone
ciliary zonule
ciliated cell
ciliated columnar epithelium
ciliated epithelium
ciliospinal center
cimicosis
CIN (cervical intraepithelial neoplasia)
    classification
Cinna-Biotecx protocol
circinata, psoriasis
circinate
circle
    arterial
    articular vascular
circle of Willis artery
circular electrode mark
circular fiber
circular fold
circular layer
circular muscle coat
circular sinus
circular sulcus
circular swirl
circular syncytium
circular vortex
circulating anticoagulant
circulating blood
circulating leukocyte
circulating lymphocyte
circulation
    capillary
    collateral
    cross
    extracorporeal
    increased local
circulatory collapse
circulatory compromise
circulatory disorder
circulatory impairment

circulatory stasis
circulatory system
circumanal gland
circumcised
circumcision
circumference
circumferential cartilage
circumferential fibrocartilage
circumferential lamella
circumflex artery
circumflex branch
circumflex fibular artery
circumflex nerve
circumflex scapular artery
circumflex vein
circum-marginate
circumoral pallor
circumpennate muscle
circumrenal
circumscribe
circumscribed cerebral atrophy
circumscribed pleurisy
circumscribed pyocephalus
circumtonsillar abscess
circumvallate papilla
circumventricular organ
circus senilis
cirrhosis
    acholangic biliary
    acute juvenile
    alcoholic
    atrophic
    bacterial
    biliary
    calculus
    cardiac
    Charcot
    congestive
    Cruveilhier-Baumgarten
    decompensated
    diffuse septal
    fatty

cirrhosis *(continued)*
    hepatic
    Indian childhood
    Laënnec
    macrolobular
    microlobular
    malarial
    metabolic
    micronodular
    multilobular
    nutritional
    periportal
    pigment
    pipe stem
    portal
    posthepatitic
    postnecrotic
    primary biliary
    pulmonary
    secondary biliary
    septal
    stasis
    syphilitic
    Todd
    toxic
    unilobular
    vascular
cirrhosis of liver
cirrhosis of lung
cirrhotic gastritis
cirrhotic inflammation
cirsoid aneurysm
cirsoid placenta
cirsoid varix
cistern
    basal
    cerebellomedullary
    chyle
cisterna of endoplasmic reticulum
cisternal puncture
citrate
citrate test

citrated plasma
Citrobacter
Citrobacter amalonaticus
Citrobacter diversus
Citrobacter freundii
citrovorum factor
citrulline test
Civinini canal
Civinini ligament
CK-BB (CK$_1$) isoenzyme
CK enzyme (also, CPK)
CK isoenzyme
CK-MB isoenzyme (CK$_2$)
CK-MM (CK$_3$) isoenzyme
cL (centiliter)
Cladosporium
Cladosporium bantianum
Cladosporium carrionii
Cladosporium cladosporioides
Cladosporium trichoides
Cladosporium werneckii
Clado ligament
clam digger's itch
Clapton line
Clara cell
Clarite mounting medium
Clark classification of malignant
   melanoma
Clarke cell
classical hemophilia
classical osteosarcoma
classic dengue
classic interstitial pneumonia
classic phenylketonuria
classification (see also *grade*, *stage*)
   Arneth c. of polymorphonuclear
     neutrophils
   Astler-Coller modification
     of Dukes c. of carcinoma
   Bethesda PAP smear c.
   Breslow c. of malignant melanoma
   Broders tumor index

classification *(continued)*
   Brooker periarticular heterotopic
     ossification (PHO)
   burns
   Butchart staging c.
   Caldwell-Moloy c.
   CDC c. for HIV infection
   chemotherapy code
   Child c. of hepatic risk criteria
   Child-Pugh A, B, C
   Child-Turcotte
   CIN (cervical iantraepithelial
     neoplasia)
   Clark c. of malignant melanoma
   DeBakey aortic c.
   Delbet fracture c.
   Denver chromosome c.
   diabetes mellitus c.
   Dubin and Amelar varicocele c.
   Dukes c. of carcinoma
   Erlanger and Gasser peripheral
     nerve c.
   FAB c. of acute nonlymphoid
     leukemia
   FIGO staging of adenocarcinoma
     of endometrium
   Floyd peripheral nerve c.
   Frykman c. of hand fractures
   Gell and Coombs hypersensitivity
     reactions
   HIV c. of children
   Hoehn and Yahr staging
     of Parkinson disease
   House-Brackmann facial weakness
   Hunt and Hess neurological c.
   Hyams grading of esthesioneuro-
     blastoma
   International C. of Diseases
     for Oncology (ICD-O)
   Jackson and Parker c. of Hodgkin
     disease
   Jansky human blood groups

classification *(continued)*
    Jewett c. of bladder carcinoma
    Judet epiphyseal fracture c.
    Karnofsky status c.
    Keith-Wagener c. of retinopathy
    Kiel c. of non-Hodgkin lymphoma
    Klatskin tumor c.
    Lancefield c. of hemolytic
      streptococci into groups
    leukemia c.
    Lukes-Butler c. of
      non-Hodgkin lymphoma
    Lukes-Collins c. of non-Hodgkin
      lymphoma
    microinvasive carcinoma c.
    Modic disk abnormality c.
    morphologic c.
    MSTS (Musculoskeletal Tumor
      Society) staging system
    multiaxial
    murmur grades
    Neer shoulder fractures I, II, III
    NYHA (New York Heart
      Association) c. of congestive
      heart failure
    Olerud and Molander fracture c.
    osteoarthritis grading
    Pauwels femoral neck fracture
    Rappaport lymphoma
    Reese-Ellsworth c. of retinoblastoma
    Rye c. of Hodgkin disease
    Singh-Vaughn-Williams arrhythmia
    TNM (tumor size, nodal involve-
      ment, metastatic progress) c.
    van Heuven anatomic c. of diabetic
      retinopathy
    Wiberg c. of patellar types
    Wolfe breast carcinoma c.
Claudius cell
clavate papilla
clavicle bone
clavicle, midpoint of

clavicular artery
clavicular facet
clavicular notch
clavicular part
clavipectoral fascia
clavipectoral triangle
clay-colored stool
clean-catch urine
clean-catch urine specimen
clean-voided urine specimen
clearance
    creatinine
    insulin
    urea
clear cell
clear cell adenocarcinoma of cervix
    or vagina
clear cell carcinoma of vagina
clear cell carcinoma of vagina and
    cervix among DES daughters
clearing factor
clearing of tissue specimen
clear margin
clear medium
clear tissue
clear urine
cleavage
    adequal
    determinate
    discoidal
    enamel
    equatorial
cleavage cavity
cleavage cell
cleavage line
cleavage spindle
cleaved cell
CLED (cystine, lactose, electrolyte
    deficient)
cleft
    anal
    branchial

cleft *(continued)*
  cholesterol
  facial
  first visceral
  gill
  pudendal
cleftlike space
cleft lip
cleft palate
cleistothecia
climbing fiber
clinical diagnosis
Clinistix
Clinitest
clinoid plate
clinoid process
clitoral artery
clitoral hypertrophy
clitoris
  angle of
  crus of
  deep artery of
  frenulum of
  glans of
  prepuce of
clival meningioma
CLL (chronic lymphocytic leukemia)
cloacal membrane
cloacal plate
clomiphene test
clone
cloning
clonogenic cell
clonorchiasis
Clonorchis sinensis
C-loop, duodenal
Cloquet canal
Cloquet fascia
Cloquet ganglion
Cloquet gland
Cloquet ligament
Cloquet space

closed comedo
closed gland
closed loop
closed-loop obstruction
closing membrane
Clostridium
Clostridium bifermentans
Clostridium botulinum
Clostridium butyricum
Clostridium cadaveris
Clostridium difficile (slang "C. diff")
Clostridium difficile toxin assay
Clostridium histolyticum
Clostridium innocuum
Clostridium novyi
Clostridium paraputrificum
Clostridium perfringens
Clostridium putrificum
Clostridium ramosum
Clostridium septicum
Clostridium sordellii
Clostridium sphenoides
Clostridium sporogenes
Clostridium subterminale
Clostridium tertium
Clostridium tetani
Clostridium welchii
closure of skull, failure of
clot
  agonal
  antemortem
  blood
  chicken
  chicken fat
  currant jelly
  distal
  external
  friable
  heart
  internal
  laminated
  marantic

clot *(continued)*
  organized
  passive
  plastic
  postmortem
  proximal
  retraction of
  spider-web
  stratified
  washed
clot lysis test
clot retraction test
clotting factor
clotting time (also, coagulation)
  activated
  Lee-White
  plasma
clot tube
cloudy gray streaks in lens
cloudy "snowflake" opacities
cloudy swelling
cloudy urine
clubbed finger
clubbed penis
clubbing of digits
clublike dermal papillae
club-shaped bacillus
clue cell
clump cell
clumped chromatin
clumping of cells
clumping of white blood cells
clumps and nests
cluster of cells with large nuclei
cluster of differentiation (CD)
Clutton joint
cm (centimeter)
cmol (centimole)
CMT (cervical motion tenderness)
c-myc protein
CNS (central nervous system) tumor
CO (carbon monoxide)

"coag" (slang for coagulation)
coagulase-negative staphylococcus
coagulase test
coagulate
coagulated protein
coagulation
  acquired disorder of
  blood
  diffuse intravascular (DIC)
  congenital disorder of
  disseminated intravascular (DIC)
  electric
  massive
coagulation defect
coagulation factor
  failure to form
  factor I (fibrinogen)
  factor II (prothrombin)
  factor III (tissue thromboplastin)
  factor IV (calcium)
  factor V (proaccelerin)
  factor VI (stable)
  factor VII (proconvertin)
  factor VIII (antihemophilic)
  factor IX (plasma thromboplastin
    component)
  factor X (Stuart-Prower)
  factor XI (plasma thromboplastin
    antecedent)
  factor XII (Hageman)
  factor XIII (fibrin stabilizing)
coagulation factor assay
coagulation necrosis
coagulation of tissue by excessive heat
coagulation panel
  bleeding time
  clot retraction
  clotting time
  partial thromboplastin time
  plasma assay
  platelet count
  prothrombin time

coagulation time (also, clotting)
   activated
   Lee-White
   plasma
coagulation time test
coagulopathy
coarctate retina
coarctation of aorta
coarse azurophilic granules
coarse basophilic stippling in
   cytoplasm of neutrophils
coarse features
coarsely granular
coarsening of hair
coarsening of skin
coat
   buffy
   choroid
   circular muscle
   longitudinal muscle
cobalamin
cobalt, radioactive
cobblestone appearance
cobblestone granulations of conjunctiva
Cobelli gland
Coca-Cola urine
coccal infection
cocci (pl. of coccus)
coccidioidal meningitis
coccidioidin test
Coccidioides immitis
coccidioidin skin test
coccidioidomycosis
coccidiosis
coccobacillus
coccus (pl. cocci), gram-negative
coccygeal body
coccygeal bone
coccygeal ganglion
coccygeal gland
coccygeal joint
coccygeal muscle

coccygeal nerve
coccygeal part
coccygeal plexus
coccygeal sinus
coccygeal vertebra
coccygeal whorl
coccygeus muscle
coccyx, tip of
cochlea, aqueduct of
cochlear aqueduct
cochlear area
cochlear artery
cochlear canal
cochlear canaliculus
cochlear duct
cochlear hair cell
cochleariform process
cochlear joint
cochlear labyrinth
cochlear nerve
cochlear nucleus
cochlear part
cochlear recess
cochlear root
cockscomb (also, coxcomb)
cockscomb of cervix
cockscomb papilloma
Code 500
Code Blue
codfish vertebra
codocyte
codominant gene
coeliac (also celiac)
coenzyme factor
cofactor
coffee-grounds material
coffin bone
coffin formation
coffin joint
cohesion
cohesive
coiled artery

coil gland
coin lesion
coin lesion of lungs
coil of intestine
coil of jejunum
coinfection with hepatitis B
cold abscess
cold agglutinin pneumonia
cold agglutinins
cold cone biopsy
cold cup biopsy
cold erythema
cold hemolysin
cold, injury due to
cold nodule
cold pressure test
cold-rigor point
coldsore (herpes simplex)
cold-target DNA
cold water calorics
coli
    E. (*Escherichia*)
   melanosis
   taeniae
colibacillemia
colibacillosis, enteric
coli granuloma
colic, appendicular
colic artery
colic flexure
colic impression
colic omentum
colic plexus
colic sphincter
colic surface
colic vein
coliform bacilli
coliform bacteria
colistin
colitis
   collagenous
   granulomatous

colitis *(continued)*
   hemorrhagic
   ischemic
   microscopic
   radiation
   regional
   transmural
   ulcerative
collagen bundle
collagen disease
collagen fiber
collagen fibril
collagenic fibers, matrix of
collagenous connective tissue
collagenous fiber
collagen pus
collar bone
collar-button abscess
collar chain
collateral artery
collateral branch
collateral branches of intercostal nerve
collateral circulation
collateral digital artery
collateral eminence
collateral fissure
collateral ligament
collateral radial artery
collateral route
collateral sulcus
collateral trigone
collateral ulnar artery
collateral vessel
collecting system
collecting tubule
collecting vessel
collenchyma cells
Colles fascia
Colles ligament
Colles space
colliculi of midbrain
colliculitis

colliculus
  facial
  seminal
colliquation
  ballooning
  reticular
colliquative diarrhea
colliquative necrosis
colliquative proteinuria
colloidal gel
colloidal gold test
colloid body
colloid corpuscle
colloid degeneration
colloid goiter
colloid material
colloid system
coloboma iridis
colon
  anterior band of
  ascending
  descending
  distal
  free band of
  giant
  iliac
  inflammation
  irritable
  lateral reflection of
  lead-pipe
  left
  mesosigmoid
  midsigmoid
  pelvic
  perisigmoid
  right
  sigmoid
  transverse
colon adenocarcinoma
colon polyp
colon bacillus
colonic abscess

colonic adenoma
colonic diverticulitis
colonic diverticulum
colonic fistula
colonic loop
colonic myenteric plexus
colonic pit
colonic polyp
colonies, bacterial
colonization infection
colonization of urinary tract
colony count, urine
colony-stimulating factor (CSF)
color and caliber of stool
color and consistency of skin
color and distribution of head and body
  hair
Colorado tick fever
Colorado tick fever virus
coloration
colorectal mucosa
colorimetry
colorless gas
colorless reaction
Coloscreen test for occult blood in
  stool
colostomy
colostrum corpuscle
colovaginal fistula
colovesical fistula
colposcope
colposcopic diagnosis
Columbia blood agar
column
  affinity
  anal
  anterolateral
  Bertin
  branchial efferent
  renal
  variceal
columnar cell

columnar epithelial cells
columnar epithelium
columnar layer
columnar metaplasia
columnar metaplasia of epithelium
columnar sustentacular cells
column cell
column of Bertin
column typing
coma
   agrypnodal
   alcoholic
   alpha
   diabetic
   hepatic
   hyperosmolar nonketotic
   irreversible
   Kussmaul
   metabolic
   uremic
coma scale
coma vigil
Comamonas terrigena
combined pregnancy
combined sclerosis
combined system disease
Combistix
combustion of carbon-containing fuels
comedo (pl. comedones)
   closed
   open
comedo-type DCIS (ductal carcinoma
   in situ)
comedocarcinoma
comedomastitis
comedo nevus
comma bundle
comma degeneration
comma tract (interfascicular fasciculus)
comminuted fracture
commissural cell
commissural fiber

commissural neuron
commissure, anterior labial
committed cell
common acute lymphoblastic leukemia
   antigen (CALLA)
common atrioventricular canal
common basal vein
common bile duct (CBD)
common bile duct stone
common cardinal vein
common carotid artery
common carotid plexus
common cold virus
common duct
common duct stone
common facial vein
common fibular nerve
common gall duct
common hepatic duct
common iliac artery
common iliac lymph node
common iliac node
common interosseous artery
common palmar digital nerve
common peroneal nerve
common plantar digital artery
common plantar digital nerve
common ring tendon
common synovial flexor sheath
common tendinous ring
communicans
   gray ramus
   white ramus
communicating artery
community-acquired infection
community-acquired pneumonia
compact bone
compact osteoma
compact tissue
companion artery of sciatic nerve
companion lymph node
companion vein

compartment
  infracolic
  supracolic
compatibility testing (cross-match)
compensatory atrophy
compensatory hyperplasia
compensatory hypertrophy
competent cell, immunologically
competitive binding assay
complement, C_3
complementary hypertrophy
complementary strand
complement chemotactic factor
complement fixation (CF) test
complement-fixing antibody
complement-mediated depletion
complete abortion
complete blood count (see *CBC*)
complete protein
complex
  aberrant
  AIDS dementia
  AIDS-related (ARC)
  amyotrophic lateral sclerosis–
    parkinsonism–dementia
  antigen-antibody
  antigenic
  apical
  atrial
  auricular
  avidin-biotin (ABC)
  avidin-biotin peroxidase
  avidin-biotinylated peroxidase
    Carney
  caudal pharyngeal
  C_1 q immune
  Eisenmenger
  gastroduodenal artery
  HLA (human lymphocyte antigen)
  immune
  junctional
  Meyenburg

complex *(continued)*
  MHC (major histocompatibility)
  nipple-areola
  streptavidin-biotin peroxidase
  Tacaribe
  thrombin-antithrombin III (TAT)
  triangular fibrocartilage
  von Meyenburg
complications of abortion
component
composite articulation
composite joint
composite odontoma
composition, homogeneous
compound aneurysm
compound articulation
compound gland
compound granule cell
compound joint
compound lipid
compound nevus
compound pregnancy
compound protein
compound tubuloalveolar gland
compressible cavernous body
compression atrophy
compression myelitis
compressor muscle
concanavalin A
concave abdomen
concealed penis
concentrated human red blood
  corpuscle
concentration
  mean corpuscular hemoglobin
  minimum inhibitory (MIC)
  minimum lethal (MLC)
concentration test, Fishberg
concentration test for renal function
concentric atrophy
concentric lamella
concentric rings

concentrically laminated concretions
concentrically laminated mass
conception, products of
concha (pl. conchae)
  inferior nasal
  middle nasal
  superior nasal
conchal cartilage
conchal crest
conchiolin osteomyelitis
conchoidal body
concretion
  bile
  fecal
  prostatic
concretion of abnormal substances
concussion, cerebral
concussion myelitis
condensing osteitis
conducting bronchiole
conducting system
conduction, atrioventricular
condylar articulation
condylar axis
condylar canal
condylar emissary vein
condylar fossa
condylar joint
condylar process
condyle cord
condyle path
condyloid articulation
condyloid canal
condyloid foramen, anterior
condyloid joint
condyloid process
condyloma (pl. condylomata)
  cervical
  flat
  pointed
condyloma acuminatum (pl. acuminata)
condyloma latum (pl. condylomata lata)

condylomatous
cone
  arterial
  retinal
cone-and-plate viscometer
cone biopsy of cervix
cone cell
cone disk
cone fiber
configuration
  back-to-back
  biventricular
  stellate
cone granule
confluent articulation
confluent reticulated papillomatosis
confocal epifluorescence microscope
confocal laser scanning microscopy
confocal microscopy
congenital adrenal hyperplasia
congenital agammaglobulinemia
congenital aneurysm
congenital anomaly
congenital baldness
congenital cataract
congenital defect
congenital deficiency of galactosylceramidase
congenital erythropoietic porphyria
  (CEP)
congenital goiter
congenital hemolytic anemia
congenital hemolytic jaundice
congenital malaria
congenital malformation of the eye
congenital megacolon
congenital methemoglobinemia
congenital nephritis
congenital nevus
congenital porphyria
congenital pulmonary arteriovenous
  fistula

congenital rubella pneumonitis
congenital syphilis
congenital toxoplasmosis
congential hemolytic anemia
congested kidney
congestion
  active
  cardiac
  centrilobular
  cerebral
  chronic passive
  functional
  hepatic
  hypostatic
  intravascular
  neurotonic
  passive
  pulmonary
  splenic
  vascular
  venous
congestion of tissues with blood
congestive cirrhosis
congestive heart failure
conglobate gland
conglutinating complement absorption
  test (CCAT)
Congolian red fever
Congo red stain test for amyloidosis
congruent point
conical bulging of cornea
conical masses
conical papilla
conidia, diamond-shaped
Conidiobolus coronatus
Conidiobolus incongruus
conization of cervix
conjoined tendon
conjoint tendon
conjugate axis
conjugate foramen
conjugate ligament

conjugated antigen
conjugated bile acid
conjugated bilirubin
conjugated protein
conjugative plasmid
conjunctiva
  cobblestone granulations of
  edema of
  lymphocytic aggregations of
  mucopurulent exudate of
  papillary hypertrophy of
conjunctival artery
conjunctival cul-de-sac
conjunctival gland
conjunctival layer
conjunctival ring
conjunctival sac
conjunctival scrapings
conjunctival test
conjunctival varix
conjunctival vein
conjunctivitis
  granulomatous
  inclusion (of newborn)
  noninfectious
  ulcerative
  vernal
connecting canal
connecting cartilage
connecting tubule
connective tissue
  areolar
  dense
  fibril
  loose
  peribronchial
  regular
  reticular
  subcutaneous
connective-tissue cell
connective-tissue covering of cartilage
connective-tissue disorder

connective-tissue fiber
connective-tissue matrix
connective-tissue nevus
connective-tissue stroma
Conn syndrome
conoid ligament
conoid process
conoid tubercle
consecutive aneurysm
consent, autopsy
consistency of stool
consolidation, pulmonary
consolidative pneumonia
constituents of umbilical cord
constitutive protein
constricting
constrictive pericarditis
contact area zone
contact dermatitis
contact patch test
contact-type dermatitis
contagiosum
   impetigo
   molluscum
contagious ecthyma (orf)
contagious pustular dermatitis
contamination
contents
   abdominal
   bowel
   digestive tract
   gastric
   intestinal
continuous capillary
contour line
contracted kidney
contracted pelvis
contracted tendon
contractile fiber cells
contractile vacuole
contraction band
contraction band necrosis

contraction, peristaltic
contraction stress test (CST)
contracture deformity
contracture, Volkmann
contrast medium (pl. media)
contrasuppressor cell
control
   negative
   positive
control gene
contused wound
contusion, cerebral
contusion of brain
contusion of muscle
contusion pneumonia
conus
convalescent serum
convergence, angle of
convex border of stomach
convexity, cortical
convexity meningioma
convoluted bone
convoluted gland
convoluted part
convoluted seminiferous tubule
convoluted tubule
convolution
   ascending frontal
   ascending parietal
   callosal
convulsant threshold
Cook aspiration biopsy needle
cooled-knife method
Cooley anemia
Coomassie blue
Coombs test
   direct
   indirect
Cooper ligament
COPD (chronic obstructive pulmonary disease)
Cope needle

copious discharge
copious rice-water diarrhea
copious watery diarrhea
Coplin jar
copper (Cu)
   excessive absorption of
   impaired excretion of
copper-containing plasma globulin
copper grid
copper line
copper poisoning
copper sulfate method
copper-wire artery
coprine toxin
Coprinus cinereus
coproporphyrin test
coproporphyrin, urinary excretion of
coracoacromial ligament
coracobrachial muscle
coracoclavicular ligament
coracohumeral ligament
coracoid process
coracoid tuberosity
cor bovinum
cord
   condyle
   dental
   false vocal
   gangliated
   genital
   germinal
   hepatic
   medullary
   spermatic
   spinal
   three-vessel umbilical
   two-vessel umbilical
   umbilical
   vocal
cordate pelvis
cord bladder
cordiform pelvis

cordis, apex
cordlike arrangements of cells
cordlike trunk
cords in parallel bundles
cord structure
corduroy artery
core, necrobiotic
corium
corkboard
corkscrew artery
corkscrew-shaped bacterium
cornea
   conical bulging of
   fibrosis in
   inflammation of the
   opaque
   vascularization in
corneal cell
corneal corpuscle
corneal layer
corneal lens
corneal margin
corneal opacity
corneal scarring
corneal section
corneal space
corneal tube
corneal ulcer
corneal ulceration
Corner-Allen test
corneum, stratum
corniculate cartilage
corniculate tubercle
corniculopharyngeal ligament
cornification
cornified layer
cornmeal-Tween 80 agar
cornu (pl. cornua), sacral
cornual myelitis
cornual pregnancy
cornua of spinal cord
cornua of uterus

coronal plane
coronal pulp
coronal section
coronal suture
coronal zone
corona of glans
coronary arteriosclerosis
coronary artery embolism
coronary artery of heart
coronary artery of stomach
coronary band
coronary bone
coronary groove
coronary ligament of knee
coronary ligament of liver
coronary node
coronary plexus
coronary sinus
coronary sulcus
coronary tendon
coronary valve
coronary vein
coronavirus
coroner's autopsy
coroner's case
corporis, tinea
corpse
corpse fat
cor pulmonale
corpus albicans
corpus cavernosum
corpuscle
  amylaceous
  amyloid
  articular
  axile
  axis
  basal
  blood
  bone
  bridge
  bulboid

corpuscle *(continued)*
  cartilage
  cement
  chyle
  colloid
  colostrum
  concentrated human red blood
  corneal
  Dogiel
  dust
  exudation
  fat
  genital
  ghost
  Hassall
  malpighian
  Meissner
  pus
  Zimmermann
corpuscular lymph
corpus luteum
corpus luteum cyst
corpus spongiosum
corpus spongiosum penis
correlated atrophy
Corrigan line
Corrigan pneumonia
corrugated
corrugator muscle
cortex (pl. cortices)
  adrenal
  auditory
  bone
  cerebellar
  cerebral
  dysgranular
  frontal
  lymphatic
  ovarian
  pale
  renal
Corti arch

cortical arch
cortical artery
cortical atrophy
cortical bone
cortical convexity
cortical cyst
cortical defect
cortical hormone
cortical nodule
cortical osteitis
cortical part
cortical plate
cortical substance
cortical surface
cortical tissue
Corti canal
Corti cell
corticobinding globulin (CBG)
corticosterone test
corticobulbar tract
corticomedullary demarcation
corticomedullary junction
corticonuclear fiber
corticopontine tract
corticoreticular fiber
corticospinal fiber
corticospinal tract
corticosteroid-binding globulin
corticosterone test
corticostriatal-spinal degeneration
    cell
corticotropic hormone
corticotropin-releasing factor
corticotropin-releasing hormone
Corti fiber
Corti ganglion
Corti pillar
Corti rod
cortisol, free
cortisol hormone
Corti tunnel
Corynebacterium acnes

Corynebacterium bovis
Corynebacterium diphtheriae
Corynebacterium equi
Corynebacterium haemolyticum
Corynebacterium minutissimum
Corynebacterium pseudodiphtheriticum
Corynebacterium pseudotuberculosis
Corynebacterium ulcerans
Corynebacterium xerosis
coryza
cosmetic dermatitis
costal angle
costal arch
costal arch reflex
costal artery
costal bone
costal cartilage
costal facet
costal groove
costal margin
costal notch
costal part
costal pit
costal pleura
costal pleural reflection
costal pleurisy
costal process
costal surface
costal surface of lung
costal tuberosity
costeocartilaginous
costoaxillary vein
costocentral articulation
costocentral joint
costocervical artery
costocervical trunk
costocervical trunk artery
costochondral articulation
costochondral joint
costochondral junction
costoclavicular ligament
costoclavicular line

costocolic ligament
costodiaphragmatic recess of pleura
costomediastinal recess
costomediastinal sinus
costophrenic angle
costophrenic septal line
costosternal articulation
costosternal joint
costotransverse articulation
costotransverse foramen
costotransverse joint
costotransverse ligament
costovertebral angle (CVA)
costovertebral articulation
costovertebral joint
costovertebral junction
costovertebral ligament
costoxiphoid ligament
cothromboplastin
cotton-fiber embolism
cotton-mill fever
cotton-wool patch, spot
Cotunnius canal
Cotunnius space
cotyledon, basal plate
cotyloid cavity
cotyloid joint
cotyloid ligament
cotyloid notch
couch grass
cough
    paroxysmal
    whooping
coughing up blood from respiratory
    tract
cough plate
Coumadin anticoagulant
coumarin anticoagulant
Councilman body
Councilman chisel
Councilman lesion
counseling, genetic

count
    absolute
    absolute neutrophil (ANC)
    Addis
    CD4 (T4) lymphocyte
    cell (of cerebrospinal fluid)
    cell (of urine)
    colony (of urine)
    complete blood (CBC)
    differential
    differential white blood
    differential white blood cell
    indirect platelet
    lamellar body density (LBD)
    platelet
    red blood cell (RBC)
    reticulocyte
    urine colony
    white blood cell (WBC)
counter, B-emission
counterimmunoelectrophoresis (CIE)
counterstain
counting cells
Courvoisier gallbladder
cover cell
covering, fascial
covering of spermatic cord
covering of umbilical cord
coverslip
CO_2–withdrawal seizure test
cow kidney
cowl muscle
Cowper gland
Cowper ligament
coxa
coxal articulation
coxal bone
coxal joint
coxcomb (see *cockscomb*)
Coxiella burnetii
coxofemoral articulation of Buisson
Coxsackie virus (also, coxsackievirus)

coxsackievirus A
coxsackievirus B
coxsackievirus myocarditis
C-peptide (connecting peptide)
CPK (creatine phosphokinase)
(also, CK, creatine kinase)
CPK-MB (CK_2) isoenzyme
C_3 proactivator
CPT (Current Procedural Terminology) codes
C_1q immune complex
crackling
cramp, muscle
cranial base
cranial bone
cranial capacity
cranial cavity
cranial flexure
cranial fontanelle
cranial fossa
cranial meninges
cranial meningocele
cranial nerves (I through XII)
cranial part of accessory nerve
cranial root
cranial sinus
cranial suture (joint)
cranial synchondrosis
cranial synostosis
cranial vault
cranial vertebra
craniofacial angle
craniofacial axis
craniofacial notch
craniometric point
craniopharyngeal canal
craniopharyngeal duct
craniopharyngioma
craniosacral system
craniovertebral articulation
crater arc
C-reactive protein (CRP)

crease
    ear lobe
    inguinal
    midline abdominal
    palmar
    skin
    torso
crease wound
creatine kinase (CK)
creatine phosphokinase (CPK)
creatinine clearance
creatinine test
creatinine, urinary
creeping eruption
cremasteric artery
cremasteric fascia
cremaster muscle
crenated
crepitant
crepitation
crepitus
crescent, articular
crescent cell
crescentic border
crescentic lobule
crescent of cardia
crescent of foramina
crescent-shaped structure
crest
    acoustic
    acousticofacial
    alveolar
    ampullary
    arched
    arcuate
    articular
    basilar
    buccinator
    conchal
    deltoid
    dental
    ethmoidal

crest *(continued)*
   falciform
   frontal
   ganglionic
   gingival
   iliac
   pubic
   sacral
   urethral
CREST syndrome
   calcinosis
   Raynaud phenomenon
   esophageal dysfunction
   sclerodactyly
   telangiectasia
cresyl blue
cresyl blue brilliant
cresyl fast violet
cretinism
Creutzfeldt-Jakob disease
creviced appearance
crevicular epithelium fluid
cribrate cell
cribriform
cribriform area
cribriform bone
cribriform fascia
cribriform pattern
cribriform plate
cribriform tissue
cricoarytenoid articular capsule
cricoarytenoid articulation
cricoarytenoid joint
cricoesophageal tendon
cricopharyngeal diverticulum
cricopharyngeal ligament
cricopharyngeal part
cricopharyngeal sphincter
cricosantorinian ligament
cricothyroid artery
cricothyroid articular capsule
cricothyroid articulation

cricothyroid joint
cricothyroid ligament
cricothyroid membrane
cricothyroid muscle
cricotracheal ligament
cricotracheal membrane
cricovocal membrane
Crigler-Najjar syndrome
Crimean-Congo hemorrhagic fever
   virus
Crimean fever
crisscrossing cords
crista galli
crista terminalis
"crit" (slang for hematocrit)
criteria, Broder
Crithidia luciliae
critical angle
critical organ
CRM (cross-reacting material)
cRNA (complementary RNA)
Crohn disease
cromolyn sodium
Crooke cell
Crooke hyaline degeneration
Crooke-Russell band
cross-bridges
cross-circulation
crossed embolism
crossed eye
crossed pyramidal tract
crossed reflex
cross-infection
crossing over (also, crossover)
cross-linking
crossmatch
   HLA (human lymphocyte antigen)
   major
   minor
   pretransplant
   type and
crossmatching

crossover (also, crossing over)
cross-reacting agglutinin
cross-reacting antibody
cross-reacting material (CRM)
cross-reactivation
cross-reactivity
cross-reference
cross-resistance
cross-section (noun, verb)
cross-sectional (adj.)
cross-sensitization
croup-associated virus (CA v.)
croupous inflammation
croupous lymph
croupous membrane
croupous nephritis
croupy
crown cavity
crown, ciliary
crown-heel length
crown-rump length
crown tubercle
CRP (C-reactive protein)
^{51}Cr red cell survival
CRST syndrome (see *CREST*)
crucial anastomosis
cruciate eminence
cruciate ligament
cruciate ligament of atlas
cruciate ligament of knee
cruciate ligament of leg
cruciate muscle
cruciform eminence
cruciform ligament
cruciform part
crumbly
crura (plural of crus)
crura of diaphragm
crura of penis
crural arch
crural canal
crural fossa

crural nerve
crural ring
crural septum
crural sheath
crural triangle
cruris, tinea
crurotalar articulation
crus (pl. crura)
  lateral
  left
  medial
  right
crush kidney
crush syndrome
crus penis, crus of penis
crust (scab)
crusting center
crust of exudate
Cruveilhier atrophy
Cruveilhier-Baumgarten cirrhosis
Cruveilhier fascia
Cruveilhier joint
Cruveilhier ligament
cryofibrinogen
cryoglobulin
cryostat
crypt
  anal
  enamel
  epithelium
  ileal
  Lieberkühn
  Morgagni
  tonsillar
crypt abscess
cryptitis, anal
cryptococcal meningitis
cryptococcosis
Cryptococcus
Cryptococcus albidus
Cryptococcus laurentii
Cryptococcus luteolus

Cryptococcus neoformans
Cryptococcus neoformans pneumonia
cryptogenic pyemia
cryptorchidism
cryptosporidiosis
Cryptosporidium
crystal (pl. crystals)
  asthma
  blood
  Böttcher
  calcium
  calcium pyrophosphate dihydrate
    (CPPD)
  Charcot-Leyden
  cholesterol
  coffin lid
  dumbbell
  hydroxyapatite
  liquid
  Lubarsch
  thorn-apple
  urate
  Virchow
  whetstone
crystal violet
crystal violet stain
crystallization
crystalloid
crystals in urine
crystals of calcium salts
Crystodigin
CSF (cerebrospinal fluid)
CSF glucose
CSF protein
CST (contraction stress test)
cu mm (cubic millimeter)
Cu (copper)
cubic centimeter (cc)
cubic millimeter (cu mm or mm³)
cubital articulation
cubital bone
cubital fossa

cubital joint
cubital lymph node
cubital nerve
cubital tunnel
cubitoradial articulation
cubitus valgus
cuboidal articular surface
cuboidal epithelial cell
cuboidal epithelium
cuboidal glandular cell
cuboid bone
cuboid cell
cuboideonavicular articulation
cuboideonavicular joint
cuboideonavicular ligament
cuff
  musculotendinous
  rectal muscle
  rotator
  suprahepatic caval
cuffing, perivascular
cuirass, tabetic
cul-de-sac, conjunctival
cul-de-sac of Douglas
cul-de-sac smear
Culex mosquito
Cult-Dip Plus bacteriological culture
  test
culture
  abscess
  aerobic
  anaerobic
  arterial line
  bacterial
  blood
  cell
  cervical
  cerebrospinal fluid
  diphtheria
  disk
  fungal
  mixed leukocyte

culture *(continued)*
   mixed lymphocyte (MLC)
   nasopharyngeal
   radioisotopic
   Sabouraud
   spinal fluid
   sputum
   stool
   throat
   tissue (TC)
   Tween-albumin broth
   urine
   Vero cell
   viral
culture and sensitivity (C&S)
cultured cells of human lympho-
   blastoid line
culture medium (pl. media)
   agar
   bacterial
   laked sheep blood, kanamycin,
     vancomycin
   sheep red blood cells (sRBC)
   sRBC and phenylethyl alcohol
   tryptic soy agar with sRBC,
     colistin, and nalidixic acid
cuneate fasciculus
cuneate nucleus
cuneiform bone, first
cuneiform cartilage
cuneiform lobe
cuneiform tubercle
cuneocerebellar tract
cuneocuboid joint
cuneocuboid ligament
cuneometatarsal articulation
cuneometatarsal joint
cuneonavicular articulation
cuneonavicular joint
cuneonavicular ligament
cup ear
cupola, pleural

cupular blind sac
cupulate part
curdlike discharge
curdlike excrescence
curdy pus
curet (also, curette)
curet lesion
curettage
   endocervical
   endometrial
curetting
curled edge
Curling ulcer
currant jelly clot
currant jelly stool
current, electrotonic
Curschmann spiral
cursory examination
Curtis–Fitz-Hugh syndrome
curvature
   angular
   anterior
   backward
   gingival
curvature of stomach
   greater
   lesser
curve
   anti-Monso
   buccal
   glucose tolerance
   sigmoid
curve of duodenum
curving of diaphyses
Curvularia geniculata
Curvularia lunata
Curvularia pallescens
Curvularia senegalensis
Curvularia verruculosa
Cushing disease
Cushing phenomenon
Cushing syndrome

Cushing ulcer
cushion of auditory tube
cushion, polar
cusp
    anterior
    aortic
    noncoronary
    posterior
    septal
    valve
cusp angle
cuspidate tooth
cuspid tooth
cusp of valve
Custer cells
custocolic fold
cutaneomucous muscle
cutaneous abscess
cutaneous angiomata
cutaneous atrophy
cutaneous bleb
cutaneous branch
cutaneous cervical nerve
cutaneous cyst
cutaneous defect
cutaneous ellipse
cutaneous emphysema
cutaneous erosion
cutaneous fissure
cutaneous gland
cutaneous horn
cutaneous larva migrans
cutaneous leishmaniasis
cutaneous lymphangioma
cutaneous muscle
cutaneous nerve
cutaneous nodule
cutaneous papilloma
cutaneous pigmentation
cutaneous pit
cutaneous plaque
cutaneous ridge

cutaneous schistosomiasis
cutaneous test
cutaneous tissue
cutaneous tuberculin test
cutaneous tumor
cutaneous twig
cutaneous ulcer
cutaneous vein
cutaneous wound
cutaneous zone
cuticle
    acquired
    dental
    enamel
cutis anserina (goose flesh)
cutis hyperelastica
cutis marmorata (marble skin)
cutis laxa
    acquired
    congenital
cutis rhomboidalis nuchae
cutis verticis gyrata (gyrate scalp)
cut surface
cutter tissue
Cuvier, canal of
CVA (cerebrovascular accident)
CVA (costovertebral angle)
C vitamin
CVP (central venous pressure) catheter
C wave
cyanide–nitroprusside test
cyanide poisoning
cyanide test
cyanmethemoglobin
cyanocobalamin
cyanosis
cyanotic induration
cyanotic kidney
cyclical changes
cyclic AMP (adenosine monophos-
    phate)
cyclodextrin agar

cylindrical cells
cylindrical punch
cylindric epithelium
cylindroid aneurysm
cyst
   acoustic
   Baker
   Bartholin
   benign
   bland
   Blessig
   blue dome
   bone
   branchial
   branchial cleft
   bronchogenic
   calcification of
   cerebral
   chocolate
   corpus luteum
   cortical
   cutaneous
   dentigerous
   dermoid
   endometrial
   epidermal
   epidermal inclusion
   epithelial
   fluid-filled
   follicular
   functional ovarian
   ganglion
   germinal inclusion
   hemorrhagic
   hydatid
   inclusion
   joint
   lutein
   mammary
   meibomian
   mesothelial
   milk-filled

cyst *(continued)*
   morgagnian
   mucous
   müllerian
   multilocular
   multiloculated
   myxoid
   nabothian
   neoplastic
   non-neoplastic
   ovarian
   ovarian follicular
   pancreatic
   parasite
   paratubal
   parovarian
   pearl
   pericardial
   pilar
   pilonidal
   pineal
   pituitary
   primordial
   prostatic
   renal
   retention
   sebaceous
   serosal
   solitary bone
   tarsal
   testicular
   theca-lutein
   thin-walled
   thyroglossal duct
   unilocular
   wolffian
cyst adenocarcinoma
   mucinous
   serous
cystadenoma
Cysteine Albimi media
cysteine proteinase

cysteine test (see *cystine*)
cystic adenomatoid malformation
cystic artery
cystic degeneration
cystic duct
cystic duct lumen
cysticercosis
cystic eye
cystic fibrosis
cystic fistula
cystic fluid
cystic gall duct
cystic goiter
cystic kidney
cystic lymph node
cystic mastitis
cystic medial necrosis
cystic meningioma
cystic mole
cystic ovary
cystic plexus
cystic polyp
cystic swelling in a meibomian gland
cystic teratoma
cystic vein
cystine (also, cysteine)
cystine, amino acid
cystine calculi in urinary tract
cystine, lactose, electrolyte deficient
   (CLED)
cystine metabolism abnormalities
cystine stones
cystinuria
cystitis
   acute hemorrhagic
   hemorrhagic
   honeymoon
   interstitial
   radiation
cystocholedochal junction
cystochrome system
cystoduodenal ligament

cystohepatic triangle
cystoid degeneration
cystosarcoma phyllodes
cyst wall
Cytobrush
cytochromes
cytocrine secretion
cytogenetics
cytoid body
cytokeratin immunoreactivity
cytokine
cytokinesis
cytological biopsy
cytologically bland leiomyoma
cytologic atypia
cytologic diagnosis
cytologic report
cytologic smear
cytology
   cervical
   exfoliative
cytolysis
cytolysosome
cytomegalic cell
cytomegalic inclusion disease virus
cytomegalovirus
cytomegalovirus disease
cytomegalovirus encephalitis
cytomegalovirus pneumonitis
cytometer
   ARGUS flow
   CA II flow
   Cytoron Absolute flow
   ELITE Analyzer flow
   Epics Profile II flow
   FACScan flow
   PAS III flow
cytometry
cytopathic
cytoplasm
   eosinophilic
   eosinophilic homogeneous

cytoplasm *(continued)*
   foamy
   granular
   pale
   scanty
cytoplasmic bridge
cytoplasmic granule
cytoplasmic inclusion
cytoplasmic inclusion body
cytoplasmic matrix
cytoplasmic/nuclear ratio
cytoplasmic ratio
cytoplasmic staining
cytoplasmic stippling
cytoplasmic vacuole
Cytoron Absolute flow cytometer
cytoskeletal pathology

cytosol
cytosolic concentration
cytosolic fraction
cytospin preparation
Cytospray
cytotoxic cell
cytotoxic T cell
cytotoxic T lymphocyte
cytotoxicity
   antibody-dependent cell-mediated
     (ADCC)
   complement-mediated
   lymphocyte-mediated
cytotropic antibody test
cytotrophoblast
cytotrophoblastic cell
CZE (capillary zone electrophoresis)

D, d

D (delta)
D (dorsal)
dacryocyte (teardrop cell)
Dactylaria
Dade Paramax analyzer
dag (decagram)
DAKO AEC substrate/chromogen
DAKO glycergel
DAKO liquid DAB substrate/
    chromogen
DAKO target retrieval solution
daL (decaliter)
Dalen-Fuchs nodule
dam (decameter)
damage
    irreparable
    predator
damaged nerve tissue
damaged tissue
damol (decamole)
dancer's foot malformation
Dane and Herman keratin stain
Dane particle
Danlos-Ehlers syndrome
Danysz phenomenon
DA pregnancy test
Darier disease

dark cells
darkfield examination
darkfield microscope
dark green stool
dark stool
dark urine
Darrow red stain
dartoid tissue
dartos muscle
Darwin auricular tubercle
darwinian ear
darwinian tubercle
datum plane
Daudi cell
daughter cell
Davenport stain
Davidoff cell
Davidsohn differential absorption test
dawn phenomenon
Dawson encephalitis
Day test
DBP (vitamin D-binding protein)
DCC (deleted in colon carcinoma)
    tumor suppressor gene
D cell of pancreas
DCIS (ductal carcinoma in situ)
d-dimer (or D-dimer) test

dead
  brain
  pronounced
dead bowel
dead fetus in utero (DFU)
dead nerve
dead pulp
dead space
dead tooth
dead tract
deafness due to otosclerosis
deamidizing enzyme
death
  apparent
  black
  brain
  cell
  cerebral
  cot
  crib
  fetal (early, intermediate, late)
  functional
  genetic
  liver
  local
  molecular
  natural
  programmed cell
  SIDS (sudden infant d. syndrome)
  somatic
  sudden cardiac
  sudden infant d. symdrone (SIDS)
  unattended
  unsuspected cause of
  voodoo
death syndrome, sudden infant (SIDS)
DeBakey aortic classification
debilitated patient
debrancher (debranching) enzyme
debrancher (debranching) factor
Debré phenomenon
debrided

debridement tissue
debris
  amorphous
  cellular
  chemical
  fibrin
  fibrinous
  foreign
  keratin
  laminated keratotic
  necrotic
  pasty
  semisolid sebaceous
decagram (dag)
decalcification
decaliter (daL)
decamer
decameter (dam)
decamole (damol)
decapitation factor
Decaprime II
decay
decedent
decidua
  basal
  parietal
decidual cell
decidual fissure
deciduate placenta
deciduous membrane
deciduous skin
decigram (dg)
deciliter (dL)
decimeter (dm)
decimole (dmol)
decolorizer (see *stain*)
decompensated cirrhosis
decomposition
decoy cells
decubitus ulcer
deep artery of clitoris
deep auricular artery

deep brachial artery
deep cell
deep cervical artery
deep dorsal sacrococcygeal ligament
deep epigastric artery
deep external pudendal artery
deep fascia
deep fascia of penis
deep femoral artery
deep iliac circumflex artery
deep lingual artery
deep lingual vein
deep lymph vessel
deeply pigmented lesions in retina
deep palmar arch artery
deep penis artery
deep perineal pouch
deep plantar artery
deep plexus
deep posterior sacrococcygeal ligament
deep temporal artery
deep transverse metacarpal ligament
deep transverse metatarsal ligament
deep volar branch of ulnar artery
defect
    acquired
    aortic septal
    atrial septal
    birth
    coagulation
    congenital
    cortical
    fibrous cortical
    filling
    luteal phase
    neural tube
    pear-shaped
    pressure cone
    retention
    salt-losing
    septal
    ventricular septal

defective synthesis of hemoglobin
defective virus
deferens, ductus
deferent canal
deferent duct
deferential artery
deferential plexus
defibrinated blood
deficiency
    acquired immune
    adenosine deaminase
    adrenal cortical
    biotin-dependent carboxylase
    cobalamin
    congenital
    galactokinase
    immune
    iron
    oxygen
    plasma clotting factor
    platelet
    protein C
    thiamine
    transcobalamin 2
    vitamin
deficient production of red blood cells
definitive diagnosis
deformans
    osteitis
    osteochondrodystrophia
deformity
    Akerlund
    Arnold-Chiari
    bell clapper
    bone
    boutonnière
    contracture
    gibbous
    Erlenmeyer flask
    funnel-like
    gunstock
    Haglund

deformity *(continued)*
    J-sella
    keyhole
    lobster-claw
    Madelung
    mermaid
    parachute
    phrygian cap
    reduction
    seal-fin
    silver-fork
    Sprengel
    swan-neck
    torsional
    whistling
    Whitehead
deformity of bony digits
degenerate blood clot
degenerated blood
degenerating fibrils within neurons
degenerating neurons
degeneration
    Abercrombie
    adipose
    adiposogenital
    albuminous
    Alzheimer neurofibrillary
    amyloid
    angiolithic
    ascending
    atheromatous
    atrophic pulp
    axonal
    ballooning
    black
    bone
    bone marrow
    brain
    breast
    calcareous
    carneous
    cerebromacular (CMD)

degeneration *(continued)*
    cerebroretinal
    colloid
    comma
    corticostriatal-spinal
    Crooke hyaline
    cystic
    cystoid
    descending
    Doyne familial colloid
    Doyne honeycomb
    dystrophic
    earthy
    elastoid
    esophageal
    fascicular
    fatty
    fibrillary
    fibrinoid
    fibrinous
    fibroid
    gelatiniform
    glassy
    glistening
    glycogenic
    Gombault
    granulovacuolar
    gray matter
    heart
    hematohyaloid
    hepatic
    hepatolenticular
    hyaline
    hydropic
    lipoidal
    liquefaction
    liver
    macular
    malignant
    Mönckeberg
    mucinoid
    mucinous

degeneration *(continued)*
  mucoid
  mucous
  muscular
  myelinic
  myxomatous
  nerve
  nerve cell
  nerve tissue
  neuronal
  Nissl
  optic
  otic
  pancreas
  parenchymatous
  periodontal
  pigmental
  pigmentary
  primary progressive cerebellar
  progressive
  red
  renal tubular
  retinal
  retrograde
  rim
  Rosenthal
  sclerotic
  secondary
  senile
  solar
  spinal
  spongiform
  spongy
  Stargardt macular
  striatonigral
  subacute combined
  testicular
  thyroid
  trabecular
  transneuronal
  traumatic
  Türck

degeneration *(continued)*
  vacuolar
  wallerian
  Zenker waxy
degeneration of retinal ganglion cells
degeneration of sarcoplasm, vacuolar
degeneration of white substance of
  spinal cord
degenerative arthritic change
degenerative atrophy
degenerative changes
degenerative disk disease
degenerative joint disease (DJD)
degenerative liver
degenerative nephritis
degenerative osteoarthritis
degenerative spine disease
degenerative spondylosis
degenerative spur
deglutition mechanism
deglutition pneumonia
Degos disease
Dehio test
dehydration
dehydration fever
dehydrocholate test for speed of blood
  circulation
dehydroepiandrosterone (DHEA) test
dehydroepiandrosterone sulfate
  (DHEA-SO$_4$) test
dehydrogenase, alpha-ketoglutarate
deiterospinal tract
Deiters cell
Dejerine-Landouzy dystrophy
Dejerine-Landouzy muscular
  dystrophy
Dejerine-Sottas atrophy
Dejerine-Thomas atrophy
Delafield fluid
Delafield hematoxylin
Delafield hematoxylin stain
Delafield solution

delayed resolution of pneumonia
Delbet fracture classification
deletion
    chromosomal abnormality of
    interstitial
    terminal
delicate
delimited
delineate
delineation
delirium
delivery, postmortem
delomorphous cell
Del Rio Hortega method
delta-aminolevulinic acid
delta antigen (delta-Ag)
delta band
delta cell
delta granule
delta hepatitis (hepatitis D)
delta wave
deltoid artery
deltoid crest
deltoid eminence
deltoideopectoral trigone
deltoid impression
deltoid ligament
deltoid muscle
deltoid reflex
deltoid region
deltoid tuberosity
demarcation, corticomedullary
demifacet
demilune body
demilune cell
demineralized material
demyelinating disease of brain
demyelination and gliosis in central
   nervous system
demyelination of cerebral white matter
demyelination, segmental
demyelinization

denatured protein
dendrite, apical
dendritic cell
dendritic keratitis
dendritic process
dendritic reticular cell
denervated muscle atrophy
dengue
   classic
   hemorrhagic
   Philippine
dengue hemorrhage fever
dengue-like disease
dengue shock syndrome
dengue virus
Denis Browne superficial inguinal
    pouch
Denonvilliers fascia
Denonvilliers ligament
dens
dense connective tissue
density, bone mineral
dental abscess
dental alveolus
dental arch
dental artery
dental articulation
dental bulb
dental canal
dental caries
dental cord
dental crest
dental cuticle
dental fiber
dental follicle
dental groove
dental lamina
dental lymph
dental material
dental mottling
dental neck
dental nerve

dental plaque
dental polyp
dental process
dental pulp
dental ridge
dental root
dental root canal
dental sac
dental shelf
dental tubercle
dental tubule
dental tumor
dentate fascia
dentate fissure
dentate gyrus
dentate ligament of spinal cord
dentate line
dentate margin
dentate nucleus
dentate suture
dentatothalamic tract
denticulate hymen
denticulate ligament
dentigerous cyst
dentin
dentin globule
dentinal fiber
dentinal fluid
dentinal papilla
dentinal pulp
dentinal sheath
dentinal tubule
dentinocemental junction
dentinoenamel junction
dentoalveolar abscess
dentoalveolar articulation
dentoalveolar gomphosis
dentoalveolar joint
dentofacial zone
dentogingival lamina
denture basal surface
denture-bearing area

denture cell
denture foundation area
denture foundation surface
denture impression surface
denture occlusal surface
denture polished surface
denture-supporting area
denture-supporting structure
Denucé ligament
denudation
denude
denuded
Denver chromosome classification
Denys-Leclef phenomenon
D enzyme
11-deoxycortisol hormone
    (Compound S)
11-deoxycorticosterone (DOC)
deoxyribonuclease (DNase) test
deoxyuridine suppression test
deparaffinization
dependent edema
dependent lividity
Depex mounting solution
depigmentation
depigmented lesion
depletion of colloid
depletion of fat stores
deposit, albuminous
deposition
    collagen
    fibrin
    hemosiderin
    melanin
    pigment
deposition of calcium salts in kidney
    tissue
deposition of mineral salts
deposition of mucoid material in
    muscle
deposition of mucoid material in
    subcutaneous tissue

deposition of unconjugated bilirubin
deposition of yellow or brown pigment
   granules in cytoplasm
depressed ejection fracture
depressed marrow
depressor fiber
depressor muscle
depressor nerve
depressor reflex
depth
de Quervain disease
de Quervain thyroiditis
derived protein
dermabrasion
dermal bone
dermal chromatophores
dermal lymphatic involvement
dermal melanocytoma
dermal microabscess
dermal nevus
dermal papilla (pl. papillae)
dermal sinus
dermal stria
dermal system
dermal tissue
dermal wart
dermatitis
   actinic
   allergic
   allergic contact
   ammonia
   Ancylostoma
   ashy
   atopic
   berlock
   blastomycetic
   brown-tail moth
   bubble gum
   cercarial
   chemical
   contact
   contact-type

dermatitis *(continued)*
   contagious pustular
   cosmetic
   dhobie mark
   diaper
   eczematous
   exfoliativa neonatorum
   exfoliative
   exudative
   exudative and lichenoid
   exudative discoid
   factitial
   grass
   industrial
   infectious eczematous
   insect
   irritant
   Jacquet
   Leiner
   lichenoid
   livedoid
   mango
   marine
   meadow
   meadow grass
   nickel
   nummular eczematous
   occupational
   onion mite
   papular (of pregnancy)
   papulovesicular
   perfume
   periocular
   perioral
   photoallergic contact
   phototoxic
   pigmented purpuric lichenoid
   plant
   poison ivy
   poison oak
   poison sumac
   precancerous

dermatitis *(continued)*
    primary irritant
    proliferative
    radiation
    rat-mite
    rhus
    sabra
    sandal strap
    scaly erythematous
    Schamberg
    schistosome
    seborrheic
    solar
    stasis
    swimmer's
    trefoil
    uncinarial
    verminous
    vesicular
    washerman's mark
    x-ray
dermatitis aestivalis
dermatitis atrophicans
dermatitis bullosa
dermatitis bullosa striata pratensis
    (grass)
dermatitis calorica
dermatitis combustionis (burn)
dermatitis congelationis (frostbite)
dermatitis gangrenosa infantum
dermatitis herpetiformis
dermatitis hiemalis
dermatitis medicamentosa (drug
    eruption)
dermatitis nodosa
dermatitis nodularis necrotica
dermatitis papillaris capillitii
dermatitis pediculoides ventricosus
dermatitis repens
dermatitis simplex
dermatitis vegetans
dermatitis venenata

dermatitis verrucosa
dermatofibroma
dermatofibrosarcoma
dermatofibrosarcoma protuberans
dermatofibrosis
dermatofibrosis lenticularis disseminata
dermatome
dermatomic area
dermatomycosis
dermatomyositis
dermatopathology
Dermatophilus
Dermatophilus congolensis
dermatophytic fungi
dermatophytid
dermatophytosis
dermatosis (pl. dermatoses)
    acarine
    acute febrile neutrophilic
    ashy
    Bowen precancerous
    chronic bullous
    dermolytic bullous
    digitate
    dyschromic
    industrial
    scaly
    transient acantholytic
    ulcerative
dermis
    papillary
    papillary layer of
    reticular
dermoepidermal interface
dermoepidermal junction
dermoid cyst
dermoid system
dermolytic bullous dermatosis
dermotropic virus
DES (diethylstilbestrol)
descemetocele
Descemet membrane

descending aorta
descending aorta artery
descending artery
descending branch of occipital artery
descending branch of uterine artery
descending colon
descending degeneration
descending duodenum
descending lymphangitis
descending neuritis
descending nucleus
descending palatine artery
descending part
descending pyelonephritis
descending scapular artery
descending thoracic aorta
descending tract
Deschamps needle
desiccate
desiccation
Desjardins point
desmoplakin protein
desmoplasia
desmoplastic malignant melanoma
desmoplastic response
desmoplastic stroma
desmosomal junction
desquamated cells
desquamation
desquamative interstitial pneumonia
desquamative pneumonia
destruction of tissue
detached retina
detachment, retinal
determinate cleavage
detrusor muscle
development, abnormalities of
developmental age
developmental anomaly
developmental groove
developmental line
Deventer pelvis

deviating eye
Devic disease
devitalized pulp
devitalized tissue
devoid
dewaxed
dewy appearance
dexamethasone single dose overnight
     suppression test
dexamethasone suppression test
dextran sulfate
dextrocardia
dextrose test
Dextrostix
DFA-TP test (direct fluorescent anti-
     body-*Treponema pallidum* test)
DF-2 bacillus
DFU (dead fetus in utero)
dg (decigram)
D hemoglobin
D hepatitis
dhobie mark dermatitis
DI (diabetes insipidus)
diabetes
     adult onset
     borderline
     brittle
     bronze
     calcinuric
     chemical
     drug-induced
     gestational
     growth-onset
     insulinopenic
     juvenile onset
     ketosis-prone
     ketosis-resistant
     latent
     lipoatrophic
     lipogenous
     maturity-onset
     maturity-onset d. of youth (MODY)

diabetes *(continued)*
  maternal
  metahypophysial
  Mosler
  neurogenic
  obesity-associated
  overt
  pancreatic
  phosphate
  preclinical
  pregnancy
  puncture
  renal
  renal amino acid
  secondary
  starvation
  steroid
  steroidogenic
  subclinical
  thiazide
  type I insulin-dependent
  type II non-insulin-dependent
  uncontrolled
  vasopressin-resistant
  Young
diabetes innocens
diabetes insipidus (DI)
diabetes intermittens
diabetes mellitus (DM)
  adult-onset
  juvenile-onset
  type I, IDDM (insulin-dependent
    diabetes mellitus)
  type II, NIDDM (non-insulin-
    dependent diabetes mellitus)
  type II, NIDDM, non-obese
  type II, NIDDM, obese
diabetes mellitus classification
diabetes neonatorum
diabetic acidosis
diabetic amyotrophy
diabetic Charcot foot

diabetic colitis
diabetic coma
diabetic dermopathy
diabetic encephalopathy
diabetic foot
diabetic gangrene
diabetic gastroparesis
diabetic glomerulosclerosis
diabetic ketoacidosis
diabetic lipemia
diabetic microangiopathy
diabetic mother
diabetic myelopathy
diabetic nephropathy
diabetic neuroarthropathy of foot
  and ankle
diabetic neuropathy
diabetic peripheral neuropathy
diabetic polyneuropathy
diabetic polyradiculopathy
diabetic retinitis
diabetic retinopathy (DR)
diabeticogenic hormone
diabetic peripheral vascular insufficiency
diabetic third nerve palsy
diabetic ulcer
diabetogenic factor
diaceturia
diacetyl test for urea
diagnosis (pl. diagnoses)
  admitting
  antenatal
  clinical
  colposcopic
  cytologic
  definitive
  differential
  discharge
  empirical
  fetal
  final

diagnosis *(continued)*
  frozen section
  genetic
  gross
  histologic
  histopathological
  initial
  microscopic
  neonatal
  operative
  pathologic
  physical
  postoperative
  preliminary
  prenatal
  prenatal genetic
  preoperative
  presumptive
  principal
  provisional anatomic
  tentative
  ultrasound
  working
diagnosis by exclusion
diagnostic cascade
Diagnostic and Statistical Manual III—
  Revised (DSM-III-R)
diagnosis related group (DRG)
diagnostic imaging
diagnostic laparoscopy
diagnostic procedure
diagnostic radiation
diagnostic test
diagonal band of Broca
dialysis encephalopathy
diameter, anteroposterior
diaminobenzidine tetrahydrochloride
diamond-shaped conidia
diamond-shaped incision
Di antigen
diapedesis
diaper dermatitis

diaper rash dermatitis
diaphragm
  aponeurotic portion of
  arcuate ligaments of
  Bucky
  central tendon
  crus of
  dome of
  leaves of
  pelvic
  Potter-Bucky
  thoracoabdominal
  twigs to pelvic
  urogenital
diaphragmatic arch
diaphragmatic fascia
diaphragmatic hernia
diaphragmatic ligament
diaphragmatic node
diaphragmatic pleura
diaphragmatic pleurisy
diaphragmatic surface of liver
diaphragm of sella turcica
diaphyseal center
diaphyseal dysplasia
diaphysis (pl. diaphyses), curving of
diarrhea
  bacillary
  bloody
  chronic bacillary
  colliquative
  copious rice-water
  copious watery
  Dientamoeba
  dysenteric
  explosive
  lienteric
  mucous
  serous
  watery
diarrheal disease
diarrheal stool

diarthrodial cartilage
diarthrodial joint
diaspirin-cross-linked hemoglobin
   (CDLHb)
Dibothriocephalus latus
DIC (disseminated intravascular
   coagulation)
dichroic reflector
dichromate, potassium
dichuchwa
Dick intracutaneous test
Dick test for scarlet fever susceptibility
dicrotic notch
dicrotic pulse
dicrotic wave
didelphia, uterine
didelphic uterus
Diego blood group
Dientamoeba diarrhea
Dientamoeba fragilis
diener (morgue attendant)
Dientamoeba fragilis
dietary fat
Dieterle silver stain
dietetic neuritis
dietetic proteinuria
diethylstilbestrol (DES)
Dieulafoy lesion
Dieulafoy triad
Dieulafoy vascular malformation
differential count
   bone marrow
   leukocyte
   synovial fluid
   white blood cell
differential diagnosis
differential renal function test
differential sugars
differential test for infectious
   mononucleosis
differential threshold
differential ureteral catheterization test

differential white blood cell count
differentiated
differentiation, cluster of (CD)
diffuse abscess
diffuse dermal neutrophil infiltration
diffuse esophageal spasm
diffuse fibrotic reaction
diffuse ganglion
diffuse goiter
diffuse hair loss
diffuse idiopathic atrophy of skin
diffuse interstitial fibrosis
diffuse large cell lymphoma
diffuse lymphoma
diffuse meningoencephalitis
diffuse mixed small and large cell
   lymphoma
diffuse myelitis
diffuse necrosis
diffuse opacities
diffuse pleurisy
diffuse psoriasis
diffuse sclerosing osteomyelitis
diffuse septal cirrhosis
diffuse small cleaved cell lymphoma
diffuse toxic goiter
diffusely
diffusion capacity of lungs for
   carbon monoxide (DL_{CO})
diffusion capacity of lungs for
   oxygen (DLO_2)
diffusion capacity of lungs for
   single-breath ($DLCO_{SB}$)
diffusion capacity of lungs for
   steady state ($DLCO_{SS}$)
diffusion, double
digastric fossa
digastric groove
digastric impression
digastric muscle
digastric notch
digastric triangle

DiGeorge anomaly
digestive enzyme
digestive fluid
digestive tract
digestive tube
digit
   accessory
   webbed
digital artery
digital collateral artery
digital fossa
digital joint
digital process of fat
digital pulp
digital reflex
digital vein
digital web
digital whorl
digit, accessory
digit articulation
digitate dermatosis
digitation
dihydrotestosterone (DHT) test
1,25-dihydroxycholecalciferol assay
   (1,25-OH-D$_3$)
dihydroxyphenylalanine (DOPA)
dilatation
   cardiac
   cavitary
   gastric
   idiopathic
   post-stenotic
   prognathic
dilatation of duct or vessel
dilate
dilated
dilation, digital
dilator muscle
dilator pupillae
"dils" (dilutions)
diluent
diluted whole blood clot lysis

dilutional hyponatremia
dilution, serial
dimensions of specimen
diminution
dimorphic fungus
dineric interface
dinitrophenol poisoning
dinitrophenylhydrazine test
dioxide, carbon
DIP (desquamative interstitial
   pneumonia)
DIP (distal interphalangeal) joint
DiPAS-positive granule
diphtheria bacillus
diphtheria culture
diphtheria test
diphtheritic membrane
diphtheritic myocarditis
diphtheroids
diplococci, gram-negative intracellular
   (GNID)
diplococcus of Morax-Axenfeld
diplococcus of Neisser
Diplococcus pneumoniae
diploic artery
diploic canal
diploic vein
diploid nucleus
diplopia
dipslide, Uricult
dipstick
   Clinistix
   Combistix
   Glucostix
   Ketodiastix
   Labstix
   Multistix
   N-Multistix
   Uristix
direct antiglobulin test
direct bilirubin
direct Coombs test

direct embolism
direct fluorescent antibody–*Treponema*
  pallidum (DFA-TP) test
direct immunofluorescence
direct inguinal hernia
direct pyramidal tract
direct radioimmunoassay
direct-reacting bilirubin
direct transfusion
disarray
disc (from Latin *discus*) (see *disk*)
discernible
discharge
  cheesy
  copious
  curdlike
  foul
  frothy
  purulent
  serosanguineous
  scant
discharge diagnosis
discharging tubule
discission needle
discoid lupus erythematosus (LE)
discoidal cleavage
discoloration
discontinuation test
discrete objects
discrete tumor
discrete yellow masses in pus
disease
  Addison
  Albers-Schoenberg
  Alexander leukodystrophy
  allogeneic
  Alzheimer
  anhydride-induced immunologic
    respiratory
  anti-glomerular basement
    membrane (anti-GBM) antibody
  aorticorenal

disease *(continued)*
  Armanni-Ebstein
  autoimmune (collagen)
  Besnier-Boeck
  Besnier-Boeck-Schaumann
  Blount
  Boeck
  Bowman
  Bornholm
  bowel
  Bowen
  Brill-Zinsser
  Brinton
  Bruton
  Buerger
  Calvé-Perthes-Legg
  Canavan
  Canavan–van Bogaert–Bertrand
  cardiac
  cat-scratch
  celiac
  Chagas
  choked disk
  Christian-Hand-Schüller
  Christmas
  collagen
  combined system
  Creutzfeldt-Jakob
  Crohn
  Cushing
  cytomegalovirus
  Darier
  degenerative joint
  Degos
  demyelinating
  dengue-like
  de Quervain
  Devic
  diarrheal
  Duhring
  Ebola
  Ebstein-Armanni

disease *(continued)*
  endocrine
  Fabry
  fibrocystic breast
  fifth
  foot, hand, and mouth
  Freiberg
  Gaucher
  Gilchrist
  Glanzmann
  glycogen storage
  Graves
  Grover
  Hailey-Hailey
  Hallopeau
  hand, foot, and mouth
  Hand-Schüller-Christian
  Hansen
  Hartnup
  Hashimoto
  hemoglobin
  hemolytic d. of newborn
  hepatic
  highly contagious sexually
    transmitted
  Hirschsprung
  Hodgkin
  hyaline membrane
  hydatid cyst
  idiopathic
  infectious
    communicable
    contagious
    transmissible
  inflammatory bowel
  Jakob-Creutzfeldt
  Jüngling
  Kaposi
  Kawasaki
  Kienböck
  Kimmelstiel-Wilson
  Köhler (Koehler)

disease *(continued)*
  Krabbe
  Legg-Calvé-Perthes
  legionnaire's
  lethal
  Letterer-Siwe
  Lichtheim
  life-threatening
  linear IgA bullous
  lumpy skin
  Lyme
  Majocchi
  maple syrup urine
  marble bone
  Marburg
  Marie-Strümpell
  Merzbacher-Pelizaeus
  metastatic
  Mondor
  Morquio
  mouth, foot, and hand
  myeloproliferative
  neurodegenerative
  Niemann-Pick
  nonvenereal skin
  Norwalk
  Osgood-Schlatter
  Osler-Weber-Rendu
  osteochondritis dissecans
  Paget
  Panner
  Parkinson
  Pelizaeus-Merzbacher
  pelvic inflammatory (PID)
  Perthes-Legg-Calvé
  Peyronie
  Pick-Niemann
  Pick
  Pompe
  Pott
  primary
  progressive

disease *(continued)*
   pulseless
   Quervain (also, de Quervain)
   reactive airways
   Recklinghausen (also, von
      Recklinghausen)
   renal
   Rendu-Osler-Weber
   respiratory syncytial
   Ritter
   Runeberg
   Sachs-Tay
   Scheuermann
   Schilder
   Schlatter-Osgood
   Schoenberg-Albers
   Schüller-Christian-Hand
   secondary
   Senear-Usher
   sexually transmitted (STD)
   sickle cell
   silo filler's
   Simmonds
   Siwe-Letterer
   smallpox-like
   Still
   storage
   streptococcal (of newborn)
   Strümpell-Marie
   Sweet
   systemic
   Takayasu
   Tay-Sachs
   thromboembolic
   Unna
   vascular
   von Gierke
   von Recklinghausen
   von Willebrand
   Weber-Rendu-Osler
   Weil
   Wilson-Kimmelstiel

disease *(continued)*
   Wilson
   woodworker lung's
   woolsorter's
   Zinsser-Brill
diseased kidney
dish, Petri
disk (Greek *diskus*) (also, *disc*)
   A
   acromioclavicular
   acromioclavicular joint
   anal
   anisotropic
   articular
   blastodermic
   Bowman
   cervical vertebral
   choked
   chorionic
   ciliary
   cone
   culture
   distal radioulnar joint
   embryonic
   emery
   germ
   germinal
   H
   hair
   Hensen
   herniated
   I
   intercalated
   intervertebral
   isotropic
   lumbar vertebral
   mandibular
   Merkel tactile
   noncontained
   optic
   placental
   Placido da Costa

disk *(continued)*
  protruded
  Q
  radioulnar
  Ranvier
  ruptured
  sequestered
  slipped intervertebral
  sternoclavicular joint
  temporomandibular joint
  thoracic vertebral
  transverse
  triangular
  vertebral
disk diffusion test for antibiotic
  sensitivity in bacteria
disk electrophoresis
disk kidney (disk-shaped)
disk sensitivity method
disorganization of connective tissue
disparity angle
disproportionately short limbs
disruption of nerve tracts
dissecans, osteochondritis
dissecting aneurysm of abdominal aorta
dissecting aneurysm of thoracic aorta
dissecting cellulitis of scalp
dissecting needle
dissection tubercle
disseminated condensing osteopathy
disseminated cutaneous gangrene
disseminated gonococcal infection
disseminated inflammation
disseminated intravascular coagulation
  (DIC)
disseminated lupus erythematosus (LE)
disseminated myelitis
disseminated tuberculosis
Disse space
dissociation
  albuminocytologic
  bacterial

distal bile duct
distal bulbar septum
distal clot
distal colon
distal convoluted tubule
distal duodenum
distal esophageal ring
distal interphalangeal (DIP) joint
distally
distal part
distal radioulnar articulation
distal radioulnar joint
distal surface
distal tibiofibular joint
distend
distended gallbladder
distention
distention of fibroblasts and
  macrophages by mucoid material
distinct
distortion of cells
distortion of fibrils within cell
  processes
distributing artery
disturbance
  metabolic
  respiratory
disuse atrophy
disuse osteoporosis
diurese
diuresis
diuretic agent
diuretic drug
diverging meniscus
diverticulitis
  colonic
  Meckel
diverticulum (pl. diverticula)
  bladder
  colonic
  cricopharyngeal
  esophageal

diverticulum *(continued)*
  Meckel
  metanephric
  pulsion
  traction
  urethral
  Zenker
diving goiter
division, mitotic
divisum, pancreas
DJD (degenerative joint disease)
dL (deciliter)
dm (decimeter)
DM (diabetes mellitus)
dmol (decimole)
DNA (deoxyribonucleic acid)
DNA analysis
DNA gap
DNA marker
DNA ploidy
DNA probe
DNA sequencing electrophoresis
DNA tumor virus
DNA tumor virus protein
DNA virus
DNA, wild-type
Döderlein bacillus (also, Doederlein)
dog-bite infections
Dogiel cells
Dogiel corpuscles
Döhle body (also, Doehle)
dolichopellic pelvis
dolorogenic zone
Dombrock blood group
dome cell
dome of diaphragm
dome of liver
dominance
dominant gene
dominant hemisphere
dominant trait
Donath-Landsteiner antibody

Donath-Landsteiner test for
  paroxysmal cold hemoglobinuria
donor blood
donor cells
donor kidney
donor organ
donor serum
donor sperm
Donovan bodies in monocytes
Donovania granulomatis
DOPA (dihydroxyphenylalanine) stain
d'orange, peau
Dorello canal
Dorothy Reed cell
dorsal (D)
dorsal antebrachial cutaneous nerve
dorsal aorta
dorsal arch, venous
dorsal artery
dorsal branch of posterior intercostal
  artery
dorsal calcaneocuboid ligament
dorsal carpal artery
dorsal carpal ligament
dorsal carpometacarpal ligament
dorsal cuboideonavicular ligament
dorsal cuneocuboid ligament
dorsal cuneonavicular ligament
dorsal interosseous artery
dorsal lingual vein
dorsal mesogastrium
dorsal metacarpal artery
dorsal metacarpal ligament
dorsal metatarsal ligament
dorsal nasal artery
dorsal nerve of penis
dorsal pancreatic bud
dorsal point
dorsal primary ramus
dorsal radiocarpal ligament
dorsal ramus (pl. rami) nerve
dorsal sacroiliac ligament

dorsal talonavicular bone
dorsal talonavicular ligament
dorsalis pedis
dorsal artery
dorsally
dorsi, latissimus
dorsispinal vein
dorsolateral fasciculus
dorsolateral placode
dorsolateral tract
dorsomedial hypothalamic nucleus
dorsomedial nucleus
dorsum of foot reflex
dorsum of penis
dorsum pedis reflex
dorsum sellae
dot-blot hybridization
dots
   Gunn
   Horner-Trantas
   Marcus Gunn
   Maurer
   Schüffner
   Trantas
   Ziemann
double-crush syndrome
double diffusion procedure
double gallbladder
double glucagon test
double-inlet left ventricle of heart
double-inlet right ventricle of heart
double-labeling immunocytochemistry
double-layered sheets of peritoneum
double-mouthed uterus
double-outlet left ventricle of heart
double-outlet right ventricle of heart
double penis
double pleurisy
double pneumonia
double-pointed needle
double tertian malaria
double uterus

double vagina
doughnut kidney
Douglas
   cul-de-sac of
   pouch of
Douglas abscess
Douglas fold
Douglas ligament
Douglas pouch suppuration
Douglas rectouterine pouch
Downey cell
Down syndrome
Doyne familial colloid degeneration
Doyne honeycomb degeneration
DR (diabetic retinopathy)
Drabkin solution
dracontiasis (Guinea worm)
Dracunculus medinensis
Dragendorff test for bile
drenching sweats
Dresbach syndrome
Dreulofoy lesion
dried-out material
dried smears of urine
drift, antigenic
dromedary kidney
droplet nucleus
droplet, respiratory
drop metastases
dropsy
drug, diuretic
drug fever
drug-induced diabetes
drug-induced hemolytic anemia
drugs of abuse, test on venous blood
   for
drum membrane
drusen
dry abscess
dry gangrene
dry joint
dry necrosis

dryness of mouth
dry pericarditis
dry pleurisy
dry scales (dandruff)
dry scaling
DSM-III-R (Diagnostic and Statistical Manual III—Revised)
DUB (dysfunctional uterine bleeding)
Dubin and Amelar varicocele classification
Dubin-Johnson syndrome
Dubois abscess
Duchenne-Aran muscular atrophy
Duchenne muscular dystrophy
Ducrey bacillus
Ducrey intradermal test
duct (see also *ductule*)
  aberrant
  aberrant bile
  accessory hepatic
  accessory pancreatic
  alveolar
  amniotic
  arterial
  Bartholin
  beaded hepatic
  bile
  biliary
  branchial
  bucconeural
  canalicular
  carotid
  choledochous
  cochlear
  common
  common bile (CBD)
  common gall
  common hepatic
  craniopharyngeal
  cystic
  cystic gall
  deferent

duct *(continued)*
  distal bile
  efferent
  ejaculatory
  endolymphatic
  excretory
  extrahepatic bile
  frontonasal
  galactophorous
  gall
  Gartner
  genital
  hepatic
  Hering
  His
  interlobular bile
  intrahepatic biliary
  lacrimal
  left hepatic
  lymph
  lymphatic
  main pancreatic
  middle extrahepatic bile
  müllerian
  obstruction of
  pancreatic
  paramesonephric
  paraurethral
  perilobular
  preampullary portion of bile
  prepapillary bile
  prostatic
  right hepatic
  Santorini
  Stensen
  subvesical
  terminal bile
  thoracic
  thyroglossal
  vitelline
  Wirsung
ductal aneurysm

ductal carcinoma
ductal carcinoma in situ (DCIS)
ductal cell
ductal duct
duct cell
duct cell carcinoma
duct ectasia
duct epithelial atypia
ductless gland
duct lumen
duct papilloma
duct system, intrahepatic
ductular element
ductule
   aberrant
   biliary
   excretory
ductule of testis, efferent
ductus arteriosus
   patent
   remnant of
ductus deferens
   ampulla of
   artery of
Duffy blood group
Duhring disease
Duke bleeding time test
Dukes classification of carcinoma
Dukes staging for colon carcinoma
Dulbecco modified Eagle medium
dullness, superficial cardiac
dumping syndrome
Duncan placenta
Duncan ventricle, fifth ventricle
duodenal ampulla
duodenal artery
duodenal bulb, apex of
duodenal C-loop
duodenal cap
duodenal contents examination
duodenal end of dorsal pancreatic duct
duodenal end of main pancreatic duct

duodenal fold
duodenal fossa
duodenal gland
duodenal impression on liver
duodenal ligament
duodenal loop
duodenal lumen
duodenal papilla
duodenal recess
duodenal sphincter, first
duodenal stump
duodenal sweep
duodenal ulcer
duodenal vein
duodenal villi
duodenal web
duodenojejunal angle
duodenojejunal flexure
duodenojejunal fold
duodenojejunal fossa
duodenojejunal junction
duodenojejunal recess
duodenojejunal sphincter
duodenomesocolic fold
duodenorenal ligament
duodenum
   C-loop of
   curve of
   descending
   distal
   supravaterian
   suspensory muscle of
duplex kidney
DuPont ACA analyzer
Dupuytren canal
dural septa
dural sheath
dural sinus
dura mater
Duran-Reynals permeability factor
Duran-Reynals spreading factor
Duret lesion

dust-borne infection
dust cell
dust corpuscle
Dutton relapsing fever
Duverney foramen
Duverney gland
D vitamin
dwarfism
   achondroplastic
   deprivation
   Lorain-Lévi
   pituitary
   renal
   Russell-Silver
   Walt Disney
dwarf pelvis
dwarf tapeworm
D-xylose absorption test
D-xylose tolerance test
dye
   blue aniline
   phenanthridium
   synthetic azo
   Taq
   vital
dye exclusion test
dye-tagged substrate
DynaBeads
dynamic aorta
dynamic/spastic ileus
dyschromic dermatosis
dyscrasia
dysenteric algid malaria
dysenteric diarrhea
dysentery
   amebic
   bacillary
dysfunctional uterine bleeding (DUB)
dysgerminoma
dysgranular cortex
dyshidrotic eczema
dyskeratoma

dyskeratosis
dyskeratotic cells with inclusions
dysmenorrheal membrane
dysmorphic
dysmotility
dysostosis, mandibulofacial
dysphagia
dysplasia
   bone
   bronchopulmonary
   cervical
   diaphyseal
   ectodermal
   epithelial
   fibromuscular
   fibrous
   low-grade
   mammary
   metaphyseal
   mild
   moderate
   retinal
   severe
   thymic
dysplastic epithelium
dysplastic nevus
dyspnea
dyssebacia (also, dyssebacea)
dystrophic calcification
dystrophic calcinosis
dystrophic degeneration
dystrophy
   Becker
   Dejerine-Landouzy
   Duchenne muscular
   Emery-Dreifuss muscular
   Erb muscular
   Fuchs
   Fukuyama
   Gowers muscular
   infantile neuroaxonal (INAD)
   Landouzy-Dejerine muscular

dystrophy *(continued)*
    muscular (MD)
    otic
    progressive muscular (PMD)
    thoracic-pelvic-phalangeal
    vulvar
dystrophy-dystocia syndrome (DDS)

E, e

ear
   artificial
   auricula dextra
   aviator's
   Aztec
   cauliflower
   cockleshell
   constricted
   cup
   darwinian
   diabetic
   external
   glue
   hairy
   inflammation of
   inner
   middle
   Morel
   Mozart
   ossicles of
   outer
   prizefighter's
   protruding
   swimmer's
   telephone
   tin
   tropical

ear canal
eardrum
earlobe adipose tissue
early pneumonitis
ear, nose, and throat (ENT) examination
earthy degeneration
easily compressible nodule
eastern equine encephalitis antibody
"eating cell" (phagocyte)
Eaton agent
Eaton agent pneumonia
Eberth bacillus
Eberth line
Ebner gland
Ebner line
Ebner reticulum
Ebola disease
Ebola hemorrhagic fever
Ebola virus
Ebstein-Armanni disease
Ebstein lesion
eburnated bone
eburnation
ECC (endocervical curettage)
eccentric atrophy
eccentric nuclei

eccentrically
ecchymosis (pl. ecchymoses)
eccrine gland
ecdysial gland
echinococcosis
Echinococcus granulosus
echinocyte
ECHO (enterocytopathogenic human
 orphan) virus
ECHO infection
Eck fistula
ECL cell (enterochromaffin-like)
ECLT (euglobulin clot lysis time)
ECM (extracellular matrix)
E. coli (Escherichia coli)
E. coli serotype O157:H7
ectasia, ductal (of breast)
ectatic aneurysm
ecthyma, contagious
ecthyma gangrenosum
ectoblast
ectocervical surface
ectoderm
ectodermal dysplasia
ectopia
ectopically
ectopic endometrium
ectopic pregnancy
ectopic testis
ectopic tissue
ectoplasm
ectropion
eczema
 allergic
 atopic
 baker's
 chronic
 dyshidrotic
 facial
 flexural
 hand
 infantile

eczema *(continued)*
 lichenoid
 seborrheic
 stasis
 tropical
 varicose
 vascular
 weeping
 winter
eczema craquelé ("marred with
 cracks")
eczema diabeticorum
eczema epilans (with hair loss)
eczema erythematosum
eczema herpeticum (herpesvirus type 1)
eczema hypertrophicum (lichenoid
 eczema)
eczema papulosum
eczema parasiticum
eczema pustulosum
eczema rubrum
eczema squamosum
eczema tyloticum
eczema vaccinatum
eczema verrucosum
eczema vesiculosum
eczematization
eczematoid
eczematous dermatitis
eczematous plaques
eddy (pl. eddies)
edema
 ambulant
 angioneurotic
 bronchiolar
 bronze
 cardiac
 cerebral
 dependent
 epithelial
 focal
 generalized

edema *(continued)*
  gestational
  heat
  hereditary angioneurotic
  ileocecal
  inflammatory
  laryngeal
  local
  lymphatic
  lymphedema
  malignant
  massive pulmonary hemorrhagic
  osmotic
  patchy intercellular
  periorbital
  pitting
  premenstrual
  presacral
  pretibial
  pulmonary
  Quincke
  renal
  visceral
edema neonatorum
edema of parotid glands
edematous brain
edematous kidneys
edge
  ligament reflecting
  ligament shelving
  liver
  Poupart ligament shelving
Edmondson grading system
EDRF (endothelium-derived relaxing
  factor)
EDTA (ethylenediaminetetraacetic
  acid)
Edwardsiella
Edwardsiella tarda
effect
  estrogen
  isomorphic

effect *(continued)*
  mass
  Somogyi
effector cell
effects of poisoning
efferent arteriole
efferent duct
efferent ductule of testis
efferent fiber
efferent glomerular arteriole
efferent limb
efferent loop
efferent lymph vessel
efferent lymphatic vessel
efferent nerve
efferent vessel
effluvium
effort proteinuria
effusion
  bloodstained
  hemorrhagic
  pericardial
  pleural
  pleuropericardial
  serous
  subdural
EG (esophagogastric) junction
EGD (esophagogastroduodenoscopy)
EGFR (epidermal growth factor
  receptor)
egg cell
egg membrane
egg yolk agar
eggs in intestinal venules
Eglis gland
E hemoglobin
E hepatitis
Ehlers-Danlos syndrome
Ehrlich acid hematoxylin stain
Ehrlich granule
Ehrlichia canis
Ehrlichia chaffeensis

Ehrlichia sennetsu
Ehrlich neutral stain
ehrlichiosis, human granulocytic
    (HGE)
Ehrlich triacid stain
Eichhorst atrophy
Eichhorst neuritis
Eikenella corrodens (formerly
    Bacteroides corrodens, HB-1)
Eisenmenger complex
ejaculatory duct
ejection fraction
Ektachem analyzer
elastica–van Gieson stain
elastic artery
elastic cartilage
elastic fiber
elastic fibers stain (Weigert)
elasticity
elastic lamella
elastic lamina
elastic lattices
elastic layer
elastic ligature
elastic membrane
elastic skin
elastic stain
elastic tissue
elastic web
elastin
elastoid degeneration of arteries
elastosis
    nodular
    senile
    solar
elbow articulation
elbow bone
elbow joint
elbow reflex
electrical energy
electrical shock
electric coagulation

electrode pad
electrolyte
    serum
    sweat
    testing
    test on venous blood for
    urine
electrolyte balance
electrolyte metabolism
electrolyte panel
electrolytes, consisting of
    bicarbonate
    calcium
    chloride
    potassium
    sodium
electron microscope
electron microscopy
electrophoresis
    agarose gel
    capillary zone (CZE)
    carrier
    cellulose acetate
    disk
    DNA sequencing
    free
    gel
    hemoglobin
    isoenzyme
    lipoprotein
    paper
    polyacrylamide gel (PAGE)
    protein
    pulsed-field gel
    SDS-polyacrylamide gel
        (SDS-PAGE)
    serum protein
    thin-layer
    two-dimensional gel
    urinary protein
electrophoretically
electrotonic current

electrotonic junction
electrotonic synapse
element
   ductal
   ductular
   end-ductal
   epithelial
   lobular
   stromal
elementary body
elementary cell
elementary granule
elementary particle
elephantiasis
elephantoid fever
elevation, frontonasal
ELISA (enzyme-linked immunosorbent
   assay)
ELITE Analyzer flow cytometer
ellipse of skin
ellipsoid
ellipsoid joint
ellipsoidal articulation
elliptic
elliptical
elliptocyte
elliptocytosis, hereditary
Ellison-Zollinger syndrome
Ellsworth-Howard test
elongate pattern
elongated mass
elongated structure
eluate
eluent
elute
elution
EMA (epithelial membrane antigen)
emanation, actinium
embalm
embalmer
embalming fluid
embed

embedded
embedding medium
embedding of tissue specimen
emboli (pl. of embolus)
embolic phenomenon
embolic pneumonia
emboliform nucleus
embolism (also called *embolus*)
   air
   amniotic fluid
   arterial stenosis
   atheromatous
   bacillary
   bland
   bone marrow
   cancer
   capillary
   cardiogenic
   catheter-induced
   cellular
   cerebral
   cholesterol
   coronary artery
   cotton-fiber
   crossed
   direct
   fat
   fibrin platelet
   foam
   gas
   gas nitrogen
   hematogenous
   infective
   intraluminal
   lymphogenous
   massive
   miliary
   multiple
   obturating
   occluding spring
   oil
   pantaloon

embolism *(continued)*
  paradoxical
  peripheral
  plasmodium
  prosthetic valve
  pulmonary (PE)
  pulmonary venous–systemic air
  pyemic
  recurrent
  renal cholesterol
  retinal
  retrograde
  riding
  septic
  septic pulmonary
  straddling
  submassive pulmonary
  thrombus
  trichinous
  tumor
  venous
  visceral
embolus (pl. emboli)
embryo, frozen
embryonal area
embryonal carcinoma
embryonal cell carcinoma
embryonic area
embryonic axis
embryonic blastoderm
embryonic cell
embryonic development
embryonic disk
embryonic membrane
embryonic mesenchymal cell
embryonic ovary
embryonic sac
embryonic shield
embryonic thyroglossal duct
embryonic truncus arteriosus
embryonic umbilical vein
emery disk

emesis
emetic
eminence
  arcuate
  articular
  collateral
  cruciate
  cruciform
  deltoid
  facial
  frontal
  genital
  hypothenar
  iliopubic
  intercondylar
  median
  occipital
  pyramidal
  thenar
  thyroid
emiocytosis
emissary sphenoidal foramen
emissary vein
emphysema
  bullous
  centrilobular
  cutaneous
  interstitial
  panlobular
  pulmonary
  pulmonary subcutaneous
emphysematous bleb
emphysematous bulla
emphysematous lungs
empirical diagnosis
empty sella syndrome
empyema
emulsion proteinuria
en bloc
en cuirasse
en face
en masse

ENA (extractable nuclear antigen)
enamel cap
enamel cell
enamel cleavage
enamel crypt
enamel cuticle
enamel epithelium
enamel fiber
enamel fissure
enamel-forming cells
enamel lamella
enamel layer
enamel ledge
enamel membrane
enamel niche
enamel organ
enamel pearl
enamel projection
enamel pulp
enamel wall
enanthema
enarthrodial joint
encapsulated abscess
encapsulated subdural hematoma
encasing cell
encephalic vesicle
encephalitis
   acute necrotizing
   bunyavirus
   California
   cytomegalovirus
   Dawson
   Eastern equine
   hemorrhagic
   HIV
   Japanese B
   La Crosse
   measles
   mumps
   St. Louis
   Strümpell-Leichtenstern
   tick-borne

encephalitis *(continued)*
   Venezuela equine
   viral
   Western equine
encephalitogenic protein
encephalocele
encephalomalacia
encephalomyelonic axis
encephalomyelitis
encephalomyocarditis virus
encephalopathy
   AIDS
   boxer's
   dialysis
   hepatic
   HIV
   hypoxic
   Korsakoff
   metabolic
   myoclonic
   spongiform
   Wernicke
enchondral bone
enchondral ossification
encircle
encrusted
en cuirasse, carcinoma
encysted pleurisy
endarteritis, obliterative
end artery
end bud
end bulb, Krause
end-ductal element
endemic goiter
endemic hematuria
endemic typhus
endocardial fibrosis
endocardial tumor
endocarditis
   atypical verrucous
   fungal
   infective

endocarditis *(continued)*
 Libman-Sacks verrucous
 rheumatic
 Sacks-Libman
 subacute bacterial
endocardium
endocervical canal
endocervical cell
endocervical curettage
endocervical epithelium
endocervical gland
endocervical mucosa
endocervical smear
endocervical tissue
endochondral bone
endocranium
endocrine atrophy
endocrine gland
endocrine system
endoderm
endodermal cell
endodermal pouch
endoepithelial gland
endogenous fiber
endogenous infection
endogenous lipoid pneumonia
endogenous obesity
endogenous pigment
endolymphatic duct
endolymphatic sac
endometrial adenocarcinoma
endometrial atrophy
endometrial biopsy
endometrial cavity
endometrial curettage
endometrial cyst
endometrial gland
endometrial hyperplasia
endometrial polyp
endometrial sampling
endometrial smear
endometrial stroma

endometrial stromal sarcoma
endometriosis
endometritis
endometrium
 atrophic
 bland
 cystic hyperplasia of
 late secretory
 menstrual
 mixed phase
 progestational
 proliferative
 proliferative phase
 secretory
endomyocardial fibrosis
endomysial antibody
endomysium
endopelvic fascia
endoplasm
endoplasmic reticulum
end organ
endoscope
endosteum
endothelial cell
endothelial leukocyte
endothelial proliferation
endothelial relaxing factor
endothelial space
endothelial swelling
endothelial tissue
endothelin-1 peptide
endothelium
endothelium-derived relaxing factor
 (EDRF)
endothoracic fascia
endothoracic tube
endotoxin-induced mediator
endotracheal (ET) tube
end piece
end plate
end point
end-stage renal disease

energy
  electrical
  kinetic
  radiant
  thermal
en face
engorged
engorgement
  splenic
  vascular
engorgement of tissues with blood
enhanced polymer one-step method of
  labeling
enlarged marrow cavities
enlargement
  heart
  liver
  skull
  spleen
en masse
enolase, neuron-specific
ensheathing callus
ensiform appendix
ensiform cartilage
ensiform process
Entamoeba histolytica
enteric bacillus
enteric fever
enteric orphan viruses
enteric plexus
enteritis, regional
Enterobacter (formerly *Aerobacter*)
Enterobacter aerogenes
Enterobacter agglomerans
Enterobacter cloacae
Enterobacter gergoviae
Enterobacter hafniae
Enterobacter liquefaciens
Enterobacter sakazakii
enterobacterial common antigen (ECA)
enterobiasis
Enterobius vermicularis

enterochromaffin cell
Enterococcus (pl. *Enterococci*)
Enterococcus avium
Enterococcus faecalis
Enterococcus faecium
enterocolitis, pseudomembranous
enterocytopathogenic human orphan
  (ECHO) virus
enteroendocrine cell
enterogenic proteinuria
enterogenous methemoglobinemia
enteroinsular axis
enteropathy, asymptomatic
  gluten-sensitive
enterotome
enterotoxin
enterovaginal fistula
Enterovirus, enterovirus
entodermal canal
entodermal cell
entodermal cloaca
entodermal pouch
entoplasm (endoplasm)
entorhinal area
entry zone
enveloped virus
enzymatic
enzyme
  acetyl-activating
  acetylcholinesterase
  adaptive
  angiotensin converting (ACE)
  autolytic
  beta-carotene cleavage
  brancher
  branching
  CK
  D
  deamidizing
  debranching
  digestive
  extracellular

enzyme *(continued)*
   lactase
   lipase
   lipolytic
   liver (glucuronosyltransferase)
   muscle
   pancreatic
   proteinase
   proteolytic
   uroporphyrinogen-1-synthetase
enzyme activity
enzyme hyaluronidase, streptococcal
enzyme-linked immunosorbent assay
   (ELISA)
enzyme panel
"eo" (eosinophil)
eosin azure
eosin, hematoxylin and (H&E)
eosinopenia
eosinophil count
eosinophil granule
eosinophilia
eosinophilic crystalloid
eosinophilic cytoplasm
eosinophilic gastroenteritis
eosinophilic granuloma
eosinophilic homogeneous cytoplasm
eosinophilic hyaline
eosinophilic leukemia
eosinophilic leukocyte
eosinophilic meningitis
eosinophilic myocarditis
eosinophilic pneumonia
eosinophil leukocyte
eosinophil smear
eosin-phloxine
eosin stain
EP (erythrocyte protoporphyrin) test
epactal bone
epactal ossicle
epamniotic cavity
eparterial bronchus

ependyma
ependymal cell
ependymal layer
ependymal lining
ependymal zone
ephelides (freckles)
ephemeral fever
ephemeral pneumonia
epicanthal fold
epicardial
epicardium
epicolic lymph node
epicondyle
epicranial aponeurosis
epicranial muscle
epicranius
Epics Profile II flow cytometer
epidemic cerebrospinal meningitis
epidemic hemorrhagic fever
epidemic keratoconjunctivitis
epidemic keratoconjunctivitis virus
epidemic parotitis
epidemic pleurodynia
epidemic typhus
epidermal atrophy
epidermal carcinoma
epidermal cyst
epidermal growth factor
epidermal growth factor receptor
   (EGFR)
epidermal growth factor–urogastrone
epidermal hyperplasia
epidermal inclusion cyst
epidermal ridge
epidermal tissue
epidermal ulceration
epidermic cell
epidermidization
epidermis
   centrally slightly thickened
   pigmented
   superficial

epidermoid carcinoma
epidermolysis bullosa, acquired
Epidermophyton
Epidermophyton floccosum
Epidermophyton stockdaleae
epididymis
   appendix of
   body of
   edema of
   inflammation of
   interstitial congestion of
   ligament of
   lobule of
   sinus of
   tail of
epididymitis
epidural abscess
epidural cavity
epidural hemorrhage
epidural space
epifluorescence
epigastric angle
epigastric artery
epigastric fold
epigastric fossa
epigastric lymph node
epigastric reflex
epigastric region
epigastric vein
epiglottic cartilage
epiglottic tubercle
epiglottis
epiglottiditis
epihyal bone
epihyal ligament
epi-illumination
epilation
epileptogenic zone
epinephrine
epineurium
epiotic center
epipapillary membrane

epipericardial ridge
epiphyseal artery
epiphyseal cartilage
epiphyseal cartilage plate
epiphyseal cartilaginous zone
epiphyseal ischemic necrosis
epiphyseal line
epiphyseal plate
epiphysis (pl. epiphyses)
   annular
   atavistic
   capital
   hypertrophy of
   pressure
   slipped
   stippled
   traction
epiphysis cerebri
epiphysis of long bone
   bulky
   irregularly calcified
   knobby
epiploic abscess
epiploic appendage
epiploic appendices
epiploic foramen, node of
epipteric bone
episcleral artery
episcleral lamina
episcleral space
episcleral tissue
episcleral vein
epispadias
epistaxis
episternal bone
epistropheus
epithelial adenoma
epithelial body
epithelial bridging
epithelial cast
epithelial cell
epithelial choroid layer

epithelial cyst
epithelial dysplasia
epithelial edema
epithelial element
epithelial hyperplasia
epithelial keratinization
epithelial lamina
epithelial layer
epithelial lining
epithelial membrane antigen (EMA)
epithelial neoplasm
epithelial nests
epithelial plug
epithelial reticular cell
epithelial tissue
epithelial "pearls" of keratinous debris
epithelioid cell
epithelioid granulomas
epithelioma, basal cell
epitheliosis
epithelium
  acetowhite
  Barrett
  ciliated
  ciliated columnar
  ciliated respiratory-type
  columnar
  columnar metaplasia of
  crypt
  cuboidal
  cylindric
  dysplastic
  enamel
  endocervical
  germinal
  glandular
  junctional
  keratinizing squamous
  low columnar
  metaplastic squamous
  nonkeratinizing
  perineural

epithelium *(continued)*
  pseudostratified
  pseudostratified columnar
  respiratory
  secretory
  simple
  simple columnar
  simple cuboidal
  simple squamous
  squamous
  squamous cell
  stratified
  stratified columnar
  stratified cuboidal
  stratified squamous
  stratified transitional
  surface
  tall columnar
  transitional
epithelium adenocarcinoma
epithelium fluid
epithelium-lined mastoid air cell
epithelium-lined tubular structure
epitrichial layer
epitrochlear node
epituberculous infiltration
epitympanic recess
epitympanic space
epivaginal connective tissue
Epon embedding medium
Eppendorf tube
Epstein-Barr virus
Epstein nephrosis
epulis
Eq (equivalent)
equatorial cleavage
equatorial plate
equina, cauda
equine encephalitis
  Eastern
  Venezuelan
  Western

equivalent (Eq)
ERA (estrogen receptor assay)
Erb atrophy
Erdheim cystic medial necrosis
Erb muscular dystrophy
erectile nodule
erectile tissue
erector muscle of penis
erector muscle of spine
erector spinal reflex
Erlanger and Gasser peripheral nerve
    classification
Erlenmeyer flask deformity
erogenous zone
erosion
    cervical
    cutaneous
    tumor
erosion of epiphyseal bone
erosive
E-rosette test
erotogenic zone
eruption
    pruritic
    purpuric cutaneous
erysipelas
erysipeloid
Erysipelothrix rhusiopathiae
erythema
    cold
    Jacquet
    "slapped cheek"
erythema ab igne
erythema and scaling, papular
erythema chronicum migrans
erythema infectiosum (fifth disease)
erythema marginatum
erythema migrans
erythema multiforme
erythema nodosum
erythema nodosum leprosum
erythema simplex

erythematosus
    discoid lupus
    lupus (LE)
    systemic lupus (SLE)
erythematous lesion
erythematous patches, itchy
erythrasma, Baerensprung
erythroblast
erythroblastosis fetalis
erythrocyte
    broken-down
    incubation
    nucleated
    sickle-shaped
    teardrop-shaped
erythrocyte adherence test
erythrocyte agglutinin
erythrocyte antigen
erythrocyte fragility
erythrocyte index
erythrocyte maturation factor
erythrocyte progenitor cell
erythrocyte protoporphyrin (EP) test
erythrocyte sedimentation rate (ESR)
erythrocytopenia
erythrocytosis
erythroderma
erythrohepatic porphyria
erythroid cell
erythroid hyperplasia of bone marrow
erythroplasia of Queyrat
erythropoiesis
erythropoietic hormone
erythropoietic porphyria
erythropoietin
eschar at site of mite bite
Escherich bacillus
Escherichia coli (E. coli)
Escherichia fergusonii
Escherichia hermannii
Escherichia vulneris
esophageal A ring

esophageal acid infusion test
esophageal artery of aorta
esophageal artery of inferior thyroid
esophageal atresia
esophageal B ring
esophageal body
esophageal candidiasis
esophageal degeneration
esophageal diverticulum
esophageal gland
esophageal groove
esophageal hiatal hernia
esophageal hiatus
esophageal impression
esophageal inlet
esophageal lumen
esophageal mucosal ring
esophageal opening
esophageal plexus of nerves
esophageal ring, distal
esophageal spasm, diffuse
esophageal sphincter
   hypertensive
   inferior
esophageal stenosis
esophageal varix (pl. varices)
esophageal vein
esophageal web
esophagitis
esophagogastric (EG) junction
esophagogastric orifice
esophagogastric vestibule
esophagogastroduodenoscopy (EGD)
esophagosalivary reflex
esophagospasm
esophagostenosis
esophagotracheal (ET) junction
esophagus
   achalasia of
   Barrett
   B ring of
   nutcracker

espundia
ESR (erythrocyte sedimentation rate)
essential amino acid
essential fatty acid (EFA)
essential fever
essential hematuria
essential hypertension
essential proteinuria
essential pruritus
Essick cell band
established cell line
esterase
   alpha naphthol
   C1
   leukocyte (LE)
   naphthol-ASD chloroacetate
esthesiodic system
estradiol hormone
estradiol test
estriol (E_3) hormone
   free
   total
estrogen
   serum
   total
   urinary
estrogen effect
estrogen level, urine
estrogen receptor assay (ERA)
estrogenic hormone
estrogenic stimulation
estrone (E_1) test
ethanol intoxication
ethanolism
ethidium bromide
ethmoidal air cell
ethmoid, alae of
ethmoidal artery
ethmoidal bulla
ethmoidal cell
ethmoidal crest
ethmoidal foramen

ethmoidal groove
ethmoidal labyrinth
ethmoidal notch
ethmoidal process
ethmoidal roof of nasal cavity
ethmoidal sinus
ethmoidal vein
ethmoid angle
ethmoid bone
ethmoid canal
ethmoid infundibulum
ethmoidolacrimal suture
ethmoidomaxillary suture
ethmovomerine plate
ethyl alcohol
ethylenediaminetetraacetic acid
  (EDTA)
ET-NANB (enterically transmitted
  non-A, non-B) hepatitis
Eubacterium alactolyticum
Eubacterium lentum
Eubacterium limosum
euglobulin clot lysis
euglobulin clot lysis time (ECLT)
euglobulin lysis test
euglycemia
eukaryosis
euplastic lymph
European blastomycosis
eustachian canal
eustachian tube
eustachian valve
evanescent
eversion, cervical
Ewingella
Ewing sarcoma
Ewing tumor
ExacTech blood glucose meter
examination
  cursory
  darkfield
  duodenal contents

examination *(continued)*
  external
  gross
  internal
  microscopic
  physical
  postmortem
  urine
exanthem (also, exanthema)
  Boston
  maculopapular
  mosquito-borne febrile
  papular
  pustular
  vesicular
  viral
exanthema subitum
exanthematous fever
exanthematous necrosis
excavatum, pectus
excessive absorption and impaired
  excretion of copper
excessive intake of iron
excessive loss of water due to diuresis
excessive loss of water due to sweating
excessive loss of water due to vomiting
exchange transfusion
excise
excision
excisional biopsy
excitable area
excitable cell
excitor nerve
excitoreflex nerve
excoriation
excrescence
  curdlike
  nodular
excretion of 5-hydroxyindoleacetic acid
  (5-HIAA), urinary
excretion of carbon dioxide,
  pulmonary

excretion of coproporphyrin, urinary
excretion of delta-aminolevulinic acid
excretion of hydrogen ion, renal
excretion of water, increased renal
excretion, urinary 17-ketosteroid
excretory duct
excretory ductule
excretory gland
excretory system
executive profile
exercise bone
exfoliate
exfoliation
exfoliativa neonatorum, dermatitis
  (staphylococcal scalded skin
  syndrome)
exfoliative cytology
exfoliative dermatitis
exhaustion atrophy
exhaustive blood grouping
Exner-Call bodies
exoccipital bone
exocelomic membrane
exocervical tissue
exocrine gland
exocytosis
exodic nerve
exogenous fiber
exogenous obesity
exogenous pigment
exogenous pneumonia
Exophiala dermatitidis
Exophiala heteromorpha
Exophiala jeanselmei
Exophiala spinifera
exophthalmic goiter
exophthalmos-producing substance
exophytic
expansion arch
expansion of duct or vessel
expansion of the cerebral ventricles
expiration

expire
expired
exploratory biopsy
exploratory laparotomy
explosive diarrhea
exsanguination transfusion
Exserohilum rostratum
exstrophy of bladder
extension, gland neck
extensor aponeurosis
extensor carpi ulnaris sheath
extensor retinacular
externa muscularis
externa
  otitis
  theca
external acoustic meatus
external anal sphincter
external auditory canal
external auditory meatus
external biliary ductule
external carotid artery
external clot
external collateral ligament of wrist
external ear
external examination
external genitalia
external hemorrhoid
external iliac lymph node
external intercostal membrane
external intercostal muscle
external ligament
external maxillary artery
external oblique muscle
external oblique reflex
external os, cervical
external pillar cell
external pubic artery
external pudendal artery
external pudendal branches
  of femoral artery
external pudendal vein

external ring, apex of
external spermatic artery
external urethral opening
external urethral orifice
extracapsular ligament
extracellular enzyme
extracellular fluid
extracellular matrix (ECM)
extracellular tissue
extrachromosomal gene
extracorporeal circulation
extractable nuclear antibody
extractable nuclear antigen (ENA)
extradural abscess
extradural hemorrhage
extraembryonic blastoderm
extraembryonic celom
extraembryonic mesoderm
extrahepatic bile duct
extrahepatic biliary duct
extrahepatic biliary system
extraintestinal
extramedullary hematopoiesis
    in liver and spleen
extranodal
extraosseous osteosarcoma
extraperitoneal fascia
extraperitoneal fat
extraperitoneal organ
extraperitoneal tissue
extrapyramidal motor system
extrauterine pregnancy
extravasate
extravasated blood
extravasation of erythrocytes
extravascular fluid
extravisual zone
extremity arteries
extrinsic allergic alveolitis
extrinsic factor
extrinsic sphincter
extruded disk

exuberant granulation tissue
exuberant hypertrophic granulation
    tissue
exudate
    fibrinous
    fibrin-rich
    foamy
    frothy
    hemorrhagic
    neutrophilic
    purulent
    purulent subarachnoid
    serous
    stringy mucous
    subarachnoid
    viscous greenish
exudate in alveoli, mucopurulent
exudation cell
exudation corpuscle
exudation of fibrin-rich fluid
exudative dermatitis
exudative discoid and lichenoid
    dermatitis
exudative inflammation
exudative inflammation of glomeruli
exudative nephritis
exudative pharyngitis
exudative pleurisy
exudative tuberculosis
exude
ex vivo
eye
    aphakic
    artificial
    black
    congenital malformation of
    crossed
    cystic
    deviating
    epiphyseal
    following
    inflammatory conditions of

eye *(continued)*
    innermost coat of
    lifeless
    neoplasm of
    pannus of
    parietal
    pink
    pseudophakic
    shrunken

eyeball
eye-closure reflex
eye-ear plane
eye fundus
eyelid
    inflammation of
    lower
    upper
eye tumor

F, f

F (Fahrenheit)
FA (fluorescent antibody) test
FAB (formalin ammonium bromide)
FAB (French, American, British)
    classification of acute nonlymphoid
    leukemia
fabella bone
Fabry disease
face
    en
    labial artery of
    moon
facet
    articular
    atlas
    capitate
    clavicular
    corneal
    costal
    flat
    hamate
    inferior articular
    inferior costal
    Lenoir
    locked
    lunate
    scaphoid

facet *(continued)*
    squatting
    superior articular
    superior costal
    transverse costal
facetectomy
facet for head of rib
facet for tubercle of rib
facet joint
facial angle
facial artery
facial atrophy
facial axis
facial bone
facial canal
facial cleft
facial colliculus
facial eczema
facial eminence
facial herpes simplex
facial hirsutism
facial lymph node
facial muscle
facial nerve
facial plane
facial plexus
facial reflex

facial root
facial surface
facial triangle
facial vein
facies, moon
FACS (fluorescence-activated cell sorter)
FACScan
FACScan flow cytometer
FACSGal assay system
FACSort flow cytometer
FACSprep automated staining system
FACStrak flow cytometer
FACSVantage cell sorter
factitial dermatitis (self-inflicted lesions)
factitious purpura
factor
  ABO
  accelerator
  adrenal weight
  adrenocorticotropic releasing
  angiogenesis
  antiacrodynia
  antialopecia
  antianemic
  antiberiberi
  anti-black-tongue
  anticomplementary
  antidermatitis
  antihemophilic
  antihemophilic globulin (AHG, factor VIII)
  antihemorrhagic
  antineuritic
  antinuclear
  antipellagra
  antisterility
  atrial natriuretic (ATF)
  augmenting
  B-cell differentiating
  B-cell stimulatory

factor (continued)
  beta
  blood (see coagulation)
  branching
  B_T
  C
  CAMP (Christie, Atkins, Munch-Petersen)
  capillary permeability
  Castle intrinsic
  Christmas (factor IX)
  citrovorum
  clearing
  clotting
  coagulation, blood
    I (fibrinogen)
    II (prothrombin)
    III (tissue thromboplastin)
    IV (calcium)
    V (labile; proaccelerin)
    VI (stable)
    VII (proconvertin)
    VIII (antihemophilic globulin, AHG)
    IX (Christmas; plasma thromboplastin component)
    X (Stuart-Prower)
    XI (plasma thromboplastin antecedent)
    XII (Hageman)
    XIII (fibrin stabilizing)
  coenzyme
  colon-stimulating (CSF)
  complement chemotactic
  corticotropin-releasing
  debranching
  diabeticogenic
  Duran-Reynals permeability
  Duran-Reynals spreading
  endothelial relaxing
  endothelium-derived relaxing (EDRF)

factor *(continued)*
  epidermal growth
  erythrocyte maturation (EMF)
  extrinsic
  fertility
  fibrin-stabilization (FSF)
  filtrate
  Fitzgerald
  Flaujeac
  Fletcher
  follicle-stimulating hormone
    releasing
  G
  galactagogue
  galactopoietic
  glass
  glucose tolerance
  glycotropic
  gonadotropin-releasing (GRF)
  granulocyte-macrophage colony-
    stimulating
  growth
  growth hormone-releasing (GH-RF)
  Hageman (HF)
  human antihemophilic
  hyperglycemic-glycogenolytic
  immunogenetic
  immunoglobulin-binding (IBF)
  inhibition
  initiation
  insulin-antagonizing
  insulin-like growth
  intrinsic
  ischemia-modifying
  labile (V)
  Laki-Lorand
  LE (lupus erythematosus)
  lethal
  leukocytosis-promoting
  leukopenic
  lipotropic
  L-L

factor *(continued)*
  luteinizing hormone/follicle-
    stimulating hormone-releasing
    (LH/FSH-RF)
  lymph node permeability
  macrophage-activating
  macrophage colony-stimulating
  mammotropic
  melanotropin-releasing
  mesodermal
  migration-inhibitory (MIF)
  monocyte derived neutrophil
    chemotactic (MDNCF)
  multi-colon-stimulating (multi-CSF)
  myocardial depressant
  natural killer cell stimulating
    (NKSF)
  nephritic
  nerve growth (NGF)
  neural
  neutrophil activating
  neutrophil chemotactant
  osteoclast activating
  pellagra-preventing
  plasma clotting
  plasma labile
  plasma thromboplastin antecedent
    (XI)
  plasma thromboplastin component
    (IX)
  platelet
  platelet-activating
  platelet-aggravating
  platelet-derived growth
  predisposing
  proaccelerin (V)
  proconvertin (VII)
  prolactin-inhibiting
  prolactin-releasing
  protein
  Prower-Stuart
  psi

factor *(continued)*
   relaxation
   releasing (RF)
   resistance
   resistance-inducing
   resistance-transfer
   Rh
   rheumatoid (RF)
   risk
   secretor
   sex
   sigma
   somatotropin-releasing (SRF)
   somatotropin releasing-inhibiting
     (SRIF, SIF)
   stable (VI)
   stringent
   Stuart
   Stuart-Prower (X)
   T cell growth
   termination
   testis-determining (TDF)
   thymic lymphopoietic
   thyroid-stimulating hormone-
     releasing (TSH-RF)
   thyrotoxic complement-fixation
   thyrotropin-releasing (TRF)
   tissue
   transfer
   transforming
   transforming growth
   tumor angiogenic (TAF)
   tumor necrosis (TNF)
   uterine relaxing (URF)
   von Willebrand
   Williams
Fahrenheit scale (F)
failure
   adrenal
   bone marrow
   cardiac
   hepatic

failure *(continued)*
   multiple organ
   multisystem
   pituitary
   renal
   respiratory
failure of long-bone growth
failure of skull closure in the midline
failure to thrive
fair-skinned person
falciform cartilage
falciform crest
falciform ligament
falciform lobe
falciform margin
falciform process
falciform retinal fold
falcine meningioma
falciparum malaria
fall-and-rise phenomenon
fallopian aqueduct
fallopian arch
fallopian artery
fallopian canal
fallopian hiatus
fallopian ligament
fallopian neuritis
fallopian pregnancy
fallopian tube
Fallot, tetralogy of
false aneurysm
false colonic obstruction
false coxa
false glottis
false hematuria
false joint
false macula
false membrane
false mole
false negative
false pelvis
false positive

false positive RPR
false pregnancy
false proteinuria
false rib
false ringbone
false suture
false vertebra
false vocal cord
falx cerebelli
falx cerebri
falx meningioma
familial adenomatous polyposis (FAP)
familial disorder
familial hepatitis
familial hypercatabolism
familial hypophosphatemic osteomalacia
familial lipodystrophy
familial nonhemolytic jaundice
familial polyposis
Fananás cell
Fanconi syndrome
fan-shaped mesentery
fan-shaped muscle
FAP (familial adenomatous polyposis)
Farber test
farmer's lung
Farr test
fascia (pl. fasciae)
   anal
   antebrachial
   anterior rectus
   axillary
   bicipital
   brachial
   broad
   buccopharyngeal
   Camper
   cervical
   clavipectoral
   Cloquet
   Colles
   cremasteric

fascia *(continued)*
   cribriform
   Cruveilhier
   deep
   Denonvilliers
   dentate
   diaphragmatic
   endopelvic
   endothoracic
   extraperitoneal
   Gerota
   iliac
   lateral oblique
   obturator
   obturator internus
   parietal pelvic
   pelvic
   perineal
   psoas
   renal
   rim of
   Scarpa
   subcutaneous
   superficial
   thoracolumbar
   visceral pelvic
   Waldeyer
fasciae latae, tensor
fascia iliaca
fascial covering
fascia lata (pl. fasciae latae)
fascial layer
fascial sheath
fascia of abdomen
fascia of arm
fascia of penis, deep
fascia transversalis
fascicle, interlacing
fascicular degeneration
fascicular sarcoma
fasciculata zona
fasciculation

fasciculus (pl. fasciculi)
  calcarine
  central tegmental
  cuneate
  dorsolateral
  fronto-occipital
  nerve
fasciitis, necrotizing
Fasciola gigantica
Fasciola hepatica
fasciolar gyrus
fascioliasis
fasciolopsiasis
Fasciolopsis buski
fashion, pagetoid
fast blue
fast green
fastidious
fastigiobulbar tract
fasting blood glucose
fasting blood sugar
fasting chemistry panel
fasting triglyceride level, normal
fast red
fast smear
fat
  brown
  corpse
  dietary
  digital process of
  extraperitoneal
  fecal
  free (FF)
  intracellular
  ischiorectal pad of
  microvesicular
  pericolonic
  perirectal
  perirenal
  preperitoneal
  properitoneal
  protective layer of

fat *(continued)*
  renal
  subcutaneous
fat body
fat cell
fat content
fat-containing chyme
fat-digesting enzyme
fat embolism
fat globule
fatigability
fatigue fever
fat-induced hyperlipidemia
fat in stool
fat lobule
fat marrow
fat necrosis
fat pad
  antimesenteric
  ischiorectal
fat stores, depletion of
fat-storing cell
fatty acid
  activated
  aliphatic
  essential
  free nonesterified
  medium chain
  nonesterified, free
  omega-3
  short chain
  straight-chain
  total
  unesterified free
  unsaturated
fatty acid profile
fatty acid synthase complex
fatty acid thiokinase
fatty areolar tissue, subperitoneal
fatty atrophy
fatty change
fatty cirrhosis

fatty degeneration of liver
fatty granule cell
fatty heart
fatty infiltration of liver
fatty kidney
fatty meal
fatty metamorphosis
fatty nevus
fatty pigment
fatty renal capsule
fatty stool
fatty superficial layer
fatty tissue
fatty vacuole
fauces (pl. of faux)
    anterior pillar of
    arch of
faucial reflex
faucial tonsil
faux (pl. fauces)
fava bean
favism
favus
Fazio-Londe atrophy
FBA (fecal bile acid)
FBD (fibrocystic breast disease)
Fe (iron)
febrifuge
febrile agglutinin panel
febrile agglutinins
febrile antigen
febrile proteinuria
fecal abscess
fecal bile acid (FBA)
fecal concretion
fecal fat test
fecalith
fecal material
fecal urobilinogen
feces, mass of inspissated
$FeCO_2$ (fraction of expired carbon
    dioxide)

Felix-Weil test
feltlike
female genital tract (FGT) cytologic
    smear
female hormone
female pattern alopecia
female pelvis
female, perimenopausal
female prostate
female reproductive system
feminization
femoral aneurysm
femoral arch
femoral artery
femoral articulation
femoral bone
femoral canal
femoral circumflex artery
femoral-femoral bypass graft
femoral fossa
femoral head
femoral hernia
femoral ligament
femoral muscle
femoral neck
femoral nerve
femoral opening
femoral plexus
femoral-popliteal bypass graft
femoral reflex
femoral region
femoral ring
femoral septum
femoral sheath
femoral triangle
femoral vein
femoroabdominal reflex
femoropatellar joint
femorotibial joint
femtogram (fg)
femtoliter (fL)
femtometer (fm)

femtomole (fmol)
femur (pl. femora)
   apex of
   body of
   greater trochanter of
   head of
   lesser trochanter of
   neck of
   nutrient artery of
fenestrated capillary
fenestrated membrane C
fenestrated sheath
fermentation test for sugar in urine
fern test
ferning
Ferrata cell
Ferrein canal
Ferrein ligament
ferric ammonium sulfate
ferric chloride
ferric chloride test
ferritin, serum
ferritin test
ferrocyanide salt
ferrohemoglobin solubility test
ferrozine
fertility factor
fertilization ex vivo
fertilization in vitro (IVF)
fertilization in vivo
fertilization membrane
fertilized ovum
fetal alcohol syndrome
fetal chromosome analysis
fetal death
   early
   intermediate
   late
fetal diagnosis
fetal hemoglobin (hemoglobin F)
fetal hypoxia
fetalis, erythroblastosis

fetal lobe
fetal maturity
fetal membrane
fetal placenta
fetal small parts
fetal tissue
fetal viability
fetal zone
fetoglobulin, alpha-
fetomaternal transfusion
fetoprotein
   alpha$_1$-
   fucosylated alpha
fetus
   aborted
   amorphous
   calcified
   growth-retarded
   harlequin
   HLA-compatible
   impacted
   macerated
   maturity of
   mummified
   nonstressed
   nonviable
   paper-doll
   parasitic
   placenta of
   presentation of
   previable
   retained dead
   small parts of
   stressed
   stunted
   tissue of
   umbilical artery in
   viable
fetus papyraceus
fetus sanguinolentus
Feulgen method of staining
Feulgen stain

fever
 absorption
 acute rheumatic (ARF)
 Aden
 aestivoautumnal
 African hemorrhagic
 African tick-borne
 algid pernicious
 ardent
 Argentinian hemorrhagic
 arthropod-borne relapsing
 artificial
 aseptic
 Australian Q
 black
 blackwater
 blue
 Bolivian hemorrhagic
 bouquet
 boutonneuse
 brass founder's
 Brazilian spotted
 breakbone
 bullous
 Bunyamwera
 Burdwan
 Bwamba
 cachectic
 camp
 canicola
 Carter
 catarrhal
 cat-bite
 cat-scratch
 catheter
 Central European tick-borne
 Charcot intermittent
 Colorado tick
 Congolian red
 cotton-mill
 Crimean-Congo hemorrhagic
 dehydration

fever *(continued)*
 dengue hemorrhagic
 drug
 Dutton relapsing
 Ebola hemorrhagic
 elephantoid
 enteric
 ephemeral
 epidemic hemorrhagic
 essential
 exanthematous
 fatigue
 Fort Bragg
 Gambian
 glandular
 harlequin
 Haverhill
 hay
 hemorrhagic
 herpetic
 icterohemorrhagic
 inanition
 jail
 jungle
 Katayama
 Kenya
 Kew Gardens
 Korean hemorrhagic
 Lassa
 Malta
 Manchurian
 meningotyphoid
 Mexican spotted
 miliary
 milk
 monoleptic
 nodal
 Omsk hemorrhagic
 Oroya
 papular
 parathyroid
 parenteric

fever *(continued)*
  parrot
  periodic
  petechial
  pharyngoconjunctival
  Philippine hemorrhagic
  phlebotomus
  pinta
  polymer fume
  Pontiac
  pretibial
  puerperal
  pyogenic
  Q
  quartan
  rat-bite
  redwater
  relapsing
  remittent
  rheumatic
  Rocky Mountain spotted
  Ross River
  San Joaquin Valley
  Saõ Paulo
  scarlet
  septic
  spirillary rat-bite (sodoku)
  steroid
  streptobacillary rat-bite
  syphilitic
  Texas
  Thai hemorrhagic
  tick-borne
  typhoid
  undulant
  uveoparotid
  valley
  viral hemorrhagic
  vivax
  yellow
  Zika
fever, chills, and circulatory collapse

fever of unknown origin (FUO)
fever-producing substance
fg (femtogram)
FGT (female genital tract) cytologic
  smear
F hemoglobin
fiber
  A
  accelerator
  afferent
  alpha
  anastomosing
  anastomotic
  arcuate
  argyrophilic
  association
  augmentor
  B
  beta
  C
  cardiac muscle
  cholinergic
  chromatic
  circular
  climbing
  collagen
  collagenous
  commissural
  cone
  connective-tissue
  corticobulbar
  corticonuclear
  corticopontine
  corticoreticular
  corticospinal
  dental
  dentinal
  depressor
  efferent
  elastic
  enamel
  endogenous

fiber *(continued)*
  exogenous
  intercrural
  interlacing
  interlacing tendinous
  matrix of collagenic
  motor
  muscle
  myocardial
  nerve
  pain
  postganglionic
  preganglionic
  preganglionic sympathetic
  Purkinje
  reticular
  sensory
  Sharpey
  skeletal muscle
  sling muscle
  unmyelinated postganglionic
  yellow elastic
fiber of Remak
fibril
  collagen
  connective tissue
  degeneration
  nerve
fibril distortion within cell processes
fibrillar protein
fibrillar structure, delicate
fibrillary bacteria
fibrillary degeneration
fibrin breakdown products
fibrin clot
fibrin debris
fibrin deposition
fibrin in bronchi
fibrin, insoluble
fibrinocartilaginous ring
fibrinogen, plasma protein
fibrinogen uptake

fibrinopurulent inflammation
fibrinoid degeneration
fibrinoid necrosis
fibrinoligase
fibrinolysin
fibrinolysis
fibrinolytic purpura
fibrinopeptide A
fibrinous debris
fibrinous degeneration
fibrinous exudate
fibrinous inflammation
fibrinous pericarditis
fibrinous pleurisy
fibrinous pleuritis
fibrinous pneumonia
fibrinous polyp
fibrin platelet embolism
fibrin-rich exudate
fibrin-rich fluid, exudation of
fibrin split products
fibrin-stabilizing factor
fibrin thrombus
fibroadenoma of breast
fibroadipose tissue
fibroareolar tissue
fibroblast
fibroblastic meningioma
fibroblastic osteosarcoma
fibrocartilage
  circumferential
  intra-articular plates of
  triangular
fibrocartilaginous joint
fibrocartilaginous pad
fibrocartilaginous ring
fibrocartilaginous tissue
fibrocollagenous
fibrocystic breast
fibrocystic breast disease (FBD)
fibrocyte
fibroelastic band

fibroelastic cartilage
fibroelastic septa
fibroepithelial papilloma
fibroepithelial polyp
fibrofatty connective tissue
fibrofatty layer
fibrofatty stroma, tissue
fibrohyaline tissue
fibroid (pl. fibroids)
   intramural
   pedunculated
   uterine
fibroid degeneration
fibroid myocarditis
fibroid uterus
fibrolipomatous nephritis
fibroma, ovarian
fibromatosis
fibromuscular band
fibromuscular dysplasia
fibromuscular pelvic floor
fibromuscular stroma
fibromuscular tissue
fibromyelinic plaque
fibromyoma, uterine
fibroplasia, retrolental
fibroplastic process
fibroplastic proliferation
fibrosa cystica, osteitis
fibrosarcoma
fibrosing granulation tissue
fibrosing inflammation
fibrosing osteochondroma
fibrosis
   cystic
   diffuse interstitial
   endocardial
   endomyocardial
   idiopathic interstitial
   interstitial
   interstitial pulmonary
   leptomeningeal

fibrosis *(continued)*
   mediastinal
   nodular subepidermal
   pericentral
   periductal
   perimuscular
   periportal
   pipestem
   pulmonary
   replacement
   retroperitoneal
   subadventitial
   subintimal
   subserosal
   Symmers
fibrosis in cornea
fibrosus, annulus
fibrotic band
fibrotic patches
fibrotic pattern
fibrotic reaction
fibrotic stricture of urethra
fibrous adhesion
fibrous ankylosis
fibrous apex
fibrous arch
fibrous articulation
fibrous band
fibrous capsule of kidney
fibrous cartilage
fibrous connective tissue
fibrous cortical defect
fibrous dysplasia
fibrous goiter
fibrous induration
fibrous joint
fibrous layer
fibrous matrix
fibrous mediastinitis
fibrous membrane
fibrous meningioma
fibrous myocarditis

fibrous nodules
fibrous obliteration
fibrous odontoma
fibrous pericardium
fibrous plaque
fibrous pneumonia
fibrous protein
fibrous reaction
fibrous renal capsule
fibrous ring
fibrous scar
fibrous scar tissue
fibrous septa
fibrous sheath
fibrous skeleton
fibrous stroma
fibrous tissue
fibrous tubercle
fibrovascular adhesion
fibrovascular stroma
fibrovascular tissue
fibula
    apex of
    nutrient artery of
fibular artery
fibular articular surface
fibular bone
fibular circumflex artery
fibular collateral ligament of ankle
fibular lymph node
fibular margin
fibular notch
fibular surface
fibular vein
Ficoll gradient
Ficoll-Hypaque separation
Fiedler myocarditis
field
    auditory
    dark
    Flechsig
    high-power

field *(continued)*
    low-power
    morphogenic
    myelinogenic
    visual
    Wernicke
field of Forel
fièvre boutonneuse
fifth disease (erythema infectiosum)
FIGLU excretion test
FIGO (International Federation of
    Gynecology and Obstetrics)
FIGO grade
FIGO grade of adenocarcinoma of
    endometrium
FIGO staging of adenocarcinoma of
    endometrium
FIGO staging of cervical carcinoma
figure, mitotic
filament
    actin
    branching
filamented neutrophil
filament-forming bacillus
filamentous mass
filariasis (elephantiasis)
filiform papilla (pl. papillae)
Filley method
filling defect
Filobasidiella neoformans
Filovirus, filovirus
filter
    band-pass
    LeukoNet
    Millipore
    Nuclepore
filtrate factor
filtration angle
filtration fraction
filtration, glomerular
filtration of fluid specimen
filtration space

fimbria (pl. fimbriae), ovarian
fimbriated fold
fimbriodentate sulcus
final diagnosis
fine needle
fine-needle aspiration (FNA)
fine-needle aspiration biopsy (FNAB)
finger
   base of
   bolster
   clubbed
   sausage
   spade
   speck
   trigger
   webbed
fingerlike dermal papillae
fingernail
fingerprint whorl
fingerstick puncture
fingerstick specimen
finger-thumb reflex
Finkeldey-Warthin giant cell
Finn chamber patch test
FiO$_2$ (fractional inspired oxygen
   concentration)
first cranial nerve
first cuneiform bone
first duodenal sphincter
first parallel pelvic plane
first permanent molar
first-set phenomenon
first-set rejection
first ventricle of cerebrum
first visceral cleft
first-voided specimen
first-voided urine specimen
FISH (fluorescence in situ
   hybridization)
Fishberg concentration test for renal
   function
fish-mouth cervix

Fishman-Doubilet test for diagnosis
   of pancreatitis
fishtank granuloma
fissure
   abdominal
   anal
   antitragohelicine
   brain
   calcarine
   callosomarginal
   cerebellar
   cerebral
   chronic
   collateral
   cutaneous
   decidual
   dentate
   glaserian
   horizontal
   oblique
   oral
   palpebral
   short palpebral
fissure of lung
Fissuricella filamenta
fistula
   abdominal
   arteriovenous
   biliary
   branchial
   bronchobiliary
   bronchocavitary
   bronchoesophageal
   bronchopleural
   cholecystoduodenal
   colonic
   colovaginal
   colovesical
   congenital pulmonary arteriovenous
   cystic
   Eck
   enterovaginal

fistula *(continued)*
  fecal
  gastric
  gastrocolic
  gastroduodenal
  genitourinary
  hepatopleural
  H-type
  orofacial
  parietal
  perineovaginal
  pilonidal
  rectovaginal
  rectovesical
  sigmoidovesical
  tracheoesophageal
  urethrovaginal
  vesical
  vesicouterine
  vitelline
fistulous tracts
Fite-Faraco stain
Fitzgerald factor
Fitz-Hugh–Curtis syndrome
fixation, complement (CF)
fixative (see also *fluid, solution, stain*)
  absolute alcohol
  acetic acid
  acetone
  Altmann solution
  B5
  Bouin picroformol-acetic
  buffered formalin
  Carnoy solution
  Champy
  chlorpalladium
  chromic acid
  Delafield solution
  Flemming solution
  formaldehyde
  formalin
  formalin-alcohol

fixative *(continued)*
  formalin-ammonium bromide
  formol-calcium
  formol-Müller solution
  formol-saline
  formol-Zenker
  FU-48 Zenker solution
  Gendre solution
  glacial acetic acid
  glutaraldehyde
  Golgi osmiobichromate
  Helly
  Helly Zenker-formalin solution
  Hermann
  Jores solution
  Kaiserling solution
  Karnowsky
  Luft potassium permanganate
  Marchi
  Maximow solution
  methanol
  Michel transport
  Millonig phosphate-buffered
    formalin
  Müller solution
  neutral (buffered) formalin
  Orth
  osmic acid
  osmium tetroxide
  Park-Williams
  periodate-lysing-paraformaldehyde
  picric acid
  picroformol
  potassium bichromate (or
    dichromate)
  Regaud
  Schaudinn
  Tellyesniczky solution
  Thoma
  Zamboni
  Zenker-formol
  Zenker solution

fixator muscle
fixed interval of time
fixed macrophage
fixed time interval
fL (femtoliter)
flabby myocardium
flabby tissue
flaccid
flaccid membrane
flaccid paralysis, irreversible
flagellate cell
flagellum
flail joint
flame cell
flammeus nevus
flange, buccal
flank bone
flank scar
flank stripe, properitoneal
flap, raised
flask-shaped phialides
flask-shaped ulcer of colonic mucosa
flat abdominal muscles
flat bone
flat cell
flat condyloma
flat facet
flat genital wart
flat muscle
flat pelvis
flat plaque
flattened stool
flattening of gyri of brain
flatus
Flaujeac factor
flavivirus
Flavobacterium meningosepticum
flea-bitten kidney
flea-borne typhus
Flechsig field
Flechsig primordial zone
fleecy masses

Fleischer-Kayser ring
Flemming solution
fleshy mole
fleshy texture
Fletcher factor
Flexner bacillus
flexor canal
flexor reflex
flexural eczema
flexure
  caudal
  cephalic
  cerebral
  cervical
  cranial
  duodenojejunal
  hepatic
  left colic
  left colonic
  right colic
  right colonic
  sigmoid
  splenic
floating cartilage
floating gallbladder
floating kidney
floating organ
floating patella
floating protein
floating rib
floating section
floating spleen
floating stool
floating villus
floccular fossa
flocculation
flocculonodular lobe
flocculus, accessory
Flood ligament
floor
  bladder
  fibromuscular pelvic

floor *(continued)*
   inguinal
   pelvic
floor cell
floor of inguinal region
floor of nasal cavity
floor of thorax
flora
   bacterial
   normal
florid
florid cirrhosis
flotation bath
flow cytometer (see *cytometer*)
flow cytometry
flow microfluorimetry
Flower bone
Floyd peripheral nerve classification
fluid
   amniotic
   articular
   ascitic
   bloody
   body
   Bouin
   cavitary
   cerebrospinal
   clear
   cystic
   Delafield
   dentinal
   digestive
   edema
   embalming
   extracellular
   extravascular
   frothy
   gelatinous
   intercellular
   interstitial
   intracellular
   joint

fluid *(continued)*
   loculated
   low-viscosity
   lymphatic
   meconium-stained amniotic
   natural body
   pericardial
   pericardial effusion
   peritoneal
   peritoneal effusion
   pleural
   pleural effusion
   prostatic
   protein-rich
   seminal
   serosanguineous
   serous
   spinal
   straw-colored
   synovial
   testing
   thoracentesis
   transcellular
   turbid
   viscous
   Zenker
fluid-filled cleft
fluid-filled cyst
fluid-filled papule
fluid-filled sac
fluid-filled vacuole within lens
fluid material
fluid protein
fluid specimen, filtration of
fluid wave
fluke (trematode)
   liver
   lung
fluorescein isothiocyanate (FITC)
fluorescence
   homogeneous
   nuclear rim

fluorescence *(continued)*
  nucleolar
  speckled
fluorescence-activated cell sorter
  (FACS)
fluorescence in situ hybridization
  (FISH)
fluorescence microscope
fluorescent antibody (FA) test
fluorescent antibody technique
fluorescent antinuclear antibody test
  (FANA)
fluorescent cytoprint assay
fluorescent dye
fluorescent lighting
fluorescent microscopy
fluorescent polarization
fluorescent-tagged antibody
fluorescent *Treponema pallidum*
  absorption test
fluorescent treponemal antibody
  (FTA) test
fluorescent treponemal antibody
  absorption test (FTA-ABS)
fluoride intoxication
fluoride poisoning
fluoride test
fluorochrome
fm (femtometer)
F method of staining
fmol (femtomole)
FNA (fine-needle aspiration)
FNAB (fine-needle aspiration biopsy)
foam cell
foam embolism
foamy cytoplasm
foamy exudate
foamy fluid
foamy histiocyte
foamy stool
focal edema
focal fibrotic reaction

focal glomerular sclerosis
focal hemorrhage
focal hepatic necrosis
focal hepatocellular necrosis with
  hemorrhagic cyst
focal inflammation
focal myocytolysis of heart
focal necrosis
focal osteolysis
focal pneumonitis
focal sclerosing osteomyelitis
focal ulceration and hemorrhage
focally puckered pleura
focus (pl. foci)
folate absorption test
fold
  adipose
  alar
  amniotic
  aryepiglottic
  axillary
  caval
  cecal
  cholecystoduodenocolic
  ciliary
  circular
  circulator
  costocolic
  Douglas
  duodenojejunal
  duodenomesocolic
  epigastric
  falciform retinal
  fibriated
  gastric
  gastropancreatic
  genital
  glossopalatine
  gluteal
  Guérin
  haustral
  hepatopancreatic

fold *(continued)*
  ileocecal
  ileocolic
  inferior duodenal
  inferior transverse rectal
  inguinal
  interureteric
  Kerckring
  labioscrotal
  lateral umbilical
  medial umbilical
  mucosal
  Nélaton
  palatopharyngeal
  paraduodenal
  peritoneal
  rectal
  rectouterine
  sacrogenital
  semilunar
  sentinel
  sigmoid
  spiral
  superior duodenal
  superior transverse rectal
  vestigial
folded fundus gallbladder
folded gallbladder
fold pattern
foliaceus, pemphigus
foliate papilla
folic acid
follicle
  aggregated lymphatic
  agminated
  anovular ovarian
  atretic ovarian
  gastric
  gastric lymphatic
  graafian
  hair
  lash

follicle *(continued)*
  lymphoid
  malpighian
  nabothian
  ovarian
  pilosebaceous
  primordial
  ruptured
  thyroid
  unruptured
follicle cell
follicle-stimulating hormone (FSH)
follicle-stimulating hormone-releasing
  factor
follicular abscess
follicular adenocarcinoma
follicular adenoiditis
follicular carcinoma
follicular cell
follicular center cell lymphoma
follicular cyst
follicular epithelial cell
follicular gland
follicular goiter
follicular hormone
follicular hyperkeratosis
follicular hyperplasia
follicular lymphoma
follicular mixed small cleaved and
  large cell lymphoma
follicular mucinosis
follicular ovarian cell
follicular phase
follicular plugging
follicular predominantly large cell
  lymphoma
follicular predominantly small cleaved
  cell lymphoma
follicular tonsillitis
folliculi, liquor
folliculitis decalvans
folliculitis, keloidal

following eye
follow up (verb)
follow-up (adj.)
followup, follow-up (noun, adj.)
fomites
Fonsecaea compacta
Fonsecaea dermatitidis
Fonsecaea pedrosoi
Fontana canal
Fontana-Masson stain
Fontana methenamine-silver stain
Fontana space
fontanelle (also, fontanel)
   anterior
   anterolateral
   bregmatic
   cranial
   frontal
   Gerdy
   mastoid
   occipital
   posterior
   posterolateral
   sagittal
   sphenoid
   triangular
fonticulus (pl. fonticuli)
food-borne gastroenteritis
food faddist
food poisoning
foot
   arch of
   arcuate artery of
   articulations of
   athlete's
   Charcot
   diabetic
   digital artery of
   Madura
   perforating artery of
   phalanges of
   trench

football knee
foot fungus
foot, hand, and mouth disease
Foot reticulum stain
foramen (pl. foramina)
   alveolar
   anterior condyloid
   aortic
   apical
   arachnoidal
   blind
   carotid
   cecal
   conjugate
   costotransverse
   cranial
   emissary sphenoidal
   epiploic
   ethmoidal
   greater palatine
   greater sciatic
   intervertebral
   lesser sciatic
   node of epiploic
   nutrient (of bone)
   obturator
   pelvic sacral
   sciatic
   vertebral
foramen cecum of tongue
foramen lacerum
foramen magnum
foramen of Bochdalek
foramen of Luschka
foramen of Magendie
foramen of Winslow
foramen ovale
foramen rotundum
foramen spinosum
foramen transversarium
foramide
forced grasping reflex

forced vital capacity (FVC)
foregut
foregut artery
foreign body
foreign body giant cell
foreign body granuloma
foreign body reaction
foreign material, retained
foreign protein
Forel, field of
forensic pathology
foreskin, inflammation of
Formad kidney
formaldehyde
formaldehyde solution
formalin-alcohol
formalin ammonium bromide (FAB)
formalin, buffered neutral
formalin solution
formation
   adipocere
   callus
   capsid
   coffin
   horn cyst
   horn pearl
   keloid
   keratin pearl
   palisade
   pearl
   pseudopalisade
   rosette
   rouleaux
   syncytium
formation of abnormal hemoglobin S
formation of excessive porphyrin in
   marrow
formation of red nodules beneath skin
formative cell
formed stool
forme fruste (pl. formes frustes)
forme tardive

formol-calcium fixative
formol-Mueller solution
formol-saline fixative
formol-Zenker fixative
formol-Zenker solution
formyl-methionyl-leucryl-phenyl-
   alamine
fornix of vagina
Forssman antigen
Forssman reaction
Fort Bragg fever
forward light scatter
Foshay test for tularemia
fossa (pl. fossae)
   acetabular
   adipose
   amygdaloid
   anconeal
   anterior recess of ischiorectal
   articular
   axillary
   bony
   condylar
   crural
   cubital
   digastric
   digital
   duodenal
   duodenojejunal
   epigastric
   femoral
   floccular
   gallbladder
   glenoid
   hypochondriac
   iliac
   infrasternal
   ischiorectal
   navicular
   olecranon
   ovarian
   pararectal

fossa *(continued)*
  paravesical
  valve of navicular
fossa ovalis (pl. fossae ovalis)
fossa plane, ischiorectal
Fouchet reagent
Fouchet test for bilirubin in urine
foul discharge
foul-smelling
fourchette
Fourier transformation
foveated chest
foveola
foveolar cell
foveolar cells of stomach
foveolar gastric mucosa
F plasmid
fraction
  beta
  beta lipoprotein
  blood plasma
  depressed ejection
  ejection
  filtration
  growth
  heparin-precipitable (HPF)
  linear
  MB
  plasma
  plasma protein (PPF)
  regurgitant
  S phase
fractional inspired oxygen concentration (FiO₂)
fraction of expired carbon dioxide (FeCO₂)
fracture of bone
fracture repair
fracture site
Fraenkel typhus nodule
fragile bones
fragile X chromosome

fragile X syndrome
fragility
  capillary
  capillary hereditary
  erythrocyte
  hereditary (of bone)
  osmotic
  red blood cell
fragility test, osmotic
fragmentation myocarditis
fragmentation of cell into particles
fragmentation of cell nuclei
fragmentation of fibers
fragmented axons and dendrites
fragmented tissue
frambesia (yaws)
Francisella tularensis (formerly *Pasteurella tularensis*)
Francis test for bile acids in urine
frank blood in stool
Frankfort horizontal plane
Frankfort-mandibular incisor angle
Frankfort plane
frank blood
Frank capillary toxicosis
frank cyanosis from hypoxemia
frank hemorrhage
frank necrosis
frank perforation
frank pulmonary edema
frank pus
frank rigors
Frank-Starling curve
Frank-Starling mechanism
frank suppuration
Franseen needle
fraught with error
freckle, Hutchinson melanotic
freckle-like lesion
freckles (ephelides)
freckling, myxoma syndrome
  with facial

free band of colon
free electrophoresis
free erythrocyte protoporphyrin
free fluid
free hemoglobin
free macrophage
free radical
free thyroxine index (FTI)
free triiodothyronine test
free wall
freeze-dried
freezing microtome
Freiberg disease
Frei intracutaneous diagnostic test
fremitus, bronchial
French scale
frenulum (pl. frenula)
frenulum of clitoris
frenulum of ileocecal valve
frenulum of labia minora
frenulum of valve
frequency of stool
fresh frozen plasma
fresh frozen section
fresh normal plasma
friable clot
friable mass
friable papilloma
friction rub in knee
Friderichsen-Waterhouse syndrome
Friedländer bacillus
Friedländer pneumonia
Friedreich ataxia
fringe, costal
Frisch bacillus
Frommann line
frond
fronding sign
frondlike pattern
frontal abscess
frontal air sinus
frontal angle

frontal area
frontal artery
frontal axis
frontal bone
frontal bossing
frontal convolution
frontal cortex
frontal crest
frontal eminence
frontal fontanel
frontal horn
frontal lobe
frontal margin
frontal nerve
frontal notch
frontal plane
frontal plate
frontal pole
frontal process
frontal region
frontal section
frontal sinus
frontal suture
frontal triangle
frontal tuber
frontal vein
frontobasal artery
frontoethmoidal suture
frontolacrimal suture
frontomaxillary suture
frontonasal duct
frontonasal elevation
frontonasal process
frontonasal roof of nasal cavity
frontonasal suture
fronto-occipital fasciculus
fronto-orbital area
frontopontine tract
frontosphenoidal process
frontotemporal tract
frontozygomatic suture
Froriep induration

frostbite (dermatitis congelationis)
frosted liver
frost itch
frothy discharge
frothy exudate
frothy fluid
frozen embryo
frozen pelvis
frozen section diagnosis
frozen section, fresh
frozen sperm
fructosamine
fructose
fructose challenge test
fructose loading test
fructose tolerance test
Frykman classification of hand
    fractures
FSH (follicle-stimulating hormone)
FSH-HR (follicle-stimulating hormone-
    releasing hormone)
FTA (fluorescent treponemal antibody)
    test
FTA-ABS (fluorescent treponemal
    antibody absorption) test
FTI (free thyroxine index)
fuchsin body
fuchsinophil cell
fuchsinophil granule
fuchsinophilic granule
fucosylated alpha fetoprotein
FU-48 Zenker solution
fulgurate
fulguration
full-thickness tear
fulminant hepatitis
fulminant tuberculosis
functional congestion
functional hematuria
functional hypertrophy
functional ovarian cyst
functional proteinuria

functional residual capacity (FRC)
functioning neoplasm
functioning tumor
function, platelet
function test
fundal placenta
fundic-antral junction
fundic gland
fundic metaplasia
fundiform ligament
fundus (pl. fundi)
    bladder
    eye
    gallbladder
    gastric
    stomach
    urinary bladder
    uterine
    vaginal
fundus reflex
fundus uteri
fungal antibody
fungal body
fungal culture
fungal endocarditis
fungal infection
fungal myocarditis
fungal pneumonia
fungal scrapings
fungal smear
fungating mass
fungating neoplasm
fungemia
fungiform papillae
fungoides, mycosis
fungus (pl. fungi) (see also *pathogen*)
    dimorphic
    foot
    mold
    mosaic
    mycelial
    pathogenic

fungus *(continued)*
  slime
  yeast
  yeastlike
  zygomycetous
funguslike bacteria
fungus testis
funicular artery
funiculus, cuneate
funis
funisitis
funnel-like deformity
funnel-shaped cavity
funnel-shaped pelvis
funnel-shaped portion of hair follicle
FUO (fever of unknown origin)
furcal nerve
furuncle
furuncular
furunculoid
furunculosis
fusariotoxicosis
Fusarium moniliforme
Fusarium oxysporum
Fusarium solani
fused kidney

fused rib
fusiform aneurysm
fusiform bacillus
fusiform cell
fusiform gyrus
fusiform layer
fusiform muscle
fusion, labial
fusion of the stapes
Fusobacterium, fusobacterium
Fusobacterium gonidiaformans
Fusobacterium mortiferum
Fusobacterium mucleatum
Fusobacterium natiforme
Fusobacterium necrophorum
Fusobacterium nucleatum
Fusobacterium plauti-vincenti
Fusobacterium russii
Fusobacterium varium
fusocellular
fusospirillary
fusospirillosis
fusospirochetal
fusospirochetosis
FVC (forced vital capacity)

G, g

g (gram)
GABHS (Group A beta-hemolytic
   streptococcus)
Gaddum and Schild test
gag reflex
galactagogue factor
galactocele
galactokinase deficiency
galactophorous canal
galactophorous duct
galactopoietic factor
galactopoietic hormone
galactorrhea
galactose in tissues
galactose-1-phosphate uridyl
   transferase deficiency
galactosemia
galactose tolerance test
galactosylceramidase, congenital
   deficiency of
galea aponeurotica
Galeati gland
Galen ventricle
gallbladder
   bilobed
   body of
   Courvoisier

gallbladder *(continued)*
   dilated
   distended
   double
   fish-scale
   floating
   folded fundus
   fundus of
   hourglass
   mobile
   multiseptate
   neck of
   sandpaper
   stasis
   strawberry
   thick-walled
   thin-walled
   wandering
gallbladder bed
gallbladder bile
gallbladder calculi
gallbladder fossa
gallbladder fundus
gallbladder hydrops
gallbladder mucosa
gallbladder sludge
gallbladder stone

gallbladder villi
gallbladder wall
gall duct
Gallego method
gallstone
   cholesterol
   opacifying
   silent
Gallyas method
GALT (gut-associated lymphoid tissue)
galvanic cell
galvanic threshold
Gambian fever
gamete intrafallopian transfer (GIFT)
gametoid cell
gametokinetic hormone
Gamgee tissue
gamma angle
gamma cell
gamma counter
gamma globulins
gamma-glutamyl transferase (GGT)
gamma-glutamyl transpeptidase
   (GGTP)
gamma granule
gamma-hemolytic streptococcus
gamma loop
gamma motor neuron
gammopathy, monoclonal
Gandy-Gamma nodule
ganglia (pl. of ganglion)
gangliated cord
gangliated nerve
ganglion (pl. ganglia)
   aberrant
   acousticofacial
   aorticorenal
   auditory
   auricular
   autonomic
   basal
   cardiac

ganglion *(continued)*
   carotid
   celiac
   cervicothoracic
   ciliary
   coccygeal
   diffuse
   gasserian
   geniculate
   otic
   paravertebral
   prevertebral
   sensory
   sphenopalatine
   submandibular
   spinal
   stromal
   superior mesenteric
   sympathetic
   uterine cervical
   vestibular
ganglion artery, semilunar
ganglion cell
ganglion cyst
ganglion of Arnold
ganglion of Auerbach
ganglion of nerve
ganglion of tendon sheath
ganglion ridge
ganglionic blockade
ganglionic canal
ganglionic crest
ganglionic layer
ganglioside
gangrene
   diabetic
   dry
   gas
   wet
gangrenous granuloma
gangrenous necrosis
gangrenous pneumonia

gap
  air-bone
  anion
  anteromedian
  auscultatory
  Bochdalek
  chromatid
  isochromatid
gaping wound
Gardnerella vaginalis (formerly
  Haemophilus vaginalis or
  Corynebacterium vaginale)
Gardnerella vaginitis
gargantuan mastitis
gargoylism
Garré osteomyelitis
Gärtner bacillus
Gartner canal
Gartner cyst
Gartner duct
Gärtner phenomenon
gas
  arterial blood
  bowel
  carbon dioxide
  colorless
  formaldehyde
  nitrogen
  odorless
  pulmonary
gas abscess
gas chromatography
gas embolism
gas exchange in lungs, normal
gas exchange, pulmonary
gas gangrene
gas liquefaction
gas nitrogen embolism
gas pattern
gaseous
gases of putrefaction
gasophil granule

gasserian ganglion
gastral mesoderm
gastric achlorhydria
gastric acid secretion
gastric acid test
gastric algid malaria
gastric analysis
gastric antrum
gastric artery
gastric atrophy
gastric calculus
gastric canal
gastric carcinoma
gastric cardia
gastric channel
gastric contents
gastric fistula
gastric fold
gastric follicle
gastric function test
gastric fundus
gastric gland
gastric groove
gastric impression
gastric inhibitory polypeptide (GIP)
gastric juice
gastric lavage
gastric lymph nodes
gastric lymphatic follicle
gastric mucin
gastric mucosa
gastric mucosa atrophy
gastric obstruction
gastric omentum
gastric pacemaker region
gastric partition
gastric pit
gastric plexus
gastric polyp
gastric polyposis
gastric pouch
gastric remnant

gastric sclerosis
gastric secretion rate
gastric stump
gastric surface
gastric ulcer
gastric vein
gastric washing
gastrin hormone
gastrinoma
gastrin-secreting cell
gastrin-secretin stimulation test
gastrin test
gastritis
  acute
  antral
  atrophic
  chronic
  cirrhotic
  hemorrhagic
  hypertrophic
  necrotizing
  pseudomembranous radiation
gastrocolic fistula
gastrocolic ligament
gastrocolic omentum
gastrocolic reflex
gastrodiaphragmatic ligament
gastroduodenal artery complex
gastroduodenal fistula
gastroduodenal lumen
gastroduodenal lymph node
gastroduodenal orifice
gastroenteritis
  acute infectious
  bacterial
  Campylobacter
  eosinophilic
  food-borne
  infantile
  Norwalk
  viral
  water-borne

gastroepiploic arcade
gastroepiploic artery
gastroepiploic gland
gastroepiploic vein
gastroepiploic vessel
gastroesophageal junction
gastroesophageal laceration
gastroesophageal variceal plexus
gastroesophageal vestibule
gastrohepatic bare area
gastrohepatic ligament
gastrohepatic omentum
gastroileac reflex
gastrointestinal (GI)
gastrointestinal hormone
gastrointestinal mucosal hemorrhage
gastrointestinal plaque
gastrointestinal stoma
gastrointestinal tract
gastrointestinal tumor
gastrointestinal ulceration
gastrolienal ligament
gastro-omental artery
gastropancreatic fold
gastropancreatic ligament
gastroparesis
gastrophrenic ligament
gastrosplenic ligament
gastrosplenic omentum
Gaucher cell
Gaucher disease
gauge
gauze
Gay gland
GBIA (Guthrie bacterial inhibition assay)
GBS (Group beta-hemolytic *Streptococcus*) (also, Group B)
GC (gonorrhea)
G cell
g/dL (grams per deciliter)
GE (gastroesophageal) junction

Gegenbaur cell
gel
  acrylamide/urea
  agarose
  colloidal
  polyacrylamide
gelatiginous tissue
gelatin-chrome slide
gelatiniform degeneration
gelatinized marrow
gelatinous ascites
gelatinous infiltration
gelatinous material
gelatinous otolithic membrane
gelatinous polyp
gel diffusion precipitin test
gel diffusion reaction
gel diffusion test
gel electrophoresis
Gell and Coombs hypersentivity
  reactions
gel-like consistency
gel-like envelope
gel-like fluid
gel-like material
gel medium
gel slab
Gelvatol
gemastete cell
Gemella morbillorum
gemistocyte
gemistocytic astrocytoma
gemistocytic cell
genal gland
Gendre fixative
Gendre solution
gene (pl. genes)
  allelic
  APC (adenomatous polyposis coli)
    tumor suppressor
  antioncogene
  autosomal

gene *(continued)*
  bcl-2
  codominant
  control
  DCC (deleted in colon carcinoma)
    tumor suppressor
  dominant
  extrachromosomal
  H
  histocompatibility
  holandric
  homeobox
  homeotic
  housekeeping
  immune response
  jumping
  lethal
  mitochondrial
  modifier
  mutant
  NF (neurofibromatosis)
  NF1 tumor suppressor
  NF2 tumor suppressor
  operator
  p53 tumor suppressor
  pleiotropic
  polyphrenic
  RB1 tumor suppressor
  recessive
  regulator
  repressor
  SOS
  split
  transforming
  tumor suppressor
  V
  X-linked
  Y-linked
  Z
gene mapping
general sensory cortex
generalized morphea

generalized pustular psoriasis of
  Zambusch
generalized reticular to maculopapular
  rash
genetic amniocentesis
genetic counseling
genetic death
genetic diagnosis
genetic marker
genetic material
genetic sex of individual
genetically induced overdevelopment
Gengou phenomenon
genial (chin) tubercle
genicular artery
geniculate body
geniculate ganglion
geniculocalcarine tract
genioglossus muscle
genital branch of genitofemoral nerve
genital canal
genital carcinoma
genital cord
genital corpuscle
genital duct
genital eminence
genital fold
genital gland
genital groove
genital herpes
genital herpes simplex
genitalia
  ambiguous external
  virilization of
genital ligament
genital neoplasm
genital organ
genital ridge
genital swelling
genital system
genital tract
genital tubercle

genital ulcer
genital wart, flat
genitocrural nerve
genitofemoral nerve, genital branch of
genitoinguinal ligament
genitourinary fistula
genitourinary system
genitourinary tuberculosis
Gennari band
genoblast
genomic mutation
genotype
gentamicin
gentian orange stain
gentian violet
gentian violet stain
genu of pancreatic duct
genus (pl. genera)
geotrichosis
Geotrichum capitatum
Geotrichum fermentans
Geotrichum penicillatum
Geraghty test
Gerdy fontanelle
Gerdy interatrial loop
Gerdy ligament
Gerhardt test for acetoacetic acid
  in urine
Gerhardt test for bile pigments
  in urine
Gerlach tendon
germ cell, primordial
germ disk
germinal area
germinal cell
germinal center in lymphoid tissue
germinal cord
germinal disk
germinal epithelium
germinal inclusion cyst
germinal infection
germinal membrane

germinal pole
germinal rod
germinal spot
germinal vesicle
germination
germinative layer
germinoma
germ layer
germ membrane
germ nucleus
germ tube test
Gerota fascia
Gerrard test for glucose in urine
gestational age (GA)
gestational diabetes
gestational edema
gestational proteinuria
gestational sac
GFAP (glial fibrillary acidic protein)
GFAP antibody
GFR (glomerular filtration rate)
GGT (gamma-glutamyl transpeptidase)
GGTP liver function test
GH (growth hormone)
Ghon primary lesion
Ghon-Sachs bacillus
Ghon tubercle
ghost cell
ghost corpuscle
Giacomini, band of
Giannuzzi cell
giant Betz cell
giant cell
giant cell arteritis
giant cell carcinoma
giant cell hepatitis
giant cell monstrocellular sarcoma
giant cell myeloma
giant cell myocarditis
giant cell of bone tumor
giant cell pneumonia
giant cell sarcoma

giant cell tumor
giant chromosome
giant follicle lymphoma
giant follicular hyperplasia
giant hairy nevus
giant neutrophil
giant osteoid osteoma
giant pigmented nevus
Giardia lamblia
giardiasis
Gibberella fujikuroi
gibbous deformity
Giemsa stain
Giemsa-Wright stain
Gierke cell
Gies biuret test for proteins
GIFT (gamete intrafallopian transfer)
gigantism, pituitary
Gilchrist disease
Gilchrist skin test
gill arch skeleton
gill cleft
Gillette suspensory ligament
Gilson solution
Gimbernat ligament
Gimenez stain
gingivobuccal groove
gingiva (pl. gingivae)
gingival abscess
gingival crest
gingival curvature
gingival gland
gingival margin
gingival mucosa
gingival septum
gingival space
gingival sulcus
gingival trough
gingival zone
gingiva proper
gingivitis, necrotizing
gingivobuccal sulcus

gingivodental ligament
gingivolabial groove
gingivolabial sulcus
gingivolingual groove
gingivolingual sulcus
ginglymoid joint
ginglymus
Giordano sphincter
GIP (gastric inhibitory polypeptide)
GIP (glucose-dependent insulinotropic polypeptide)
GI (gastrointestinal) tract
gitter cell
glabrous
glacial acetic acid
glancing wound
gland
  absorbent
  accessory
  accessory lacrimal
  accessory parotid
  accessory suprarenal
  accessory thyroid
  acid
  acinar
  acinotubular
  acinous
  admaxillary
  adrenal
  aggregate
  agminate
  agminated
  Albarrán
  albuminous
  alveolar
  anal
  anteprostatic
  aortic
  apical (of tongue)
  apocrine
  aporic
  areolar

gland *(continued)*
  arterial
  arteriococcygeal
  arytenoid
  Aselli
  axillary
  axillary sweat
  Bartholin
  Bauhin
  biliary
  Blandin
  Blandin and Nuhn
  blood
  blood vessel
  Boerhaave
  Bonnot
  Bowman
  brachial
  bronchial
  Bruch
  Brunner
  buccal
  bulbocavernous
  bulbourethral
  cardiac
  carotid
  celiac
  ceruminous
  cervical (of uterus)
  cheek
  Ciaccio
  ciliary
  circumanal
  Cloquet
  closed
  Cobelli
  coccygeal
  coil
  compound
  compound tubuloalveolar
  conglobate
  conjunctival

gland *(continued)*
    convoluted
    Cowper
    cutaneous
    ductless
    duodenal
    Duverney
    Ebner
    eccrine
    ecdysial
    Eglis
    endocervical
    endocrine
    endoepithelial
    endometrial
    esophageal
    excretory
    exocrine
    follicular (of tongue)
    fundic
    fundus
    Galeati
    gastric
    gastroepiploic
    Gay
    genal
    genital
    gingival
    Gley
    globate
    glomiform
    glossopalatine
    greater vestibular
    Guérin
    gustatory
    guttural
    Harder
    Havers
    haversian
    hemal
    hemal lymph
    hemolymph

gland *(continued)*
    Henle
    hepatic
    heterocrine
    hibernating
    holocrine
    incretory
    intercarotid
    intermediate
    interscapular
    interstitial
    intestinal
    intraepithelial
    intramuscular
    jugular
    Knoll
    Krause
    labial
    lacrimal
    lactiferous
    large intestine
    large sweat
    laryngeal
    lenticular
    Lieberkühn
    Littré
    Luschka
    lymph
    lymphatic
    major salivary
    malpighian
    mammary
    mandibular
    master
    meibomian
    merocrine
    Méry
    mesenteric
    mesocolic
    mixed
    molar
    Moll

gland *(continued)*
  monoptychic
  Montgomery
  Morgagni
  mucous (lingual)
  mucus-secreting
  multicellular
  myometrial
  nabothian
  Naboth
  nasal
  Nuhn
  oil
  olfactory
  oxyntic
  palatine
  palpebral
  pancreaticosplenic
  parafrenal
  parathyroid
  paraurethral
  parotid
  pectoral
  peptic
  Peyer
  pharyngeal
  Philip
  pineal
  pituitary
  Poirier
  polyptychic
  pregnancy
  prehyoid
  preputial
  prostate
  pyloric
  racemose
  retromolar
  Rivinus
  Rosenmüller
  saccular
  salivary

gland *(continued)*
  Sandström
  saw-toothed
  Schüller
  sebaceous
  seminal
  sentinel
  seromucous
  serous
  Serres
  sexual
  Sigmund
  simple
  Skene
  small intestine (solitary)
  splenoid
  Stahr
  staphyline
  subauricular
  sublingual
  submandibular
  submaxillary
  sudoriferous
  suprarenal
  Suzanne
  sweat
  synovial
  target
  tarsal
  tarsoconjunctival
  Terson
  Theile
  thymus
  thyroid
  Tiedemann
  tongue
  tracheal
  trachoma
  triangular suprarenal
  tubular
  tubuloacinar
  tubuloalveolar

gland *(continued)*
  tympanic
  Tyson
  ultimobranchial
  unicellular
  urethral
  uropygial
  uterine
  utricular
  vaginal
  vascular
  vestibular
  Virchow
  vitelline
  vulvovaginal
  Waldeyer
  Wasmann
  Weber
  Wepfer
  Wölfer
  Wolfring
  Zeis
  Zuckerkandl
glanders
glanders bacillus
glandes (pl. of glans)
gland neck extension
gland of neck
glands of biliary mucosa
glands of Haller
glands of mouth
glands of prepuce, odoriferous
glands of Wolfring
glandular alveolus
glandular artery
glandular epithelium
glandular fever
glandular mastitis
glandular system
glandular tissue
glandulopreputial lamella
glans (pl. glandes)

glans clitoridis
glans, corona of
glans penis, inflammation of
Glanzmann disease
glaserian artery
glaserian fissure
glass factor
glass-rod phenomenon
glassy degeneration in muscle
glassy swelling
glaucoma
  chronic
  congenital
  narrow-angle
  open-angle
  posttraumatic
  wide-angle
Gleason grade
Gleason score
Gleason tumor grade
glenohumeral articulation
glenohumeral ligament
glenoid cavity
glenoid fossa
glenoid ligament
glenoid surface
glenoidal labrum
Glerke cell
Gley cell
Gley gland
glia
glia cell
glial cytoplasmic inclusion
glial fibrillary acidic protein (GFAP)
glial proliferation
glial reaction
gliding joint
glioblast
glioblastoma multiforme
glioma
gliosis
Glisson capsule

glistening degeneration
glistening masses
glitter cell
globate gland
globoid cell
globoid cell leukodystrophy
globoid material
globose
globotriaosylceramide deposition in
    arterial intima and media
globotriaosylceramide deposition in
    kidney
globotriaosylceramide deposition in
    myocardium
globular cytoplasmic inclusions
globular protein
globular proteinuria
globular valve
globule, dentin
globulin
    accelerator (AcG, ac-g)
    alpha
    alpha antitrypsin
    antihemophilic
    beta
    chickenpox immune
    copper-containing plasma
    corticosteroid-binding
    gamma
    hepatitis B hyperimmune
    thyroxine-binding (TBG)
globulin test
glomerular artery
glomerular basement membrane
    antibody
glomerular capillary membrane
glomerular filtrate (also, filtration)
glomerular filtration rate (GFR)
glomerular nephritis
glomerular selectivity test
glomerular tufts
glomerulocapsular nephritis

glomerulonephritis
    acute
    acute poststreptococcal
    chronic
    membranoproliferative
    membranous
    necrotizing
    proliferative
    segmental necrotizing
glomerulosa cell
glomerulosa zona
glomerulosclerosis
glomerulus (pl. glomeruli)
glomiform gland
glomus body
glomus cell
glossitis
glossoepiglottic ligament
glossopalatine arch
glossopalatine fold
glossopalatine gland
glottis, false
glucagon hormone
glucagon stimulation test
glucocerebrosidase deficiency
Glucocheck glucose monitoring
    machine
glucogenic storage
Glucola screen
Glucometer II
glucosamine
glucose
    blood
    body fluid
    cerebrospinal fluid (CSF)
    fasting blood
    random blood
    rapid absorption of dietary
    spinal fluid
    test
    2-hour postprandial blood
    urine

glucose-dependent insulinotropic
   polypeptide (GIP)
glucose in urine
glucose level of spinal fluid
glucose oxidase method
glucose oxidase paper strip test
glucose-6-phosphatase
glucose-6-phosphatase deficiency
glucose-6-phosphate dehydrogenase
   deficiency (G-6-PD, G6PD)
glucose test
glucose tolerance curve
glucose tolerance factor
glucose tolerance test (GTT)
glucose tolerance test with cortisone
Glucostix
glucuronic acid
glucuronosyltransferase (liver enzyme)
glucuronyl transferase, deficiency of
glue ear
glutamic oxaloacetic transaminase
   (GOT)
glutamic pyruvic transaminase (GPT)
glutamine, cerebrospinal fluid
glutamyltransferase (GGT) test
glutaraldehyde
glutathione reductase in erythrocytes
   test
gluteal aponeurosis
gluteal artery
gluteal fold
gluteal nerve
gluteal region
gluteal vessel
gluten-sensitive enteropathy
gluteofemoral
gluteoinguinal
glutethimide
gluteus maximus
glycated hemoglobin
glycerol test, free
glycerophosphate test for renal function

glycine test
glycogen
glycogen deposits in muscle
glycogenic degeneration
glycogen infiltration
glycogen nephrosis
glycogen phosphorylase kinase
glycogen starch synthase
glycogen storage disease
glycogen vacuolation
glycogen vacuoles in cytoplasm and
   nuclei of hepatocytes
glycogen vacuoles in renal tubule cells
glycogenolytic
glycogenosis
glycogeusia
glycohemia
glycohemoglobin
glycolic acid test
glycolipid pattern
glycol methacrylate
glycoprotein
   alpha acid
   CA-125
   histidine-rich (HRGP)
glycosuria
   alimentary
   renal
glycosylated hemoglobin (hemoglobin
   A_{1c})
glycosylated hemoglobin test
glycotropic factor
glycyltryptophan test for carcinoma of
   stomach
glygenolysis
glyoxylic acid test
GM activator protein
Gmelin test for bile pigments
GNID (gram-negative intracellular
   diplococci)
GMS (Gomori's methenamine-silver)
   stain

Gn-RH (gonadotropin-releasing
  hormone)
Goa antigen (Gonzales blood antigen)
goblet cell
Goethe bone
Gofman test
Gogli cell
goiter
  aberrant
  adenomatous
  Basedow
  colloid
  congenital
  cystic
  diffuse
  diving
  endemic
  exophthalmic
  fibrous
  follicular
  intrathoracic
  iodide
  lingual
  lymphadenoid
  multinodular
  nodular
  nontoxic
  parenchymatous
  perivascular
  plunging
  retrovascular
  simple
  soft
  substernal
  suffocative
  thyroid
  toxic (diffuse)
  vascular
  wandering
gold (Au)
Goldblatt hypertension
Goldblatt kidney

gold chloride
gold stain
gold test
golf-hole ureteral orifice
Golgi apparatus
Golgi epithelial cell
Golgi method of staining
Golgi osmiobichromate fixative
Golgi stain
Golgi zone
Gombault degeneration
Gombault neuritis
Gomori aldehyde fuchsin
Gomori methenamine-silver (GMS)
Gomori stain
Gomori-Takamatsu stain
gomphosis articulation
gomphosis, dentoalveolar
gomphosis joint
gonadal neoplasm
gonadotropic hormone (GTH)
gonadotropic-releasing factor (GRF)
gonadotropin
  chorionic
  human chorionic (HCG, hCG)
gonococcal ophthalmia of newborn
gonococcal perihepatitis
gonococcal salpingitis
gonococcal stomatitis
gonococcal urethritis
gonococcus (pl. gonococci)
gonorrhea (GC)
gonorrheal stomatitis
Gonzales blood antigen (Goa)
Goodpasture syndrome
Goormaghtigh cell
gooseflesh
Gordon test for globulin-albumin in
  spinal fluid
Gosset, spiral band of
GOT (glutamic oxaloacetic
  transaminase)

Gothic arch formation
Gothlin capillary fragility test
Gougerot-Blum syndrome
gout, uric acid crystals in
gouty arthritis
gouty proteinuria
Gowers muscular dystrophy
Gowers solution
G protein
GPT (glutamic pyruvic transaminase)
graafian follicle
grade (see also *classification*, *stage*)
    FIGO (International Federation of
        Gynecology and Obstetrics)
        adenocarcinoma of endometrium
    Gleason tumor
    Hyams esthesioneuroblastoma
    murmur
    osteoarthritis
    placental
grade of malignant neoplasm
gradient
    atrioventricular
    Ficoll
grading neoplasm
grading of malignancy
grading of tumor
graft, chorioallantoic
Gregerson and Boas test
Graham-Cole cholecystography
grainy texture
gram (g)
Gram iodine
Gram method
gram-negative bacilli
gram-negative bacteria
gram-negative coccus
gram-negative diplococci
gram-negative intracellular diplococci
  (GNID)
gram-negative rod
gram-positive

gram-positive bacteria
Gram solution
grams per deciliter (g/dL)
Gram stain
granular appearance
granular atrophy
granular casts in urine
granular cell
granular cell layer
granular cytoplasm
granular endoplasmic reticulum
granular induration
granular kidney
granular leukocyte
granular pneumonocyte
granular texture
granulation tissue
granulation tissue of mucous
  membrane
granulation tissue of skin
granulation, toxic
granule
    acidophil
    acidophilic
    acrosomal
    albuminous
    Alder-Reilly
    alpha
    Altmann
    amphophil
    argentaffin
    azure
    azurophil
    basal
    basophil
    basophilic cytoplasmic
    beta
    Birbeck
    Bollinger
    Chédiak-Higashi
    chromatic
    chromophil

granule *(continued)*
  chromophobe
  coarse
  coarse azurophilic
  cone
  cytoplasmic
  delta
  DiPAS-positive
  Ehrlich
  elementary
  eosinophil
  fuchsinophil
  gamma
  granule
  hemosiderin
  iodophil
  kappa
  keratohyalin
  Langerhans
  matrix
  Much
  Neusser
  Nissl
  rod-shaped
  secretory
  sulfur
  toxic
  vermiform
  Weibel-Palade
  zymogen
granule cell of connective tissue
granules of cornstarch
granuloadipose
granulocyte
granulocyte colony–stimulating factor
granulocyte–macrophage colony-
  stimulating factor
granulocytic leukemia
granulocytic sarcoma
granulocytic white cell
granulocytopenia
granulocytosis

granuloma (pl. granulomata)
  amebic
  apical
  beryllium
  candidal
  cholesterol
  coccidioidal
  coli
  eosinophilic
  epithelioid
  fishtank
  foreign-body
  gangrenous
  Hodgkin
  infectious
  inguinal
  laryngeal
  lipoid
  lipophagic
  Majocchi
  malarial
  midline
  Mignon eosinophilic
  miliary
  paracoccidioidal
  plasma cell
  pseudopyogenic
  pyogenic
  reticulohistiocytic
  rheumatic
  silicotic
  stellate
  swimming pool
  trichophytic
  umbilicus
  xanthomatous
granuloma annulare
granuloma formation
granuloma inguinale
granuloma multiforme
granuloma telangiectaticum
granuloma-theca cell tumor

granulomatosis
   allergic
   Wegener
granulomatous conjunctivitis
granulomatous hepatitis
granulomatous infection
granulomatous inflammation
granulomatous lymphoma
granulomatous myocarditis
granulomatous pannus invading
   cartilage
granulomatous pneumonia
granulomatous pneumonitis
granulomatous ulcer
granulomatous vasculitis
granulopenia
granulopoiesis
granulosa cell
granulosa cell tumor
granulosa-lutein cells
granulovacuolar degeneration
grape cell
grape-cluster shape
grapelike clusters of cysts
grass bacillus
grass dermatitis
grave prognosis
gravel particle
Graves disease
gravida
gravid uterus
Gravindex pregnancy test
gravis, myasthenia
gravitation abscess
gravity, specific (of urine)
gray (Gy) (radiation dose equal to 100
   rads)
gray hepatization stage of pneumonia
gray induration
graying of the hair
gray matter, degeneration of
gray scale

gray tumor
greasy scaling
greasy texture
great alveolar cells
great auricular nerve
great cardiac vein
great saphenous vein
great vein
great vessels, transposition of
greater curvature
greater curvature of stomach
greater multangular bone
greater omentum
greater palatine artery
greater palatine canal
greater palatine foramen
greater palatine nerve
greater peritoneal sac
greater sac of peritoneal cavity
greater trochanter of femur
greater tubercle
greater vestibular gland
green liver
Greene biopsy needle
green pus
green stool
Gregerson and Boas test for blood
   in feces
grenz zone
Gridley stain
Grigg test for proteins
grinder tissue
Griscelli syndrome
gritty material
Grocott-Gomori methenamine-silver
   nitrate stain
Grocott-Gomori stain
Grocott methenamine-silver
groove (pl. grooves)
   abomasal
   alveolingual
   alveolobuccal

groove *(continued)*
  alveololabial
  anal intersphincteric
  anterolateral
  anteromedian
  arterial
  atrioventricular (AV)
  auriculoventricular
  basilar
  bicipital
  branchial
  buccal
  carotid
  carpal
  cavernous
  central
  coronary
  costal
  dental
  developmental
  digastric
  esophageal
  ethmoidal
  gastric
  genital
  gingivobuccal
  gingivolabial
  Harrison
  infraorbital
  interatrial
  intertubercular
  interventricular
  labial
  lacrimal
  Liebermeister
  neural
  paravertebral
  radial
  radial neck
  Sibson
  spindle colonic
  ulnar

groove *(continued)*
  urethral
  venous
  Verga lacrimal
  vertebral
gross architecture
gross cystic disease
gross description of specimen
gross diagnosis
gross examination
gross examination of tissue
gross hematuria
gross lesion
grossly intact architecture
gross report
Gross test for trypsin in feces
ground-glass appearance
ground-glass-appearing cytoplasm
ground-glass cell
ground-glass pattern
ground itch (pruritus at site of skin
  invasion)
ground substance
Group A beta-hemolytic *Streptococcus*
Group B beta-hemolytic *Streptococcus*
  (GBS)
group, blood (also, blood type)
grouping, blood
group-specific
Grover disease
growth center
growth factor
growth, failure of long-bone
growth hormone
  deficiency of
  excess of
  somatotropin
growth hormone antibody
growth hormone–arginine stimulation
  test
growth hormone–glucagon stimulation
  test

growth hormone–L-dopa stimulation
  test
growth hormone–releasing hormone
  (GH-RH)
growth-onset diabetes
growth plate
growth, stunting of
Gruber fossa
grumose
grumous material
grumous tissue
Grynfeltt triangle
G-6-PD (G6PD) test
GTC (guanidine isothiocyanate)
GTC/silica beads protocol
GTH (gonadotropic hormone)
GU (genitourinary)
guaiac-negative stool
guaiac-negative test for occult blood in
  stool
guaiac-positive stool
guaiac-positive test for occult blood in
  stool
guaiac test for occult blood
Guama virus
guanidine isothiocyanate (GTC)
guanine cell
guanyl cyclase
guanyl-nucleotide-binding protein
guanylins
Guarnieri body
Guaroa virus
gubernacular canal
gubernaculum
Guérin fold
Guérin gland
Guérin sinus
Guidi canal
Guillain-Barré syndrome
guinea worm
gullet
gum, mucilaginous

gumma (pl. gummas or gummata)
gummata (pl. of gumma), tuberculous
gummatous abscess
gummatous meningitis
gums
  bleeding
  swollen
Gunn dots
Gunning-Lieben test
Gunning test for acetone in urine
gunshot wound
gunstock deformity
Günzberg test (Guenzberg)
Günz ligament (Guenz)
gustatory cell
gustatory gland
gut (intestine)
  blind
  large
  small
gut-associated lymphoid tissue (GALT)
Guthrie bacterial inhibition assay
  (GBIA)
Guthrie test for phenylketonuria
guttate
guttate morphea (white spot disease)
gutter
  lateral
  left
  paracolic
  peritoneal
  right
guttural gland
gutter wound
Gutzeit test for arsenic
Guyon canal
Gy (gray) (radiation dose equal to 100
  rads)
gynatresia
gynecoid pelvis
gynecomastia
gynecophoric canal

gyrochrome cell
gyrus (pl. gyri)
    angular
    callosal
    dentate
    fasciolar
    fusiform
    middle temporal
gyrus rectus

H, h

HAA (hepatitis associated antigen)
habitual abortion
HACEK (*Haemophilus, Actinobacillus actinomycetemcomitans, Cardiobacterium hominis, Eikenella corrodens, Kingella kingae*) gram-negative bacilli
Haemophilus
Haemophilus aegyptius
Haemophilus aphrophilus
Haemophilus ducreyi
Haemophilus haemolyticus
Haemophilus influenzae
Haemophilus influenzae meningitis
Haemophilus influenzae pneumonia
Haemophilus influenzae type b (Hib)
Haemophilus parahaemolyticus
Haemophilus parainfluenzae
Haemophilus paraphrophilus
Haemophilus segnis
Haemophilus vaginalis
Hafnia
Hafnia alvei (formerly *Enterobacter hafniae*)
Hagedorn needle
Hageman factor
Haglund deformity

HAI, HI (hemagglutination inhibition) test
HAI (hepatic arterial infusion)
Hailey-Hailey disease
hair
  auditory
  bamboo
  catagen
  color and distribution of head and body
  ingrown
  scalp
  telogen
  vellus
hair bulb
hair canal
hair cell
hair disk
hair follicle
hairlike process
hairline crack in bone cortex
hair loss
hairy cell
hairy-cell leukemia (HCL)
hairy mole
hairy nevus
Haldane apparatus

Hale iron stain
half-normal solution
halisteresis phenomenon
Haller ansa
Haller cell
Haller, glands of
Hallopeau disease
halo melanoma
halo nevus
Ham acidified serum test
Ham F-10 solution
hamartoma
hamartoma of glial tissue
hamartomatous
hamate bone
hamate, capitate
hamate facet
hamatein test
Hamburger phenomenon
Hamdi solution
Hamel test for jaundice
Hammarsten test for globulin
hammock ligament
hamster egg penetration assay
hamstring tendon
hand
   articulations of
   digital artery of
   phalanges of
H&E (hematoxylin and eosin) stain
hand eczema
hand, foot, and mouth disease
H&H (hemoglobin and hematocrit)
hand muscle
hand, phalanges of joints of
Hand-Schüller-Christian disease
hanging drop preparation
Hanks buffer
Hanks stain
Hannover canal
Hansel stain
Hansen bacillus

Hansen disease
Hantaan virus
Hantavirus
Hantavirus pulmonary syndrome
   (HPS)
hapten inhibition test
haptoglobin (Hp)
hardened pelvis
hardening of arteries
Harder gland
Harding and Ruttan test for
   acetoacetic acid
hardness scale
hard palate
hard stool
harelip
Hargraves cell
harlequin fetus
Harris and Ray test
Harris band
Harrison spot test for bilirubin in urine
Hartmann point
Hartmann pouch
Hartnup disease
Hart test for oxybutyric acid in urine
Hashimoto disease
Hashimoto thyroiditis
Hassall corpuscle
HAT (hypoxanthine, aminopterin,
   thymidine) medium
HATTS (hemagglutination treponemal
   test for syphilis) test
haunch bone
haustra
haustral fold
haustral markings
haustral pattern
haustral pouch
haustrum (pl. haustra)
HAV (hepatitis A virus)
Haverhill fever
Havers gland

haversian canal
haversian gland
haversian system
Hayem solution
hay fever
Hay test for bile salts
Hb, Hgb (hemoglobin)
HbAg (hepatitis B antigen)
H band
HB$_c$Ab (hepatitis B core antibody)
HB$_c$Ag (hepatitis B core antigen)
HB$_e$Ab (hepatitis B "e" antibody)
HB$_e$Ag (hepatitis B "e" antigen)
HBIg (hepatitis B immunoglobulin)
HB$_s$Ab (hepatitis B surface antibody)
HB$_s$Ag (hepatitis B surface antigen)
HBV (hepatitis B virus)
HbF (fetal hemoglobin)
HCG, hCG (human chorionic
    gonadotropin)
HCl (hydrochloric acid)
HCO$_3$ (bicarbonate)
HCT (hematocrit)
H disk
HDL (high density lipoprotein)
HDL cholesterol (HDLC)
HDVAg (hepatitis D virus antigen)
head
head louse (pl. lice)
head of femur
head of pancreas
head of rib
"head post" (examination of brain)
Heaf test
healing ulcer
hearing loss
heart
    aortic opening of
    apex of
    artificial
    coronary artery of
    degeneration of

heart *(continued)*
    diaphragmatic surface of
    enlargement of
    fatty
    horizontal
    inferior border of
    inflammation of
    left
    left border of
    left ventricle of
    myxedema of
    right
    right border of
    right ventricle of
    sternocostal surface of
    superior border of
    vertical
heart clot
heart disease cell
heart failure cells
heart failure classification
heart lesion cell
heart-lung transplant
heart muscle
heart-shaped pelvis
heart transplant
heat capacity
heat coagulation test
heat edema
heat, injury due to
heat instability test
heat labile
heat-labile protein
heat shock protein
heat-stable
heavy chain disease, alpha
heavy metal poisoning
heavy metal screening test
Hebra prurigo
Hecht pneumonia
heckle cell
hectogram (hg)

hectoliter (hL)
hectomole (hmol)
Hector, tendon of (heel tendon)
Hedley technique of tissue preparation
heel bone
heel tendon
heelstick
Heidenhain cell
Heidenhain iron hematoxylin
Heidenhain pouch
Heidenhain stain
Heinz body stain
Heinz cytoplasmic inclusion bodies
Hektoen, Kretschmer, and Welker
    protein
Hektoen phenomenon
HeLa cell
helical bacterium
helicine artery
Helicobacter pylori
Helicobacter pylori urease test
Heller test for albumin in urine
Heller test for blood in urine
Helly fixative
Helly Zenker-formalin solution
helmet cell
Helmholtz axis ligament
helminthic abscess
helper (T4) cell
helper/inducer T cell
helper lymphocytes
helper/suppressor cell ratio
helper T cell
helper virus
hemadsorbing virus
hemadsorption
hemadsorption test
hemadsorption virus
    type 1 (HA1 v.)
    type 2 (HA2 v.)
hemagglutination inhibition (HAI, HI)
    test

hemagglutination treponemal test for
    syphilis (HATTS)
hemal canal
hemal gland
hemal lymph gland
hemalum
hemalum stain
hemangioendothelioma
hemangioma
    capillary
    cavernous
    racemose
    sclerosing
    senile
    spider
    strawberry
    verrucous
hemangioma planum extensum
hemangiomatous nodule
hemapoiesis (hematopoiesis)
hemarthrosis
hematin test for blood
hematemesis
Hematest
hemarthrosis
hematocrit ("crit") (HCT, Hct)
hematogenous abscess
hematogenous embolism
hematogenous jaundice
hematogenous metastasis
hematogenous osteomyelitis
hematogenous pigment
hematogenous proteinuria
hematogenous pyelonephritis
hematogenous tuberculosis
hematohyaloid degeneration
hematoidin
hematologic malignancy
hematology
hematoma
    chronic subdural
    corpus luteum

hematoma *(continued)*
   encapsulated subdural
   epidural
   intramural
   organized
   subdural
   wound
hematoma formation
hematopoiesis, extramedullary
hematopoietic malignancy
hematopoietic tissue
hematoxylin
   Boehmer
   Delafield
   Gill
   Harris
   iron
   phosphotungstic acid (PTAH)
hematoxylin and eosin (H&E) stain
hematoxylin–malachite green–basic
   fuchsin stain
hematoxylin–phloxine B stain
hematuria
   acute onset
   benign recurrent
   endemic
   essential
   false
   functional
   gross
   macroscopic
   microscopic
   painful
   painless
   persistent
   primary
   renal
   terminal
   total
   urethral
   vesical
heme iron

heme-negative stool
heme-positive stool
hemiazygos vein, accessory
hemicolon
hemidiaphragm
hemin test for blood
hemisphere
   cerebellar
   cerebral
   dominant
   left
   right
hemivertebra
hemoaccess
hemoagglutination
hemobilia
hemobilinuria
hemocatheresis
hemocatheretic
Hemoccult guaiac test for occult blood
hemocholecyst
hemocholecystitis
hemochromatosis
hemoconcentration
hemoculture
hemocytometer
hemoglobin (Hb, Hgb)
   aberrant
   Bart abnormal
   defective synthesis of
   fetal
   free
   glycated
   glycosylated
   mean corpuscular
   oxygenated
   plasma
   pyridoxilated stroma-free (SFHb)
   reduced
   serial
   serum
   sickle cell

hemoglobin *(continued)*
   target cell
   unstable
   urinary
hemoglobin A
hemoglobin A_{1c}
hemoglobin A_2
hemoglobin and hematocrit (H&H)
hemoglobin anti-Lepore
hemoglobin-binding capacity
hemoglobin breakdown
hemoglobin C
hemoglobin Chesapeake
hemoglobin Constant Spring
hemoglobin D
hemoglobin disease
hemoglobin E
hemoglobin electrophoresis
hemoglobin F (fetal hemoglobin)
hemoglobin Gower-1
hemoglobin Gower-2
hemoglobin H (HbH)
hemoblobin I
hemoglobin J
hemoglobin Kansas
hemoglobin Lepore
hemoglobin M
hemoglobinometer
hemoglobinopathy, hereditary
hemoglobin Portland
hemoglobin Rainier
hemoglobin S
hemoglobin test
hemoglobinuria
   bacillary
   paroxysmal cold
   paroxysmal nocturnal
hemoglobin Yakima
hemogram
hemolymph gland
hemolymphatic cells
hemolymphatic system

hemolymphatic tissue
hemolysin
   beta
   cold
hemolysis
hemolytic anemia
hemolytic disease of newborn
hemolytic malaria
hemolytic reaction
hemolytic-uremic syndrome
hemolyze
hemolyzed blood
hemolyzed red blood cells
hemolyzing antibody
hemopericardium
hemoperitoneum
hemophilia A
hemophilia B
hemophilia, classical
hemophilic joint
hemoptysis
hemorrhage
   epidural
   extradural
   focal
   frank
   interstitial
   intra-alveolar
   punctate
   salmon-patch
   severe
   stromal
   subarachnoid
   subdural
   subserosal
hemorrhagic colitis
hemorrhagic consolidation of lung
hemorrhagic cyst
hemorrhagic cystitis
hemorrhagic dengue
hemorrhagic effusion
hemorrhagic encephalitis

hemorrhagic fever
hemorrhagic gastritis
hemorrhagic infarct
hemorrhagic malaria
hemorrhagic myelitis
hemorrhagic necrosis
hemorrhagic necrosis of alveolar septa
hemorrhagic nephritis
hemorrhagic pericarditis
hemorrhagic plague
hemorrhagic pleurisy
hemorrhagic salpingitis
hemorrhagic shock
hemorrhagic telangiectasia
hemorrhagic tendency
hemorrhoidal artery
hemorrhoidal plexus
hemorrhoid
   external
   internal
   thrombosed
hemosiderin granule
hemosiderin in hepatocytes
hemosiderin-laden macrophage
hemosiderin test
hemosiderosis
hemothorax
HEMPAS cell
Henderson-Hasselbach equation
Henke space
Henke triangle
Henke trigone
Henle, ampulla of
Henle ansa
Henle canal
Henle gland
Henle loop
Henoch-Schönlein purpura
Henoch-Schönlein syndrome
Hensen canal
Hensen cell
Hensen disk

Hensing ligament
heparin anticoagulant
heparin lock flush solution
heparin therapy, monitoring of
hepatic abscess
hepatic architecture
hepatic arterial infusion (HAI)
hepatic artery
hepatic atrophy
hepatic bed
hepatic calculus
hepatic capsule
hepatic carcinoma
hepatic cirrhosis
hepatic coma
hepatic cord
hepatic degeneration
hepatic duct
hepatic encephalopathy
hepatic failure
hepatic flexure
hepatic function test
hepatic gland
hepatic glycogen storage
hepatic hilum
hepatic ligament
hepatic lobular parenchyma
hepatic lobule
hepatic lymph node
hepatic necrosis
hepatic nerve plexus
hepatic obstruction
hepatic osteomalacia
hepatic outflow tract
hepatic parenchyma
hepatic parenchymal cell
hepatic porphyria
hepatic-renal angle
hepatic segment of liver
hepatic sinusoid
hepatic triad
hepatic vein

hepatic venous outflow
hepatic web
hepatitis
  acute parenchymatous
  alcoholic
  autoimmune
  chronic active
  chronic persisting
  coinfection with
  enterically transmitted, non-A,
    non-B (ET-NANB)
  familial
  fulminant
  giant cell
  infectious
  neonatal
  non-A, non-B (NANB)
  plasma cell
  post-transfusion
  serum
  subacute
  testing
  toxic
  transfusion
  viral
hepatitis A
hepatitis associated antigen (HAA)
hepatitis A virus (HAV)
hepatitis B
hepatitis B antigen (HBAg)
hepatitis B core antibody (HB_cAb)
hepatitis B core antigen (HB_cAg)
hepatitis B e antibody (HB_eAb)
hepatitis B e antigen (HB_eAg)
hepatitis B hyperimmune globulin
hepatitis B immunoglobulin (HBIg)
hepatitis B surface antibody (HB_sAb)
hepatitis B surface antigen (HB_sAg)
hepatitis B virus (HBV)
hepatitis C
hepatitis C virus
hepatitis D (delta) virus (HDV)

hepatitis D virus antigen (HDVAg)
hepatitis E
hepatitis E virus
hepatization
hepatobiliary
hepatobiliary tree
hepatocarcinoma
hepatocellular carcinoma
hepatocellular jaundice
hepatocolic ligament
hepatocystocolic ligament
hepatocyte
hepatoduodenal ligament
hepatoduodenal-peritoneal reflection
hepatoerythropoietic porphyria (HEP)
hepatoesophageal ligament
hepatogastric duodenal ligament
hepatogastric ligament
hepatogenous jaundice
hepatogenous pigment
hepatoiminodiacetic acid (HIDA)
hepatolenticular degeneration
hepatomegaly
hepatopancreatic ampulla, sphincter of
hepatopancreatic fold
hepatophrenic ligament
hepatopleural fistula
hepatorenal angle
hepatorenal pouch
hepatorenal recess
hepatosplenomegaly
hepatoumbilical ligament
HEp-Z cell culture preparation
hereditary abetalipoproteinemia
hereditary adult-onset leukodystrophy
hereditary alopecia
hereditary angioneurotic edema
hereditary cerebral leukodystrophy
hereditary elliptocytosis
hereditary factor
hereditary hemoglobinopathy
hereditary hemolytic anemia

hereditary hemorrhagic telangiectasia
hereditary methemoglobinemia
hereditary optic neuritis
hereditary spherocytosis
hereditary telangiectasia
Herellea vaginicola (now
    Acinetobacter calcoaceticus)
Hering, canal of
Hering duct
Hermann fixative
hermaphroditism, true
hernia
    diaphragmatic
    direct inguinal
    esophageal
    femoral
    hiatal
    incarcerated
    incarceration of
    indirect inguinal
    inguinal
    peritoneal
    strangulated
    strangulation of
    umbilical
    ventral
hernial aneurysm
hernial canal
hernia sac
herniated disk
herniated nucleus pulposus
herpangina virus
herpes
    genital
    orofacial
    traumatic
    wrestler's
herpes circinatus bullosus
herpes genitalis
herpes gestationis
herpes simplex
herpes simplex virus (HSV)

herpes ulcer
herpesvirus
    type 1
    type 2
    type 3
    type 4 (Epstein-Barr virus)
    type 5 (cytomegalovirus)
    type 6
herpes whitlow
herpes zoster
herpes zoster auricularis
herpes zoster virus (HZV)
herpetic fever
herpetic stomatitis
herpetiform
Herzberg test
Hess capillary test
Hesselbach ligament
Hesselbach triangle
heterocrine gland
heteroduplex
heterogeneous
heterologous protein
heterologous tissue
heteromeric cell
heterophil
heterophile agglutination
heterophile agglutination test
heterophile antibodies
heterophile titer
heterophilic leukocyte
heterotopic pancreas
heterotopic pregnancy
heterotopic tissue
heterozygosity
hexagonal cell
hexamer
hexosaminidase A
hexosaminidase A deficiency
Hey ligament
hg (hectogram)
H gene

hGH (human growth hormone)
HI, HAI (hemagglutination inhibition) test
5-HIAA (5-hydroxyindoleacetic acid)
hiatal (or hiatus) hernia
hiatus
 aortic
 esophageal
 fallopian
 semilunar
 sternocostal
Hib (*H. influenzae* type b)
hibernating gland
Hickey-Hare test for diabetes insipidus
hidradenitis suppurativa
hidradenoma
high density lipoprotein (HDL)
highest genicular artery
highest intercostal artery
highest thoracic artery
highest turbinated bone
high frequency blood group
high-grade malignancy
high-grade surface osteosarcoma
Highmore, antrum cardiacum of
high normal
high normal test result
high-performance liquid chromatography
high power
high-power field (hpf)
high-pressure liquid chromatography
 (HPLC)
hilar cells
hilar cell tumor of ovary
hilar lymph node
hilar plate
hilar vessel
hila (pl. of hilum)
hila of kidneys
hila of lung
Hildebrandt test for urobilin in urine

Hill-Sachs lesion
hilum (pl. hila) (formerly hilus)
 hepatic
 lips of
 renal
 splenic
hilum of kidney
hilum of lung
hilus cell
hindgut
Hines-Brown cold pressor test
hinge joint
Hinton test
hip articulation
hip joint
hippocampus, Hirano bodies in the
Hirano bodies in the hippocampus
Hirschfeld canal
Hirsch-Peiffer stain
Hirschsprung disease
hirsutism
His
 angle of
 atrioventricular node of
 atrioventricular opening of
 bundle of
His band
His bundle
His canal
His duct
His space
Hiss capsule stain
Histalog test
histamine flare test
histidine loading test
histidine-rich glycoproteins (HRGP)
histidyl-tRNA synthetase
histiocyte
 cardiac
 hyperplasia of
 sea-blue
 wandering

histiocytes in neurons
histiocytic lymphoma
histiocytoma
  benign fibrous
  malignant fibrous
histiocytosis
  nonlipid
  sinus
histochemistry
histochromatosis
histoclastic
histoclinical evaluation
histocompatibility gene
histocompatible
histocyte (histiocyte)
histodiagnosis
histodialysis
histodifferentiation
Histofine SAB-PO kit
histogenesis
histogenous
histohematogenous
histohydria
histohypoxia
histokinesis
histologic diagnosis
histologic lesion
histologic specimen
histology
Histopaque
Histopaque-1077 isolation reagent
histopathological diagnosis
histopathology
Histoplasma capsulatum
Histoplasma capsulatum antigen
  (HPA)
Histoplasma myocarditis
histoplasmin-latex test
histoplasmosis
His zone
HIV (human immunodeficiency virus)
HIVAGEN test

HIV antibody
HIV antibody test on blood
HIV Blot 2•2 test
HIV classification of children
HIV encephalitis
HIV encephalopathy
HIV-negative
HIV-positive
HIV proteins
hives
hL (hectoliter)
HLA (human lymphocyte antigen)
hmol (hectomole)
hobnail cell
hobnailed appearance of liver surface
Hoboken nodule
hockey stick
Hodgkin cell
Hodgkin disease
Hodgkin granuloma
Hodgkin lymphoma
Hoehn and Yahr staging of Parkinson
  disease
Hofbauer cell
Hoffmann atrophy
Hoffmann duct
Hoffmann test for tyrosine
Hofmann bacillus
Hofmeister test for leucine
holandric gene
Hollander gastric function test
Hollande solution
Hollenhorst plaque
Holl ligament
hollow bone
hollow needle
hollow structure
hollow viscus
Holmes silver nitrate
Holmgrén-Golgi canal
holocrine gland
holoprotein

Holz phlegmon
Holzer method
homeobox gene
homeotic gene
Homer-Wright rosette
homocystine test
homogenate
homogeneity
homogeneous casts in urine
homogeneous composition
homogeneous fluorescence
homogeneous material
homogeneous medium
homogentisic acid
homogentisic acid oxidase
homogentisic acid oxidase deficiency
homogentisuria
homoglandular
homologous protein
homologous tissue
homologue
homovanillic acid (HVA)
homozygous typing cell (HTC)
honeycombed appearance
honeycomb pattern
honeymoon cystitis
hood of cervix
hooked bone
Hooker-Forbes test
hookworm disease
Hopkins-Cole test for protein
Hopkins thiophene test for lactic acid
Hopman criteria for counting nuclei
Hopmann polyp
Hoppe-Seyler test
hordeolum
horizontal cells of Cajal
horizontal cells of retina
horizontal fissure
horizontal fissure of lung
horizontal heart
horizontal plane, Frankfort

Hormiscium dermatitidis
Hormodendrum dermatitidis
hormonal factors
hormone
  adipokinetic
  adrenocorticotropic (ACTH)
  adrenotropic
  aldosterone
  aldosterone steroid
  androgenic
  angiotensin II
  anterior pituitary-like
  antidiuretic (ADH)
  antigonadotropic
  atrial natriuretic (ANH)
  cardiac
  chemotactic sexual
  chorionic gonadotropic
  chorionic growth
  chromatophorotropic
  cortical
  corticotropic
  corticotropin-releasing
  cortisol
  cortisol steroid
  deoxycortisol
  diabeticogenic
  erythropoietic
  estradiol
  estriol
  estrogenic
  female
  follicle-stimulating (FSH)
  follicle-stimulating hormone-
    releasing (FSH-HR)
  follicular
  galactopoietic
  gametokinetic
  gastrin
  gastrointestinal
  glucagon
  gonadotropin-releasing (Gn-RH)

hormone *(continued)*
  growth
  growth hormone-releasing
    (GH-RH)
  human placental lactogen
  inappropriate antidiuretic
  inhibiting
  insulin
  interstitial cell-stimulating
  lactation
  lactogenic
  lipid-mobilizing
  lipotropic
  local
  luteinizing (LH)
  luteinizing hormone-releasing
    (LH-RH, LRH)
  luteotropic
  mammotropic
  melanocyte-stimulating
  melanotropin release-inhibiting
    (MIH)
  melanotropin-releasing (MRH)
  neurotropic
  ovarian
  pancreatic
  parathormone
  parathyroid (PTH)
  pineal
  pituitary
  pituitary gonadotropic
  placental lactogen
  progestational
  progesterone
  progesterone steroid
  prolactin
  prolactin anterior pituitary
  prolactin-inhibiting
  prolactin-releasing
  prolactoliberin
  proparathyroid
  releasing (RH)

hormone *(continued)*
  renin
  salivary gland
  sex
  somatomedin-C polypeptide
  somatotropic (STH)
  somatotropin release-inhibiting
    (SIH)
  somatotropin-releasing (SRH)
  steroid
  sympathetic
  testicular
  test on venous blood for
  testosterone
  testosterone steroid
  thyroid
  thyroid-stimulating (TSH)
  thyrotropic
  thyrotropin-releasing (TRH)
  thyroxine (T_4)
  tissue
  triiodothyronine (T_3)
  tropic
  vasopressin
hormone assay
hormone-dependent neoplasm
hormone levels
hormonelike substances
hormone receptor protein analysis
hormonosis
horn
  cicatricial
  cutaneous
  frontal
  lateral
  meniscal
  projectile
  uterine
  ventral
horn cell
horn cyst formation
Horner-Trantas dots

hornification
horn of Ammon
horn of uterus
horn pearl
horn pearl formation
horny cell
horseradish peroxidase
horseshoe crab (*Limulus polyphemus*)
horseshoe kidney
horseshoe placenta
horseshoe-shaped nucleus
horseshoe-shaped syncytium
Horsley test for glucose
Hortega cell
Hortega neuroglia stain
host cell
hot abscess
hot nodule
hour (hr)
hourglass gallbladder
hourglass pattern
hourglass stomach
House-Brackmann facial weakness
housekeeping gene
housemaid's knee
Houston, valve of
Howard test for renal function
Howell-Jolly body
Howell test for prothrombin
Howship lacuna
Hoyer canal
HPA (*Histoplasma capsulatum* antigen)
hpf (high power field)
HPV (human papillomavirus)
HPV genotyping procedure
hr. (hour)
H_2 (histamine 2)
H_2 receptor antagonist
HRGP (histidine-rich glycoproteins)
HTLV I and II (human T cell lymphoma virus)
H-type fistula

Hucker-Conn stain
Huddleson agglutination test for brucellosis
Hueck ligament
Hugh-Curtis-Fitz syndrome
Huguier canal
Huhner test
human antihemophilic factor
human chorionic gonadotropin (HCG, hCG)
human herpesvirus 3 (and 4)
human immunodeficiency virus (HIV)
human intestinal roundworm
human lymphocyte antigen (HLA)
human papillomavirus (HPV) infection
human parvovirus B19
human placental lactogen hormone
human T cell leukemia virus (HTLV)
human T cell lymphotropic virus type I (HTLV-I)
human T cell lymphotropic virus type II (HTLV-II)
humeral articulation
humeral circumflex artery
humeral joint
humeral mechanism
humeroradial joint
humeroulnar articulation
humeroulnar joint
humerus
humerus varus
humor
  aqueous
  plasmoid
  vitreous
humoral immunity
Humphry ligament
hunger osteopathy
hunger swelling
Hunner ulcer
Hunt and Hess neurological classification

Hunter canal
Hunter ligament
Hunter line
Hunter-Schreger band
Huntington chorea
Huppert-Cole test for bile pigments
Huppert test for bile pigments
Hurler syndrome
Hürthle cell
Hürthle cell adenoma
Hürthle cell carcinoma
Hürthle cell metaplasia
Hürthle cell tumor
Hurtley test for acetoacetic acid
Huschke, auditory teeth of
Huschke canal
Huschke ligament
Hutchinson plaque
Hutchinson melanotic freckle
Hutchinson teeth
HV (herpesvirus)
HVA (homovanillic acid)
hyalin
    alcoholic
    eosinophilic
    hematogenous
    Mallory
    protein
hyaline articular cartilage
hyaline body, Mallory
hyaline cartilage
hyaline casts in urine
hyaline change in renal glomeruli
hyaline degeneration
hyaline membrane
hyaline membrane disease (HMD)
hyaline necrosis
hyalinization
hyalocapsular ligament
hyaloid artery
hyaloid canal
hyaloid corpuscle

Hyams grade of esthesioneuroblastoma
hybridization
    blot-dot
    chromosome in situ
    dot-blot
    fluorescence in situ (FISH)
    Northern
hydatid
    alveolar
    sessile
    Virchow
hydatid cyst
hydatid cyst disease
hydatid disease of liver
hydatid of Morgagni
hydatid polyp
hydatid pregnancy
hydatidiform
hydatidiform mole
hydroa herpetiforme
hydrocele
hydrocelectomy
hydrocephalus
hydrochloric acid (HCl)
hydrochloric acid test
hydrogen breath test
hydrogen ion
hydrogen peroxide test for blood
hydrogen sulfide poisoning
hydrolysate, protein
hydronephrosis
hydropericardium
hydrophilic gel
hydropic degeneration
hydropic degeneration of chorionic
    tissues
hydropic degeneration of myocardial
    fibers
hydrops
hydrothorax
hydroureter
hydroxybutyric acid test

hydroxycorticoid (HC, HOC)
17-hydroxycorticosteroids (17-OHCS)
5-hydroxyindole acetic acid (5-HIAA)
    test
hydroxylamine modification
hydroxylamine test for glucose
17-hydroxyprogesterone (17-OHP)
hydroxyproline
25-hydroxyvitamin D assay (25-OH-D)
hymen
    denticulate
    imperforate
hymenal caruncles
Hymenolepis nana
hyoepiglottic ligament
hyoglossus muscle
hyoid arch
hyoid artery
hyoid bone
hyparterial bronchus
hyperadrenocorticism
hyperaldosteronism
hyperazotemia
hyperbetalipoproteinemia
hyperbilirubinemia
hypercalcemia
hypercapnia
hypercarbia
hypercatabolism
hypercellular
hyperchloremia
hypercholesterolemia
hyperchromasia
hyperchromatic cell
hyperchromatic nuclei
hyperchromatism
hyperchromia
hypercoagulable state
hyperelastosis cutis
hyperemia
    active
    passive

hyperemic
hyperferremia
hypergammaglobulinemia
hyperglobulinemia
hyperglobulinemic purpura
hyperglycemia
hyperglycemic-glycogenolytic factor
hyperglycosuria
hypergranulosis
hyper-IgE syndrome
hyperimmune
hyperinflated
hyperinsulinar obesity
hyperinsulinism
hyperinterrenal obesity
hyperkalemia
hyperkeratosis
    epidermolytic
    follicular
hyperkeratotic papilloma
hyperkeratotic plaque
hyperketonemia
hyperketonuria
hyperlipidemia
    carbohydrate-induced
    combined fat- and carbohydrate-
        induced
    endogenous
    exogenous
    essential familial
    familial
    fat-induced
    mixed
hypermagnesemia
hypermelanosis
hypermenorrhea
hypermobile kidney
hypernatremia
hypernephroma
hyperosmolality
hyperosmolar nonketotic coma
hyperostosis

hyperparathyroidism (HPT)
hyperphenylalaninemia
  malignant
  transient
hyperphosphatemia
hyperpigmentation, blotchy facial
hyperpituitarism
hyperplasia
  adaptive
  adenomatous
  adrenocortical
  angiolymphoid
  basal epithelial
  benign prostatic
  bile duct epithelium
  C-cell
  compensatory
  congenital adrenal (CAH)
  cutaneous lymphoid
  endometrial
  epidermal
  epithelial
  fibrous tissue
  focal nodular (FNH)
  follicular
  giant follicular
  histiocytes
  intravascular papillary endothelial
  lipoid adrenal
  lymphoid
  marrow
  microglandular
  mucosal
  neoplastic
  nodular adrenal
  nodular lymphoid
  nodular regenerative
  parathyroid
  pituitary
  prostatic
  pseudoepitheliomatous
  reactive

hyperplasia *(continued)*
  sebaceous
  sinus
  splenic
  Swiss-cheese
  thymus
  thyroid
  verrucous
hyperplasmic obesity
hyperplastic-appearing synovium
hyperplastic arteriolar nephrosclerosis
hyperplastic-hypertrophic obesity
hyperplastic inflammation
hyperplastic marrow
hyperplastic polyp
hyperplastic pulpitis
hyperplastic tissue
hyperpotassemia
hyperreflexia
hypersegmented neutrophil
hypersensitivity myocarditis
hypersensitivity pneumonia
hypersensitivity reaction
hypertension (HT)
  accelerated
  adrenal
  arterial (AH)
  benign intracranial (BIH)
  borderline
  essential (EH)
  Goldblatt
  idiopathic
  intracranial
  labile
  malignant
  ocular
  portal
  postpartum
  primary
  pulmonary
  renal
  renovascular

hypertension *(continued)*
  secondary
  splenovascular
  vascular
hypertensive lower esophageal
  sphincter
hypertonic
hypertonicity
hypertrichosis
hypertriglyceridemia
hypertrophic cardiomyopathy
hypertrophic gastritis
hypertrophic obesity
hypertrophic osteoarthropathy
hypertrophic pulmonary osteoarthropathy
hypertrophic scar
hypertrophic scarring
hypertrophic villi
hypertrophy
  bladder
  biventricular
  clitoral
  compensatory
  complementary
  epiphyseal
  functional
  myocardial
  physiologic
  smooth-muscle
  ventricular
  villous
  virginal
hyperuricemia
hyperventilation
hypesthesia
hypha (pl. hyphae)
  aseptate
  brown distorted
  multiseptate
  sterile
hyphae in bronchi

hyphae in nail
hyphae in scrapings
hyphae in stratum corneum
hyphae in tissues
hypoalbuminemia
hypocalcemia
hypocapnia
hypocellular
hypochloremia
hypochloremic alkalosis
hypochondriac fossa
hypochondriac region
hypochromia
hypochromic anemia
hypochromic microcytic anemia
hypodermic needle
hypodermis
hypoferremia
hypofibrinolysis
hypogammaglobulinemia
hypogastric artery
hypogastric nerve
hypogastric plexus
hypogastric region
hypogastrium
hypoglossal canal
hypoglossal nerve
hypoglossal nerve of tongue
hypoglossal trigone
hypoglycemia
hypogonad obesity
hypogonadism
hypokalemia
hypokalemic alkalosis
hypokalemic nephrosis
hypomagnesemia
hyponatremia, dilutional
hypo-osmolality
hypoparathyroidism
hypophamine, alpha-
hypopharynx
hypophosphatasia

hypophosphatemia
hypophysial (also, hypophyseal)
hypophysial artery
hypophysial fossa
hypophysial pouch
hypophysis
hypophysis cerebri
hypopigmentation
hypopituitarism
hypoplasia
hypoplasia of dental enamel
hypoplasmic obesity
hypoplastic anemia
hypoplastic lip
hypoplastic lung
hypopotassemia
hypoprothrombinemia
hypopyon
hyporeninemia
hyporrhea
hyposalemia
hyposecretion
hyposmolarity
hyposomatotropism
hypospadias
hypostasis, postmortem

hypostatic abscess
hypostatic bronchopneumonia
hypostatic congestion
hypostatic pneumonia
hyposthenuria
hypotension
hypotensive
hypothalamus
hypothenar eminence
hypothyroidism
hypothyroid obesity
hypotonic bladder
hypotonicity
hypotrichiasis
hypovolemia
hypovolemic shock
hypoxemia
hypoxia, fetal
hypoxic encephalopathy
hypsiloid ligament
Hyrtl loop
Hyrtl sphincter
hysterectomy
hysterical joint
hysteric pregnancy
HZV (herpes zoster virus)

I, i

IAPP (islet amyloid polypeptide)
iatrogenic disease
iatrogenic hyperthyroidism
iatrogenic infection
iatrogenic injury
I band
IBAS 1&2 image analyzer system
I blood group
ICA (islet cell antibody screening)
I cell (inclusion cell)
ice water calorics
ichorous pleurisy
ichorous pus
ichthyosis
icing liver
ICP (intracranial pressure) catheter
icteric
icterohemorrhagic fever
icterus index
ID (immunodiffusion)
identification of specimen
idiocy, amaurotic familial
idiogenesis
idioheteroagglutinin
idioheterolysin
idioisoagglutinin
idiopathic abnormality

idiopathic abortion
idiopathic disease
idiopathic hypertension
idiopathic hypertrophic osteo-
    arthropathy
idiopathic interstitial fibrosis
idiopathic myocarditis
idiopathic thrombocytopenic purpura
    (ITP)
idiotypic antibodies
I disk
Ig (immunoglobulin)
IgA immunoglobulin
IgD immunoglobulin
IgE immunoglobulin
IgG immunoglobulin
IgM anti-HAV antibody
IgM anti-HBc antibody
IgM antibody
IgM antibody capture enzyme
    immunoassay (MAC EIA)
IgM immunoglobulin
Ig2b kappa monoclonal antibody
ileal artery
ileal crypt
ileal inflow tract
ileal margin

ileal mucosa
ileal spout
ileitis, regional
ileoanal pouch
ileocecal edema
ileocecal fold
ileocecal junction
ileocecal orifice
ileocecal pouch
ileocecal recess
ileocecal valve
ileocolic artery
ileocolic cecal artery
ileocolic fold
ileocolic vein
ileum
    antimesenteric border of distal
    mesentery of
    terminal
ileus
    adynamic
    adynamic/paralytic
    dynamic
    dynamic/spastic
    paralytic
    spastic
iliac artery
iliac bone
iliac canal
iliac circumflex artery
iliac colon
iliac crest
iliac fascia
iliac fossa
iliac lymph node
iliac node
iliac plaque
iliac spine
iliac tubercle
iliacus muscle
iliococcygeal muscle
iliofemoral articulation

iliofemoral ligament
iliopectineal ligament
iliopsoas muscle
iliopsoas muscle abscess
iliopsoas ring
iliopubic eminence
iliosacral articulation
iliotibial band
iliotibial ligament of Maissiat
iliotrochanteric ligament
ilium bone
illumination
Ilosvay test for nitrites
IMA (inferior mesenteric artery)
imaging, diagnostic
ImM citrate buffer
immature bone
immature cell
    red blood
    white blood
immature neutrophils
immature red blood cells
immediate transfusion
immersion
imminent abortion
immobilization of bone by casting
immobilization of bone by splinting
immobilization test
immovable articulation
immovable joint
immune adhesion test
immune complex
immune complex assay
immune deficiency
immune protein
immune response gene
immune thrombocytopenic purpura
immunity
    cellular
    humoral
immunoassay, IgM antibody capture
    enzyme (MAC EIA)

immunoblastic sarcoma
immunoblot
immunoblot procedure
immunoblotting
immunocheck fluorosphere
immunocyte
immunocytochemical
immunocytochemistry
immunodeficiency disorder
immunodiffusion (ID), radial
immunoelectrophoresis
immunofixation
immunofluorescence
  direct
  indirect
immunofluorescent stain
immunogenetic factors
immunoglobulin (Ig)
  anti-D
  chickenpox
  failure to form
  IgA
  IgD
  IgE
  IgM
  monoclonal
immunoglobulin A (IgA)
immunoglobulin D (IgD)
immunoglobulin G (IgG)
immunoglobulin G/albumin ratio
immunoglobulin G synthesis rate
immunoglobulin M (IgM)
immunogold technique
immunohistochemical staining
immunohistochemistry
immunologically activated cell
immunologically competent cell
immunologic diffusion procedure
immunologic pregnancy test
immunology
immunopanning parallel method of cell
  separation

immunoperoxidase
immunoperoxidase stain
immunoperoxidase test
immunophenotypic analysis
immunoreactivity
impacted fetus
impacted fracture
impacted stool
impaction lesion
impaired excretion of conjugated
  bilirubin
impaired platelet function
impaired wound healing
imperfecta, osteogenesis
imperforate anus
imperforate hymen
impetigo, Bockhart
impetigo neonatorum
impetigo of newborn, bullous
impetiginization
IMViC metabolic tests
inadequate luteal phase
inanition
inanition fever
inapparent infection
inappropriate antidiuretic hormone
incarcerated placenta
incarceration of hernia
incarceration of loop of intestine
incasing cell (also encasing)
incise
incised ulcer
incised wound
incision
  diamond-shaped
  recently healed surgical
  spindle-shaped
  thoracoabdominal
  Y-shaped
incisional biopsy
incisive bone
incisive canal

incisive foramen
incisive papilla
incisor angle, Frankfort-mandibular
incisor canal
incisor, central
incisor teeth
incisor tissue
inclusion
   cytoplasmic
   globular cytoplasmic
   mulberry-shaped intracytoplasmic
inclusion blennorrhea
inclusion body, cytoplasmic
inclusion body myositis
inclusion cell
inclusion conjunctivitis
inclusion cyst
   epidermal
   epithelial
   germinal
   germinal epithelial
incompetence, cervical
incompetent cervix
incompetent valve
incomplete abortion
incomplete protein
incomplete resolution of pneumonia
incontinence, melanin
increased blood flow
increased renal excretion of water
incremental line
incretory gland
incubation
incubation with erythrocytes
incubator
incudomalleolar articulation
incudostapedial articulation
incus bone
indeterminate leprosy
index (pl. indices)
   Ameth
   Ayala

index *(continued)*
   cardiac
   centromeric
   erythrocyte
   free thyroxine
   icterus
   karyopyknotic
   leukopenic
   maturation
   mitotic
   nucleoplasmic
   opsonic
   phagocytic
   red blood cell
   red cell
   Robinson
   saturation
   sensitivity
   volume-corrected mitotic
India ink
India ink capsule stain
India ink preparation
Indian childhood cirrhosis
indicator
indices (pl. of index)
indifferent cell
indigo carmine
indigo carmine test for renal
   permeability
indigo red test
indirect antiglobulin test
indirect bilirubin
indirect Coombs test
indirect fluorescent antibody test
indirect hemagglutination test
indirect immunofluorescence
indirect inguinal hernia
indirect radioimmunoassay
indirect-reacting bilirubin
indirect transfusion
indiscrete nodule
indiscriminate lesion

indistinct
indole test
indolent myeloma
indophenol test
induced abortion
induced labor
induced malaria
inducer cell
indurated zone of inflammation
indurated zone of necrosis
induration
  black
  brawny
  brown
  cyanotic
  fibrous
  Froriep
  granular
  gray
  laminate
  parchment
  phlebitic
  plastic
  red
indurative mediastinitis
indurative necrosis
indurative pleurisy
indurative pneumonia
industrial dermatitis
industrial dermatosis
inevitable abortion
infantile eczema
infantile gastroenteritis
infantile pneumonia
infantum, roseola
infarction (also, infarct)
  anemic
  bilirubin
  bone
  Brewer
  calcareous
  cerebral

infarction *(continued)*
  hemorrhagic
  myocardial
  pituitary
  pulmonary
  renal
  septic
  thrombotic
  uric acid
infarcted bowel
infected abortion
infected tissue
infection
  agonal
  airborne
  animal bite
  apical
  bacterial
  candidal
  chronic
  chronic Epstein-Barr virus
  colonization
  community-acquired
  cross
  cryptogenic
  disseminated gonococcal
  dog-bite
  droplet
  dust-borne
  ECHO (enterocytopathogenic
    human orphan) virus
  endogenous
  exogenous
  focal
  fungal
  genital
  germinal
  granulomatous
  human papillomavirus (HPV)
  iatrogenic
  inapparent
  latent

infection *(continued)*
  local
  mass
  mixed
  nosocomial
  ocular
  opportunistic
  postoperative
  preexisting
  pyogenic
  recurrent upper respiratory tract
    (RURTI)
  regional spread of
  rickettsial
  Salinem
  scalp
  secondary
  secondary bacterial
  skin
  subclinical
  suppurative
  systemic
  systemic fungal
  terminal
  TORCH (toxoplasmosis, rubella,
    cytomegalovirus, herpes
    simplex)
  tunnel
  upper respiratory infection (URI
  upper respiratory tract infection
    (URTI)
  urinary tract (UTI)
  vector-borne
  Vincent
  viral
  viral respiratory (VRI)
  water-borne
  wound
infection due to gram-positive bacteria
infection due to rickettsias
infection due to RNA virus
infection due to spirochetes

infectiosum, erythema
infectious arthritis
infectious avian nephrosis
infectious disease
  communicable
  contagious
  transmissible
infectious eczematous dermatitis
infectious granuloma
infectious hepatitis
infectious jaundice
infectious mononucleosis (IM)
infectious myocarditis
infectious myositis
infectious pancreatic necrosis
infectious pancreatic necrosis virus
infectious stomatitis
infectious wart virus
infective embolism
infective endocarditis
infective myocarditis
inferior alveolar artery
inferior artery
inferior border
inferior calcaneonavicular ligament
inferior cardiac branch
inferior cerebellar artery
inferior costal cartilage
inferior deep cervical lymph node
inferior demifacet
inferior dental artery
inferior dental canal
inferior duodenal fold
inferior duodenal recess
inferior epigastric artery
inferior esophageal sphincter
inferior frontal gyrus
inferior gastroduodenal artery
inferior genicular artery
inferior gluteal artery
inferior gluteal nerve
inferior hemorrhoidal artery

inferior hypogastric nerve
inferior labial artery
inferior laryngeal artery
inferior ligament of epididymis
inferior lobe
inferior lobe bronchus
inferior longitudinal muscle of tongue
inferior margin of superior rib
inferior meatus
inferior mesenteric artery (IMA)
inferior mesenteric plexus
inferior nasal concha
inferior orbital fissure
inferior pancreaticoduodenal artery
inferior pelvic aperture
inferior phrenic artery
inferior poles
inferior profunda artery
inferior pubic ligament
inferior pubic rami
inferior pulmonary vein
inferior radioulnar joint
inferior rectal nerve
inferior rectal vein
inferior rib, superior margin of
inferior sagittal sinus
inferior six ribs
inferior surface of pancreas
inferior thoracic aperture
inferior thyroid artery
inferior thyroid, esophageal artery of
inferior tibiofibular joint
inferior tibiofibular ligament, anterior
inferior transverse rectal fold
inferior transverse scapular ligament
inferior turbinated bone
inferior tympanic artery
inferior ulnar collateral artery
inferior vena cava
inferior vesical artery
inferior wall
inferolateral surfaces of prostate

infertility
infiltrating ductal carcinoma
infiltrating plaque
infiltration (also, infiltrate)
  adipose
  calcareous
  calcium
  cellular
  epituberculous
  fatty
  gelatinous
  glycogen
  inflammatory
  lymphocytic
  lymphohistiocytic
  mononuclear cell
  neutrophilic
  paraneural
  parasitic
  perivascular
  perivascular round-cell
  plasmacytic
  punctate
  sanguineous
  serous
  small round cell
  tuberculous
  urinous
infiltration medium
infiltration of calcareous materials
  into tissues
infiltration of tissue specimen
inflame
inflamed tissue
inflammation
  acute phase of
  adhesive
  allergic
  atrophic
  catarrhal
  chronic
  cirrhotic

inflammation *(continued)*
  croupous
  diffuse
  disseminated
  ear
  exudative
  fibrinopurulent
  fibrinous
  fibrosing
  focal
  granulomatous
  hyperplastic
  hypertrophic
  interstitial
  local cutaneous
  metastatic
  necrotic
  obliterative
  parenchymatous
  proliferative
  pseudomembranous
  purulent
  repair phase of
  sclerosing
  serofibrinous
  seroplastic
  serous
  severe
  simple
  skin
  specific
  spleen
  subacute
  suppurative
  thyroid gland
  toxic
  tracheobronchial mucosal
  traumatic
  ulcerative
inflammation artery
inflammation about follicles
inflammation, causes of:

inflammation *(continued)*
  antigen-antibody reaction
  bacteria
  chemical agent
  disease-causing microorganism
  foreign body
  fungus
  parasite
  physical force
  virus
  pathogenic microorganism
  physical injury
  physical or chemical injury
    burning
    crushing
    cutting
    electrical shock
    foreign body
    freezing
    radiation
inflammation esophagus
inflammation features
  heat
  pain
  redness
  swelling
inflammatory atrophy
inflammatory bowel disease
inflammatory carcinoma
inflammatory cells
inflammatory change
inflammatory conditions
  allergic
  infectious
  toxic
  traumatic
inflammatory edema
inflammatory infiltration
inflammatory lymph
inflammatory macrophage
inflammatory myocarditis
inflammatory polyp

inflammatory pseudotumor
inflammatory reaction, smoldering
inflammatory response from living
    tissue
inflammatory response of cell
inflammatory response, self-limited
influenza
influenza virus
influenzal myocarditis
influenzal virus pneumonia
infolding
infraclavicular
infraclinoid aneurysm
infracolic compartment
infracostal artery
infraglottic
infrahepatic vena cava
infrahyoid artery
infraorbital artery
infraorbital canal
infraorbital cheek
infraorbital foramen
infraorbital groove
infrared light
infrascapular artery
infrasternal angle
infrasternal fossa
infratemporal crest
infratemporal fossa
infraumbilical mound
infundibulo-ovarian ligament
infundibulopelvic ligament
infundibulum (pl. infundibula)
infundibulum, ethmoid
infundibulum of bile duct
infundibulum of sebaceous gland
infusion
    brain-heart (BHI)
    hepatic arterial (HAI)
    saline
ingrown hair
inguinal artery

inguinal canal
inguinal crease
inguinal floor
inguinal fold
inguinal granuloma
inguinal hernia
inguinal ligament
inguinal ligament arch
inguinal lymph node
inguinal region
inguinal ring
inguinal triangle
inhalant antigen
inhalational anthrax
inhalation pneumonia
inhalation tuberculosis
inherited malformation syndromes
inhibiting antibody
inhibition factor
inhibition, hemagglutination (HI, HAI)
inhibition reaction
inhibition test
inhibitor
    alpha-trypsin
    plasminogen activator (PAI)
    platelet aggregation
    protein C (PCI)
inhibitory
initial cell
initial diagnosis
initiation factor
injection mass
injection, mucosal
injury, irreversible
inlet of esophagus
inlet, thoracic
inner cell mass
inner ear
inner membrane
innermost coat of the eye
innermost intercostal membrane
inner neural layer

inner table of skull
innocent bystander cell
innominate artery
innominate bone
innominate canaliculus
inoculation
inoculum
inorganic salt
inpacted fracture
INR (international normalized ratio)
insect dermatitis
insertion
   circum-marginate
   eccentric
   velamentous
insipidus, diabetes
in situ, carcinoma
insoluble fibrin
insoluble protein
inspiration, muscle of
inspiratory capacity
inspissated bile in hepatic canaliculi
inspissated feces, mass of
inspissated material
inspissation of semisolid material in
   tubular structure
insufficiency, renal
insula
insular artery
insulin and glucose suppression test
insulin-antagonizing factor
insulin antibody
insulin clearance test
insulin hormone
insulin hypoglycemia test
insulin-like growth factor
insulinoma
insulinopenic diabetes
insulin reaction
insulin tolerance test
insulin, 12-hour-fasting
insulin with oral glucose tolerance test

insult
   metabolic
   toxic
intact membranes
integral protein
integumentary
interalveolar septum
interarticular joint
interatrial groove
interatrial septum
interauricular arch
intercalary cell
intercalated disk
intercapillary cell
intercapital ligament
intercarotid gland
intercarpal articulation
intercarpal joint
intercarpal ligament
intercavernous sinus
intercellular bridge
intercellular canaliculus
intercellular fluid
intercellular lymph
intercellular space
interchondral articulation
interchondral joint
interclavicular ligament
interclinoid ligament
intercondylar eminence
intercornual ligament
intercostal artery
intercostal articulation
intercostal ligaments
intercostal membrane
intercostal muscle
intercostal nerve
intercostal space
intercostal vein
intercostal vessel
intercostobrachial nerve
intercrural fibers

intercuneiform articulation
intercuneiform joint
intercuneiform ligament
interdental canal
interdigitating cells
interface dermatitis
interface, dermoepidermal
interfacial canal
interferon, antiviral
interfollicular cell
interfoveolar ligament
interlacing bundles
interlacing fascicle
interlacing fibers
interlacing tendinous fibers
interlobar artery
interlobular artery of kidney
interlobular artery of liver
interlobular bile duct
interlobular biliary canal
interlobular pleurisy
intermaxillary bone
intermediary metabolism
intermediate atrial artery
intermediate bronchus
intermediate cell
intermediate cuneiform bone
intermediate gland
intermediate leprosy
intermediate lymphocytic lymphoma
intermediate tendon of diaphragm
intermesenteric plexus
intermetacarpal artery
intermetacarpal articulation
intermetacarpal joint
intermetatarsal articulation
intermetatarsal jont
intermittent malaria
intermittent proteinuria
intermixed
intermuscular septum, anal
internal abdominal ring

internal acoustic meatus
internal adhesive pericarditis
internal auditory artery
internal capsule
internal carotid artery
internal clot
internal collateral ligament of wrist
internal elastic membrane
internal hemorrhoid
internal iliac artery
internal iliac lymph node
internal iliac node
internal inguinal ring
internal intercostal membrane
internal intercostal muscle
internal jugular vein
internal malleolar artery
internal mammary artery
internal mammary
internal maxillary artery
internal oblique muscle, aponeurosis of
internal occipital crest
internal occipital protuberance
internal os, cervical
internal palpebral artery
internal pillar cells
internal plantar artery
internal pubic artery
internal pudendal artery
internal pudendal vessel
internal spermatic artery
internal thoracic artery
internal thoracic vessel
internal urethral orifice
internal vertebral plexus
International Classification of Diseases
    for Oncology (ICD-O)
international units (IU)
interosseous artery
interosseous border
interosseous cuneocuboid ligament
interosseous cuneometatarsal ligament

interosseous ligament
interosseous lunotriquetral ligament
interosseous membrane
interosseous metacarpal ligament
interosseous metatarsal ligament
interosseous nerve
interosseous sacroiliac ligament
interosseous talocalcaneal ligament
interosseous tibiofibular ligament
interparietal bone
interpeduncular cistern
interpeduncular fossa
interphalangeal articulation
interphalangeal joint
interscapular gland
intersection, tendinous
intersegmental artery
intersexuality
intersigmoid recess
interspace, dineric
interspersed
interspinous ligament
interspinous plane
intersternebral joint
interstitial atrophy
interstitial cell-stimulating hormone
interstitial cells of Cajal
interstitial cells of Leydig
interstitial cystitis
interstitial deletion
interstitial emphysema
interstitial fibrosis, diffuse
interstitial fluid
interstitial gland
interstitial hemorrhage
interstitial hypertrophic neuritis
interstitial inflammation
interstitial keratitis
interstitial mastitis
interstitial myocarditis
interstitial myositis
interstitial nephritis

interstitial pancreatitis
interstitial pattern
interstitial plasma cell pneumonia
interstitial pneumonia
interstitial pneumonitis
interstitial pregnancy
interstitial pulmonary fibrosis
interstitial salpingitis
interstitial tissue
intertarsal articulation
intertarsal joint
interterritorial matrix
intertrabecular
intertransverse ligament
intertubercular bursitis
intertubercular groove
interureteric fold
interval, fixed time
interval scale
interventricular artery
interventricular foramina
interventricular groove
interventricular septal area
interventricular septum
intervertebral articulation
intervertebral disk, slipped
intervertebral foramen (pl. foramina)
intervertebral joint
intervillous space
intestinal artery
intestinal calculus
intestinal canal
intestinal contents
intestinal gland
intestinal juice
intestinal loop
intestinal lumen
intestinal metaplasia
intestinal mucosa
intestinal obstruction
intestinal parasitism
intestinal ulcer

intestinal villi
intestinal web
intestine
  coils of
  kink in
  large
  malrotation of
  small
intima tunica
intimal
in toto
intoxication
  alcohol
  ethanol
  fluoride
  vitamin D
intra-alveolar hemorrhage
intra-articular ligament
intra-articular plates of fibrocartilage
intra-articular sternocostal ligament
intracartilaginous bone
intracartilaginous ossification
intracavernous aneurysm
intracellular bacteria
intracellular fat in cells of amniotic
  fluid
intracellular fluid
intracellular metabolism
intrachondrial bone
intracortical osteosarcoma
intracranial aneurysm
intracranial hypertension
intracranial pressure (ICP) catheter
intracranial tumor
intracutaneous test
intracutaneous tuberculin test
intracytoplasmic canal
intradermal nevus
intradermal test
intraductal papilloma
intraductal papillomatosis/epitheliosis
intradural abscess

intraepidermal carcinoma of glans
intraepidermal neutrophilic IgA
  dermatosis
intraepithelial gland
intrafollicular space
intrahaustral contraction ring
intrahepatic duct system
intrahepatic biliary duct
intrahepatic radicle
intraligamentary pregnancy
intralobular biliary canal
intraluminal acid mucin
intraluminal embolism
intramastoid abscess
intramembranous bone
intramembranous ossification
intramural fibroid
intramural portion
intramuscular gland of tongue
intraocular malignancy
intraocular melanoma
intraocular neuritis
intraosseous low-grade osteosarcoma
intraperitoneal pregnancy
intraperitoneal transfusion
intrascapular ligament
intrathoracic goiter
intrathoracic pressure
intrauterine pneumonia
intrauterine transfusion
intravascular congestion
intravascular lymph
intravascular thrombosis
intravenous (IV, I.V.)
intravenous drug abuse
intravenous narcotism
intravital microscopy
intravital stain
intrinsic factor antibody
intrinsic factor, vitamin B_{12} test
intrinsic muscle
intrinsic protein

introtus, vaginal
intubation
intussuscepted bowel
intussusception
in utero
invagination
invasion, stromal
invasive carcinoma
invasive mole
inversion
    chromosomal abnormality of
    nipple
    paracentric
    pericentric
inversion of A/G ratio
inversion of ratio
inversus, situs
inverted pelvis
in vitro
Invitrogen CDNA synthesis system
in vivo
involucrin
involucrum
involuntary muscle
involuntary reflex
involuntary sphincter of anal canal
involutional
Iodamoeba buetschlii
iodide goiter
iodinated I 125 (^{125}I) serum albumin
iodinated I 131 (^{131}I) serum albumin
iodine, Gram
iodine stain
iodine test
iodine topical solution
iodized protein
iodoform test for acetone
iodophil granule
ion
    bicarbonate
    hydrogen
    phosphate

ion-exchange chromatography
ionized calcium
ionizing radiation
iridescent virus
iridis, coloboma
iridocorneal angle
iridocyclitis
iridovirus
iris (pl. irises, irides)
iritis
    acute
    chronic
iron (Fe)
    excessive intake of
    heme
    increased absorption of
    non-heme
    reduced stainable
    stainable
iron-binding capacity of blood
iron-binding cacacity, total (TIBC)
iron-deficiency anemia
iron deposition
iron hematoxylin
iron hematoxylin stain
iron saturation
iron stain
iron stain of bone marrow
iron store
iron-sulfur protein
irradiation pneumonia
irradiation, solar
irregular bone
irregular enchondral ossification
irregular knots or clumps of degenerat-
    ing fibrils within neurons
irregularly distributed
irregularly shaped
irreparable damage
irreversible brain damage
irreversible coma
irreversible flaccid paralysis

irreversible injury
irritability of nerve cell
irritant dermatitis
irritation cell
irritative lesion
Isamine blue stain
ischemia-modifying factor
ischemia secondary to vascular
   occlusion
ischemic bowel
ischemic kidney
ischemic muscular atrophy
ischemic necrosis
ischemic zones
ischial bone
ischial spine
ischial tuberosity
ischiocapsular ligament
ischiocavernosus muscle
ischiofemoral ligament
ischiopubic ramus
ischiorectal abscess
ischiorectal fat pad
ischiorectal fossa
   anterior recess of
   apex of
   base of
   posterior recess of
ischiorectal fossa plane
ischiorectal pad of fat
ischiospongiosus muscle of penis
ischium
   ascending ramus of
   ramus of
island
   lipid
   mucosal
islet amyloid polypeptide (IAPP)
islet cell
islet cell antibody screening (ICA)
islet, pancreatic
islets of Langerhans

isoantibody
isochromosome
isocitrate dehydrogenase (ICD)
isoenzyme
   cardiac
   CK (creatine kinase)
   CK-BB (CK$_1$)
   CK-MB (CK$_2$)
   CK-MM (CK$_3$)
   CPK (creatine phosphokinase)
   LDH$_1$ (LDH1)
   LDH$_2$ (LDH2)
   Regan
   serial cardiac
isoenzyme electrophoresis
isoenzyme fractionation, CPK or C-K
isoenzyme of creatine kinase (CK)
   CK$_1$ (BB, brain)
   CK$_2$ (MB, cardiac muscle)
   CK$_3$ (MM, skeletal muscle)
isoenzyme, serum LDH (1 through 5)
isoform
isogenous nests
isolated diffuse myocarditis
isolated proteinuria
isoleucine test
isomorphic effect
isopropanol precipitation test
IsoQuick DNA isolation kit
Isosensitest agar
Isospora belli
isosthenuria
isothiocyanate, fluorescein (FITC)
isotopically tagged allergen
isotropic disk
isthmus, aortic
isthmus of auditory tube
isthmus of uterus
itch
   frost
   ground
   jock

itch *(continued)*
  lumberman's
  straw
  swimmer's
  water
  winter
itching
itchy erythematous patches
Ito cell
Ito, nevus of
Ito-Reenstierna test

ITP (idiopathic thrombocytopenic
  purpura)
^{131}I uptake (thyroid function) test
I.V. or IV (intravenous)
ivory bone
ivorylike bone
ivory osteoma
Ivy bleeding time
Ixodes dammini
Ixodes pacificus

J, j

Jackson and Parker classification of
　Hodgkin disease
Jacobson canal
Jacquemin test
Jacquet dermatitis
Jacquet erythema
Jadassohn nevus
Jadassohn-Tieche nevus
Jaffe test for creatinine and glucose
jagged bone fragments
jail fever
Jakob-Creutzfeldt disease
Jamestown Canyon virus
Jamshidi biopsy needle
Jamshidi needle
Janeway lesion
Jansky human blood group
Janus green B
Japanese B encephalitis
Japanese encephalitis virus
Jarjavay ligament
jars, Coplin
jaundice
　acholuric
　anhepatic
　breast milk
　choleric

jaundice *(continued)*
　cholestatic
　chronic acholuric
　chronic familial
　chronic idiopathic
　congenital hemolytic
　familial nonhemolytic
　hematogenous
　hepatocellular
　hepatogenous
　infectious
　neonatal
　obstructive
　physiologic
　yellow
jaw bone
jaw joint
JCV (JC virus)
jejunal artery
jejunal limb
jejunal loop
jejunal pouch
jejunum
　arterial arcades of
　coils of
　mesentery of
　windows of

jelly, Wharton
Jenner method (staining)
Jensen sarcoma
JEOL 100 CX electron microscope
Jewett classification of bladder
   carcinoma
Job syndrome
jock itch (tinea cruris)
Johne bacillus
Johnson-Dubin syndrome
Johnson test for albumin
joint (see also *articulation*)
   acromioclavicular
   amphiarthroses
   ankle
   antebrachiocarpal
   anterior intraoccipital
   arthrodial
   atlanto-occipital
   atlantoaxial
   ball-and-socket
   biaxial
   bicondylar
   bilocular
   bleeding into a
   Budin obstetrical
   calcaneocuboid
   capitate-hamate
   capitolunate
   capitular
   carpal
   carpometacarpal
   cartilaginous
   centrodistal
   Charcot
   Chopart
   Clutton
   coccygeal
   cochlear
   coffin
   composite
   compound

joint *(continued)*
   condylar
   condyloid
   costocentral
   costochondral
   costosternal
   costotransverse
   costovertebral
   cotyloid
   coxal
   cricoarytenoid
   cricothyroid
   Cruveilhier
   cubital
   cuboideonavicular
   cuneocuboid
   cuneometatarsal
   cuneonavicular
   dentoalveolar
   diarthroidial
   diarthrosis
   digit
   digital
   DIP (distal interphalangeal)
   distal radioulnar
   distal tibiofibular
   dry
   elbow
   ellipsoid
   enarthrodial
   facet
   false
   femoropatellar
   femorotibial
   fibrous
   flail
   ginglymoid
   gliding
   gomphosis
   hemophilic
   hinge
   hip

joint *(continued)*
   humeral
   humeroradial
   humeroulnar
   hysterical
   immovable
   incudomalleolar
   incudostapedial
   inferior radioulnar
   inferior tibiofibular
   interarticular
   intercarpal
   interchondral
   intercuneiform
   intermetacarpal
   intermetatarsal
   interphalangeal
   intersternebral
   intertarsal
   intervertebral
   jaw
   knee
   knuckle
   lateral atlantoaxial
   Lisfranc
   lower extremity
   lumbosacral
   lunotriquetral
   Luschka
   mandible
   manubriosternal
   median atlantoaxial
   metacarpophalangeal
   metatarsophalangeal
   midcarpal (middle carpal)
   middle radioulnar
   midtarsal
   mortise
   movable
   multiaxial
   neurocentral
   neuropathic

joint *(continued)*
   peg-and-socket
   petrobasilar
   petro-occipital
   phalangeal
   PIP (proximal interphalangeal)
   pisiform
   pisotriquetral
   pivot
   plane
   polyaxial
   posterior intraoccipital
   primary cartilaginous
   proximal interphalangeal
   proximal radioulnar
   proximal tibiofibular
   radiocarpal
   radiohumeral
   radioulnar
   rotary
   sacrococcygeal
   sacrococcygeal symphysis
   sacroiliac
   saddle
   scapholunate
   scaphotrapezoid trapezial (STT)
   scapuloclavicular
   schindyletic
   screw
   secondary cartilaginous
   shoulder
   simple
   skull-type
   socket
   spheno-occipital
   spheroid
   spiral
   sternal
   sternoclavicular
   sternocostal
   sternum
   stifle

joint *(continued)*
   STT (scaphotrapezoid trapezial)
   subtalar
   superior radioulnar
   superior tibiofibular
   suture
   symphysis cartilaginous
   synarthroses
   synchondrosis
   syndesmosis
   synovial
   talocalcaneal
   talocalcaneonavicular
   talocrural
   talonavicular
   tarsometatarsal
   tarsus
   temporomandibular
   tibiofibular
   tibiotarsal
   transverse tarsal
   triquetrohamate
   uncovertebral
   uniaxial
   unilocular
   wedge-and-groove
   weightbearing
   wrist
   xiphisternal
   zygapophyseal (zygoapophysial)
joint capsule
joint cavity
joint cyst
joint fluid
joint mice
joint tissues
Jolles test for bile pigments in urine
Jolly body
Jolly-Howell body
Jones and Cantarow urea concentration
   test
Jones fluorescein instillation test

Jones kidney stain
Jores solution
Jorissen test for formaldehyde
J-sella deformity
Judet epiphyseal fracture classification
jugal bone
jugal ligament
jugular arch
jugular foramen (pl. foramina)
jugular gland
jugular notch
jugular vein
juice
   acid-peptic
   appetite
   gastric
   intestinal
   pancreatic
jumper's knee
jumping gene
junction
   amnioembryonic
   anorectal
   cardioesophageal (CE)
   cementodentinal
   choledochoduodenal
   choledochopancreatic ductal
   corticomedullary
   costochondral
   costovertebral
   cystic-choledochal
   cystocholedochal
   dentinocemental
   dentinoenamel
   dermoepidermal
   desmosomal
   duodenojejunal
   EG (esophagogastric)
   electrotonic
   esophagogastric (EG)
   esophagotracheal (ET)
   fundoantral

junction *(continued)*
    gastroesophageal (GE)
    ileocecal
    neurocentral
    neuromuscular
    pancreaticobiliary ductal
    pyloroduodenal
    rectosigmoid
    sacrococcygeal
    sclerocorneal
    squamocolumnar
    squamocolumnar mucosal
    sternocostal
    sternomanubrial
    tracheoesophageal (TE)
    tympanostapedial
    ureteropelvic
    ureterovesical (UVJ)
    uterotubal
    uterovesical
  junctional complex

junctional epithelium
junctional nevus
jungle fever
Jüngling disease
juvenile cell
juvenile deforming metatarso-
    phalangeal osteochondritis
juvenile melanoma
juvenile muscular atrophy
juvenile neutrophil
juvenile nevus
juvenile-onset diabetes mellitus
juvenile pattern
juvenile pelvis
juvenile polyp
juvenile rheumatoid arthritis
juxtacortical osteogenic sarcoma
juxtacortical osteosarcoma
juxtacrine interaction
juxtaglomerular apparatus
juxtaglomerular cell

K, k

K (potassium)
Kaes-Bechterew, band of
Kaes line
Kaiserling fixative
Kaiserling solution
kala-azar (visceral leishmaniasis)
Kamerun swelling
Kantor and Gies test for proteins
Kaplan test for globulin-albumin
    in spinal fluid
Kaposi disease
Kaposi sarcoma
kappa chain
kappa granule
Kapsinow test for bile pigments
karatan sulfate
Karnowsky fixative
Karnovsky scale
Karnovsky status classification
karyochrome cell
karyocyte
karyokinesis
karyolysis
karyopyknotic index
karyorrhectic polymorphonuclear
    leukocyte
karyorrhexis

karyotype
karyotyping
Kasten fluorescent Feulgen stain
katal
Katayama fever
Katayama test
Kawasaki disease
Kayser-Fleischer ring in cornea
K (killer) cell
Keith-Wagener classification
    of retinopathy
Kell blood group
keloid, acne
keloidal folliculitis
keloid scar
keloid scarring
kelvin
Kelvin scale
Kemerovo virus
Kentmann test for formaldehyde
Kenya fever
kerasin
kerasin deposits in adrenal
kerasin deposits in kidney
kerasin deposits in lung
kerasin deposits in thyroid
keratan sulfate

keratic precipitates (KPs)
keratin debris
keratinization
keratinized cell
keratinized epithelial cell
keratinizing squamous epithelium
keratinizing stratified squamous
  epithelium
keratinocyte
keratinolytic
keratin pearl formation
keratin plug
keratin whorl
keratitis
  actinic
  dendritic
  interstitial
keratoacanthoma
keratocele
keratoconjunctivitis, epidemic
keratoconjunctivitis sicca
keratoconus
keratocyte
keratogenous zone
keratohyalin granule
keratomycosis
keratoprecipitates (KPs)
keratosis (pl. keratoses)
  actinic
  seborrheic
  senile
  solar
keratotic
Kerckring fold
Kerckring, valve of
keritonocyte
Kernechtrot
Kerner test for creatinine
kernicterus
ketoacidosis, diabetic
ketoaciduria
Ketodiastix

17-ketogenic steroids (17-KGS) test
ketoglutarate dehydrogenase, alpha-
ketone bodies (ketones)
ketones in urine
ketonuria
ketosis
ketosis-prone diabetes
ketosis-resistant diabetes
17-ketosteroid (17 KS) fractions
  (also, ketosteroid-17)
Ketostix
Kew Gardens fever
Keyes punch biopsy
keyhole deformity
K562 target cell
kg (kilogram)
Kidd blood group
kidney
  abdominal
  afferent vessels of
  amyloid
  arcuate artery of
  Armanni-Ebstein
  arteriosclerotic
  artificial
  Ask-Upmark
  atrophic
  biopsy of
  cake
  cicatricial
  congested
  contracted
  cow
  crush
  cyanotic
  cystic
  disk
  donor
  doughnut
  dromedary
  duplex
  edematous

kidney *(continued)*
  fatty
  fibrous capsule of
  flea-bitten
  floating
  Formad
  fused
  Goldblatt
  granular
  hila of
  horseshoe
  hypermobile
  interlobular artery of
  ischemic
  large red
  medullary sponge
  mortar
  movable
  mural
  myelin
  myeloma
  pancake
  pelvic
  polycystic
  putty
  pyelonephritic
  Rose-Bradford
  sacciform
  sclerotic
  sigmoid
  sponge
  supernumerary
  thoracic
  wandering
  waxy
kidney abscess
kidney calculus
kidney function test
kidney-shaped
kidney-shaped placenta
kidney transplant
kidney tumor

Kiel classification of non-Hodgkin
  lymphoma
Kienböck's disease
Kiernan space
killer T-cell
Killian test for carbohydrate tolerance
kilogram (kg)
kiloliter (kL)
kilometer (km)
kilomole (kmol)
Kimmelstiel-Wilson disease
kinetic energy
King-Armstrong unit
Kingella denitrificans
Kingella indologenes
Kingella kingae
kinked aorta
kinked intestine
kinked ureter
kink in bowel
Kinyoun acid-fast stain
Kinyoun carbolfuchsin stain
Kirby-Bauer test
Kirchner liquid medium
Kitasato bacillus
Kjeldahl test for nitrogen
kL (kiloliter)
Klatskin tumor classification
Klebs-Loeffler bacillus
Klebsiella
Klebsiella friedländeri
Klebsiella oxytoca
Klebsiella ozaenae
Klebsiella planticola
Klebsiella pneumoniae
Klebsiella pneumoniae ozaenae
Klebsiella pneumoniae rhinoscleromatis
Klebsiella rhinoscleromatis
Klebsiella terrigena
Kleihauer acid elution test
Kleihauer-Betke acid elution test
Kleihauer-Betke stain

Kleihauer-Betke test
Klieg eye
Klimow test for blood in urine
Klinefelter syndrome
Klumpp & Bieth method
Kluver-Barrera stain
Kluyvera
Kluyvera ascorbata
Kluyvera cryocrescens
km (kilometer)
kmol (kilomole)
Knapp test for glucose in urine
knee
    anterior cruciate deficit
    breaststroker's
    dislocated
    floating
    friction rub in
    game
    gimpy
    hamstrung
    housemaid's
    internal derangement of (IDK)
    jumper's
    locked
    Miller-Galante
    motorcyclist's
    runner's
    septic
    surfer's
    trick
    wrenched
knee articulation
knee-joint, anastomosis around
knob, aortic
knockknee
Knoll gland
knot
    net
    surfer's
    syncytial
Knott test for microfilariae in blood

knuckle
    aortic
    cervical aortic
knuckle joint
Kober test for estrogens (*not* Kobert)
Kobert test for hemoglobin (*not* Kober)
Koch bacillus
Koch phenomenon
Koch-Weeks bacillus
Kock pouch
Koebner phenomenon
Koehler disease
Koeppe nodule
KOH (potassium hydroxide)
KOH mount
KOH prep
KOH stain
KOH test
koilocytotic atypia
koilocytotic cellular change
Kokoskin modified Weber method
Kolmer test
Kondo test for indole
Koplik spots
Korean hemorrhagic fever
Korean hemorrhagic fever virus
Korotkoff test
Korsakoff encephalopathy
Koserella trabulsii
Kossa (von Kossa) stain
Kossel test for hypoxanthine
Kostmann infantile agranulocytosis
Kovalevsky canal
Kowarsky test for urine glucose
Krabbe disease
Krabbe leukodystrophy
Krause bone
Krause end bulb
Krause gland
Krause ligament
Kretschmann space
Krokiewicz urine test for bile pigment

Kronecker stain
Krukenberg tumor
Kuersteiner canal
Kühne methylene blue
Kuhnt space
Kulchitsky cell
Külz test for beta-hydroxybutyric acid
Kupffer cell
Kurthia zopfii
kuru
Kurzrok-Miller test
Kurzrok-Ratner test

Kussmaul coma
Kveim intradermal test
Kveim reaction
Kveim test for sarcoidosis
K vitamin
kwashiorkor
Kyasanur Forest hemorrhagic fever
   virus
kyphoscoliosis
kyphoscoliotic pelvis
kyphotic pelvis

L, l

L (liter)
L (lumbar)
LA (latex agglutination)
LAA (leukocyte ascorbic acid)
La autoantibody (SS-B)
Labbe triangle
Lab Tek chamber
labial artery
labial commissure
labial dysarthria
labial fusion
labial gland of mouth
labial groove
labial salivary gland
labial swelling
labial vein
labia majora
labia minora
labile factor (Factor V)
labile, heat
labile hypertension
labioglossolaryngeal paralysis
labioglossopharyngeal paralysis
labioscrotal fold
labioscrotal swelling
labium (pl. labia)
labium majus (pl. labia majora)

labium minus (pl. labia minora)
laboratory (lab) test
    precision of
    sensitivity of
labrum
    acetabular
    articular
    glenoidal
Labstix
labyrinth
    artery of
    bony
    cochlear
    ethmoidal
    Ludwig
    membranous
    osseous
    renal
    Santorini
    vestibular
labyrinthine
labyrinthitis
lacerated wound
laceration
    gastroesophageal
    V-shaped
    wound

laciniate ligament
lacis (meshwork) cell
lacrimal abscess
lacrimal apparatus
lacrimal artery
lacrimal bone
lacrimal canal
lacrimal caruncle
lacrimal crest
lacrimal duct
lacrimal fluid
lacrimal gland
lacrimal gland atrophy
lacrimal groove
lacrimal lake
lacrimal nerve
lacrimal papilla
lacrimal punctum
lacrimal sac
La Crosse encephalitis
La Crosse virus
La Crosse virus titer
lactase enzyme
lactate dehydrogenase (LDH)
lactated Ringer's solution
lactational mastitis
lactation hormone
lacteal
lactic acid
   bacillus
   blood
   cerebrospinal fluid
   plasma
   synovial fluid
lactic acid bacillus
lactic acid dehydrogenase (LDH)
lactic acid test
lactic acidosis
lactic dehydrogenase (LDH)
lactiferi, ampullae of tubuli
lactiferous gland
Lactobacillus

Lactobacillus acidophilus
Lactobacillus bifidus
Lactobacillus bulgaricus
lactogen, human placental
lactogenic hormone
lactophenol cotton blue
lactose test
lacuna (pl. lacunae)
   blood
   bone
   cartilage
   intervillous
   osseous
   penis
   resorption
lacunar abscess
lacunar cell
lacunar ligament
LAD (left anterior descending)
   coronary artery
Ladd band
Ladendorff test for blood
Laënnec cirrhosis
Laënnec pearl
Lafora body
LAK (lymphokine activated killer) cell
LAK cell phenomenon
lake
   bile
   capillary
   mucous
   venous
laked sheep blood
Laki-Lorand factor
lambdoid suture
lamella (pl. lamellae)
   articular
   circumferential
   concentric
   elastic
   enamel
   glandulopreputial

lamella of bone, articular
lamellar body density (LBD) count
lamellar body number density test
lamellar bone
lamellated (layered) pattern
lamellated blood clot
lamellated bone
lamellated thrombus
lamina
lamina cribrosa
lamina propria
laminated clot
laminated keratotic debris
laminated thrombus
laminate induration
lamina terminalis cistern
Lancefield classification of hemolytic
    streptocci into groups
Lancefield precipitation test
Lancereaux nephritis
lancet, sterile
landmark
    anatomic
    bony
Landouzy-Dejerine atrophy
Landouzy-Dejerine muscular dystrophy
Lane band
Langer line
Langerhans cell
Langerhans, islets of
Langeron iodine solution
Lange test for acetone in urine
    (*not* Lang)
Langhans cell
Langhans giant cell
Lang test for taurine *(not* Lange)
Lannelongue ligaments
Lansing virus
lanugo
Lanz point
LAP (leucine aminopeptidase)
LAP (leukocyte adhesion protein)

LAP (leukocyte alkaline phosphatase)
laparoscopy, diagnostic
laparotomy
    exploratory
    second-look
Laquer stain
large bowel
large cell carcinoma
large cell, immunoblastic lymphoma
large cell lymphoma
large cleaved cell
large cleaved cell lymphoma
large granule cell
large gut
large intestine
large intestine gland
large noncleaved cell
large noncleaved cell lymphoma
large red kidney
large sweat gland
large trunk muscle
larva migrans
    cutaneous
    visceral
larvae in mucosa of stomach
laryngeal artery
laryngeal atrophy
laryngeal edema
laryngeal gland
laryngeal granuloma
laryngeal nerve
laryngeal nodule
laryngeal part of pharynx
laryngeal polyp
laryngotracheobronchitis
larynx
    appendix of ventricle of
    infraglottic
    ventricle of
    vestibule of
LASA (lipid-associated sialic acid)
laser nephelometry

laser, pumped-dye
lash follicles
Lassa fever
Lassa virus
lata (pl. latae)
    fascia (pl. fasciae latae)
    tensor fascia (pl. latae, tensor fasciae)
Latarget nerve
latent diabetes
latent infection
latent pleurisy
latent virus
lateral alveolar abscess
lateral antebrachial cutaneous nerve
lateral aperture
lateral arcuate ligament
lateral atlantoaxial joint
lateral calcaneal artery
lateral canal
lateral circumflex artery of thigh
lateral collateral ligament of ankle
lateral costal artery
lateral costotransverse ligament
lateral crus (pl. crura)
lateral crus of superficial inguinal ring
lateral cuneiform bone
lateral cutaneous branch of intercostal
    nerve
lateral eminence
lateral epicondyle
lateral femoral circumflex artery
lateral fornix of vagina
lateral gutter
lateral horn
lateral ligament of malleus
lateral ligament of bladder
lateral lobe of prostate
lateral lumbocostal arch
lateral lumbosacral ligament
lateral malleolar ligament
lateral nasal artery
lateral oblique fascia

lateral palpebral artery
lateral palpebral ligament
lateral periodontal abscess
lateral plantar artery
lateral puboprostatic ligament
lateral recess
lateral reflection of colon
lateral sacrococcygeal ligament
lateral semicircular canal
lateral striate artery
lateral sulcus
lateral talocalcaneal ligament
lateral tarsal artery
lateral temporomandibular ligament
lateral third of inguinal ligament
lateral thoracic artery
lateral umbilical fold
lateral umbilical ligament
lateral vaginal wall smear
lateral ventricle of cerebrum
lateral wall of nasal cavity
late secretory endometrium
latex agglutination (LA)
latex agglutination test for antibody
latex beads, agglutination of
latex fixation test
latex particles coated with antigen
latissimus dorsi muscle
lattice cell
laudable pus
Lauth canal
Lauth ligament
lavage
    bronchoalveolar
    gastric
    tracheobronchial
layer
    basal
    basal cell
    blastodermic
    choriocapillary
    choroid

layer *(continued)*
  circular
  columnar
  conjunctival
  corneal
  cornified
  elastic
  enamel
  ependymal
  epithelial
  epithelial choroid
  epitrichial
  fibrous
  fusiform
  ganglionic
  germ
  germinative
  malpighian
  membranous deep
  papillary
  parietal
  prickle cell
  reticular
  subcutaneous
  subserosal
  superficial fatty
  visceral
layered
L cell
LCIS (lobular carcinoma in situ)
LCM (lymphocytic choriomeningitis)
  virus
LCT (long chain triglycerides)
LDH (lactate dehydrogenase)
LDH1 (LDH_1) isoenzyme
LDH2 (LDH_2) isoenzyme
LDL (low density lipoprotein)
LDL cholesterol (LDLC)
LE (leukocyte esterase)
LE (lupus erythematosus)
LE cell
LE cell prep (preparation)

lead (Pb)
  blood
  urinary
lead citrate
lead hydroxide stain
lead level in blood
lead level in urine
lead poisoning
lead stomatitis
leaflet, valve
leakage
leaking from vessel
leaking of red blood cells
leaky mitral valve
lean body mass
leaping atrophy
leather bottle stomach
leaves of diaphragm
leaves of mesentery
Leber optic atrophy
Lechini test for blood in urine
lecithin/sphingomyelin (L/S) ratio
Lecythophora hoffmannii
Lecythophora mutabilis
Leder stain
ledge, enamel
Lee cutting biopsy needle
Lee test for rennin
Lee tissue biopsy needle
Leeuwenhoek canal
Lee-White clotting method
Lee-White clotting time
Lee-White coagulation time
LE factor
left anterior descending (LAD)
  coronary artery
left atrium
left auricle
left border of heart
left colic artery
left colic flexure
left colon

left colonic flexure
left crus (pl. crura)
left gastric artery
left gastroepiploic artery
left gutter
left heart
left hemisphere
left hepatic vein (LHV)
left lobe of liver
left lower quadrant (LLQ)
left main bronchus
left shift on WBC count
left superior vena cava ligament
left triangular ligament
left upper outer quadrant
left upper quadrant (LUQ)
left vena cava ligament
left ventricle of heart
left ventricular hypertrophy (LVH)
Legal test for acetone
Legg-Calvé-Perthes disease
Legionella anisa
Legionella bozemanii
Legionella dumoffii
Legionella feeleii
Legionella gormanii
Legionella jordanis
Legionella longbeachae
Legionella micdadei
Legionella oakridgensis
Legionella pneumophila
Legionella sainthelensis
Legionella wadsworthii
legionellosis
legionnaire's bacillus
legionnaire's disease
Leifson flagella stain
Leiner dermatitis
leiomyoma (pl. leiomyomata)
  benign
  cytologically bland
  epithelioid

leiomyoma *(continued)*
  submucous
  subserosal
  uterine
leiomyoma uteri
leiomyosarcoma
Leishman-Donovan body
Leishmania brasiliensis (or *braziliensis*)
Leishmania donovani
Leishmania tropica
leishmaniasis
  cutaneous
  mucocutaneous
  visceral
leishmanin test
Leishman chrome cell
Leishman stain
Lendrum phloxine–tartrazine stain
length
  crown-heel
  crown-rump
lengthwise
Lennert lymphoma
lenticular ansa
lenticular artery
lenticular bone
lenticular carcinoma
lenticular glands of stomach
lenticular glands of tongue
lenticular loop
lenticulostriate artery
lentiform bone
lentiginous
lentigo
  malignant
  nevoid
  senile
  solar
lentigo maligna
lentigo maligna melanoma
Lentivirinae
Lentivirus, lentivirus

Leon virus
leopard retina
Leo test for free hydrochloric acid
LE panniculitis
Lepehne-Pickworth stain
Leporipoxvirus
lepra bacillus
lepra cell
lepromatous leprosy
lepromin test
leprosy (Hansen disease)
    borderline
    indeterminate
    intermediate
    Lucio
    tuberculoid
    water-buffalo
leprosy bacillus
leptomeningeal fibrosis
leptomeninges
Leptospira biflexa
Leptospira icterohemorrhagiae
Leptospira interrogans
leptospirosis
Leptotrichia
Leptotrichia buccalis
LES (lower esophageal sphincter)
Lesgaft space
Lesgaft triangle
lesion
    angiocentric immunoproliferative
    Armanni-Ebstein
    Baehr-Lohlein
    Bankart
    benign lymphoepithelial
    bird's nest
    blastic
    Blumenthal
    Bracht-Wachter
    bull's-eye
    cardiac valvular
    caviar

lesion *(continued)*
    central
    coin (of lungs)
    Councilman
    depigmented
    Dieulafoy
    Duret
    Ebstein
    erythematous
    flat
    freckle-like
    Ghon primary
    gross
    Hill-Sachs
    histologic
    impaction
    indiscriminate
    infiltrating
    irritative
    Janeway
    lichenoid
    linear cutaneous
    local
    Löhlein-Baehr
    lower motor neuron
    lytic
    Mallory-Weiss
    molecular
    mongolian spot-like
    napkin-ring
    necrotic
    onion scale
    onionskin
    organic
    papillary
    papular
    papulonecrotic
    partial
    peripheral
    pigmented (melanotic)
    precancerous
    primary

lesion *(continued)*
    punctate keratotic
    purulent
    radial sclerosing
    ring-wall
    satellite
    skin
    solitary
    squamous intraepithelial
    structural
    supranuclear
    systemic
    target
    total
    trophic
    tuberculoid
    upper motor neuron
    vulvar
    wire-loop
lesser curvature of stomach
lesser multangular bone
lesser omentum
lesser palatine artery
lesser palatine foramina
lesser palatine nerve
lesser pancreas
lesser peritoneal sac
lesser sac of peritoneal cavity
Lesser test
lesser trochanter of femur
lesser tubercle
LET (leukocyte esterase test)
lethal disease
lethal gene
lethal factor
Letterer-Siwe disease
leucine aminopeptidase (LAP)
leucine test
leukemia
    acute
    acute granulocytic
    acute lymphoblastic (ALL)

leukemia *(continued)*
    acute lymphocytic
    acute megakaryoblastic
    acute monocytic
    acute myeloblastic
    acute myelogenous (AML)
    acute myelomonocytic
    acute promyelocytic
    acute undifferentiated (AUL)
    adult T-cell/lymphoma (ATL)
    aleukemic
    basophilic
    B-cell type
    Burkitt-like
    chronic
    chronic lymphocytic (CLL)
    chronic myelomonocytic
    common type
    eosinophilic
    granulocytic
    hairy cell
    lymphatic
    lymphoblastic
    lymphocytic
    mast cell
    micromyeloblastic
    monocytic
    myeloblastic
    myelocytic
    myelogenous
    Naegeli monocytic
    nonlymphocytic
    null cell type
    plasma cell
    plasmacytic
    pre-B-cell type
    promyelocytic
    Rieder cell
    T-cell type
    undifferentiated
leukemia classification
leukemia cutis

leukemic
leukemid
leukemogen
leukemogenesis
leukemogenic
leukemoid reaction
leukencephalitis
leukexosis
leukin
leukoagglutinin
leukoblast
leukoblastosis
leukocidin
  Neisser-Wechsberg
  Panton-Valentine (P-V)
leukocrit
leukocyte
  acidophil
  acidophilic
  agranular
  basophilic
  beta
  circulating
  endothelial
  eosinophil
  eosinophilic
  fecal
  granular
  heterophilic
  lymphoid
  mast
  migration of
  motile
  neutrophilic
  nongranular
  nonmotile
  peripheral
  polymorphonuclear
  polymorphonuclear karyorrhectic
  Türk irritation
leukocyte acid phosphatase,
  tartrate resistant

leukocyte adherence assay
leukocyte adhesion protein (LAP)
leukocyte alkaline phosphatase (LAP)
leukocyte ascorbic acid (LAA)
leukocyte bactericidal assay
leukocyte differential count
  basophils
  eosinophils
  lymphocytes
  monocytes
  myelocytes
  neutrophils
    bands
    segs
leukocyte/erythrocyte ratio
leukocyte esterase (LE) in urine
leukocyte esterase test (LET)
leukocyte-poor red blood cells
leukocyte surface receptors
leukocythemia
leukocytic infiltration of submucosa
leukocytic sarcoma
leukocytic trapping of bacteria
leukocytoblast
leukocytogenesis
leukocytoid
leukocytolysin
leukocytolysis
leukocytolytic
leukocytoma
leukocytopenia
leukocytopoiesis
leukocytosis
  absolute
  agonal
  basophilic
  mononuclear
  neutrophilic
  pathologic
  physiologic
  pure
  relative

leukocytosis *(continued)*
  terminal
  toxic
leukocytosis-promoting factor
leukocytotactic
leukocytotaxis
leukocytotherapy
leukocytotoxicity
leukocytotropic
leukocyturia
leukoderma
  occupational
  postinflammatory
  syphilitic
leukodermatous
leukodystrophy
  globoid cell
  hereditary adult-onset
  hereditary cerebral
  Krabbe
  metachromatic
  spongiform
  sudanophilic
leukoedema
leukoencephalitis
leukoencephalopathy
  necrotizing
  progressive multifocal (PML)
  subacute sclerosing
leukoerythroblastosis
leukogram
leukokeratosis
leukokinesis
leukokinetic
leukokinetics
leukopedesis
leukopenia
leukopenic factor
leukopenic index
leukophagocytosis
leukoplakia
leukopoiesis

leukopoietic
leukopoietin
leukoprecipitin
leukorrhagia
leukorrhea
leukosarcoma
leukoscope
leukosis
leukotactic
leukotaxis
leukothrombin
leukotoxic
leukotoxicity
leukotoxin
Levaditi stain
levator muscle
level
  blood alcohol
  panic
  peak and trough
  PIVKA-II
  plasma lipoprotein
  red blood cell cholinesterase
  therapeutic
  toxic
  trough
level of umbilicus
Leventhal-Stein syndrome
Levine alkaline Congo red method
Levinson test for tuberculous meningitis
Lewis blood group
Lewis hydrophagocytosis phenomenon
Lewy body
Lewy inclusion body
Leyden neuritis
Leyden-Charcot crystal
Leydig cell
LFT, LFTs (liver function test)(s)
LH (luteinizing hormone)
LHV (left hepatic vein)
Liacopoulos phenomenon
Libman-Sacks verrucous endocarditis

lice and nits on body hair
lice and nits on pubic hair
lice and nits on scalp hair
lichen planus
lichenification
lichenoid dermatitis
lichenoid lesion
lichenoid papules
lichenoid pityriasis
Lichtheim disease
Lichtheim syndrome
Lieben-Ralfe test for acetone
Lieben test for acetone in urine
Lieberkühn crypt
Lieberkühn gland
Liebermann-Burchard test for
   cholesterol
Liebermann test for proteins
Liebermeister groove
Liebig test for cystine
lienal artery
lienophrenic ligament
lienorenal ligament
lienteric diarrhea
lienteric stool
Liesegang phenomenon
Lieutaud trigone
lifeless eye
lifelong obesity
lifesaving drugs
life span, shortening
lifestyle (noun)
life support (noun)
life-support system
life-threatening condition
life-threatening disease
Li-Fraumeni syndrome (LFS)
ligament
   accessory
   accessory plantar
   accessory volar
   alar

ligament *(continued)*
   alveolodental
   anatomy
   annular
   anococcygeal
   anterior calcaneoastragaloid
   anterior costotransverse
   anterior costovertebral
   anterior costoxiphoid
   anterior cruciate
   anterior inferior tibiofibular
   anterior longitudinal
   anterior radioulnar
   anterior talotibial
   anterior tibiotalar
   apical
   apical ligament of dens
   Arantius
   arcuate popliteal
   arcuate pubic
   arterial
   auricular
   axis
   Bardinet
   Barkow
   Bellini
   Berry
   Bertin
   Bichat
   bifurcate
   bifurcated
   Bigelow
   Botallo
   Bourgery
   broad l. of uterus
   Brodie
   Burns
   calcaneocuboid
   calcaneofibular
   calcaneonavicular
   calcaneotibial
   Caldani

ligament *(continued)*
   Campbell
   Camper
   capsular
   Carcassonne
   cardinal
   caroticoclinoid
   carpometacarpal
   casserian
   Casser
   caudal
   ceratocricoid
   cervical
   check
   cholecystoduodenal
   chondroxiphoid
   ciliary
   Civinini
   Clado
   Cloquet
   collateral
   Colles
   conjugate
   conoid
   Cooper
   coracoacromial
   coracoclavicular
   coracohumeral
   corniculopharyngeal
   coronary
   costoclavicular
   costocolic
   costotransverse
   costoxiphoid
   cotyloid
   Cowper
   cricopharyngeal
   cricosantorinian
   cricothyroid
   cricotracheal
   crucial
   cruciate

ligament *(continued)*
   cruciform
   Cruveilhier
   cuboideonavicular
   cuneocuboid
   cuneonavicular
   cystoduodenal
   deep dorsal sacrococcygeal
   deep posterior sacrococcygeal
   deep transverse metacarpal
   deep transverse metatarsal
   deltoid
   Denonvilliers
   dentate
   denticulate
   Denucé
   diaphragmatic
   dorsal calcaneocuboid
   dorsal carpal
   dorsal carpometacarpal
   dorsal cuboideonavicular
   dorsal cuneocuboid
   dorsal cuneonavicular
   dorsal metacarpal
   dorsal metatarsal
   dorsal radiocarpal
   dorsal sacroiliac
   dorsal talonavicular
   Douglas
   duodenal
   duodenorenal
   epihyal
   external
   external collateral (of wrist)
   extracapsular
   falciform
   fallopian
   femoral
   Ferrein
   fibular collateral
   Flood
   fundiform

ligament *(continued)*
  gastrocolic
  gastrodiaphragmatic
  gastrohepatic
  gastrolienal
  gastropancreatic
  gastrophrenic
  gastrosplenic
  genital
  genitoinguinal
  Gerdy
  Gillette suspensory
  Gimbernat
  gingivodental
  glenohumeral
  glenoid
  glossoepiglottic
  Günz (Guenz)
  Günzberg (Guenzberg)
  hammock
  Helmholtz axis
  Hensing
  hepatic
  hepatocolic
  hepatocystocolic
  hepatoduodenal
  hepatoesophageal
  hepatogastric
  hepatogastroduodenal
  hepatophrenic
  hepatorenal
  hepatoumbilical
  Hesselbach
  Hey
  Holl
  Hueck
  Humphry
  Hunter
  Huschke
  hyalocapsular
  hyoepiglottic
  hypsiloid

ligament *(continued)*
  iliofemoral
  iliolumbar
  iliopectineal
  iliotibial l. of Maissiat
  iliotrochanteric
  inferior calcaneonavicular
  inferior pubic
  inferior transverse scapular
  infundibulo-ovarian
  infundibulopelvic
  inguinal
  intercapital
  intercarpal
  interclavicular
  interclinoid
  intercornual
  intercostal
  intercuneiform
  interfoveolar
  internal collateral
  interosseous
  interosseous cuneocuboid
  interosseous cuneometatarsal
  interosseous lunotriquetral
  interosseous metacarpal
  interosseous metatarsal
  interosseous sacroiliac
  interosseous talocalcaneal
  interosseous tibiofibular
  interspinous
  intertransverse
  intra-articular
  intra-articular sternocostal
  intrascapular
  ischiocapsular
  ischiofemoral
  Jarjavay
  jugal
  Krause
  laciniate
  lacunar

ligament *(continued)*
  Lannelongue
  lateral arcuate
  lateral costotransverse
  lateral lumbosacral
  lateral malleolar
  lateral palpebral
  lateral puboprostatic
  lateral sacrococcygeal
  lateral talocalcaneal
  lateral temporomandibular
  lateral umbilical
  Lauth
  left superior vena cava
  left triangular
  left vena cava
  lienophrenic
  lienorenal
  Lisfranc
  Lockwood
  long plantar
  longitudinal
  lumbocostal
  lunotriquetral
  Luschka
  Mackenrodt
  Maissiat
  Mauchart
  Meckel
  medial
  medial arcuate
  medial collateral
  medial palpebral
  medial puboprostatic
  medial talocalcaneal
  medial umbilical
  median arcuate
  meniscofemoral
  middle costotransverse
  middle umbilical
  mucosal suspensory
  nuchal

ligament *(continued)*
  oblique
  oblique popliteal
  occipitoaxial
  odontoid
  orbicular
  ovarian
  palmar
  palmar carpal
  palmar carpometacarpal
  palmar metacarpal
  palmar radiocarpal
  palmar ulnocarpal
  patellar
  pectinate
  pectineal
  peridental
  periodontal
  peritoneal
  Petit
  Pétrequin
  phrenicocolic
  phrenicolienal
  phrenicosplenic
  phrenoesophageal
  phrenogastric
  phrenosplenic
  pisohamate
  pisometacarpal
  pisounciform
  pisouncinate
  plantar
  plantar calcaneocuboid
  plantar calcaneonavicular
  plantar cuboideonavicular
  plantar cuneocuboid
  plantar cuneonavicular
  plantar metatarsal
  posterior
  posterior costotransverse
  posterior costotransverse ligament
  posterior cricoarytenoid

ligament *(continued)*
- posterior cruciate
- posterior longitudinal
- posterior meniscofemoral
- posterior occipitoaxial
- posterior sacroiliac
- posterior sacrosciatic
- posterior sternoclavicular
- posterior talofibular
- posterior talotibial
- posterior tibiofibular
- posterior tibiotalar
- Poupart
- pterygomandibular
- pterygospinal
- pterygospinous
- pubocapsular
- pubocervical
- pubofemoral
- puboprostatic
- pubovesical
- pulmonary
- quadrate
- radial collateral
- radiate
- radiate sternocostal
- radiocarpal
- radiolunotriquetral
- radioscaphocapitate
- radioscapholunate
- reflected inguinal
- reflecting edge of
- reflex
- reflex inguinal
- Retzius
- rhomboid
- right triangular
- ring
- Robert
- round
- sacrodural
- sacrospinous

ligament *(continued)*
- sacrotuberous
- Santorini
- Sappey
- scapholunate
- Schlemm
- serous
- sheath
- Simonart
- Soemmerring
- sphenomandibular
- spinoglenoid
- spiral
- splenocolic
- splenorenal
- spring
- Stanley cervical
- stellate
- sternoclavicular
- sternopericardial
- stylohyoid
- stylomandibular
- stylomaxillary
- superficial dorsal sacrococcygeal
- superficial posterior sacrococcygeal
- superficial transverse metacarpal
- superficial transverse metartarsal
- superior
- superior costotransverse
- superior pubic
- superior transverse scapular
- suprascapular
- supraspinous
- suspensory
- sutural
- synovial
- talocalcaneal
- talonavicular
- tarsal
- tarsometatarsal
- temporomandibular
- Teutleben

ligament *(continued)*
  Thompson
  thyroepiglottic
  thyrohyoid
  tibial collateral
  tibiocalcaneal
  tibiofibular
  tibionavicular
  transverse
  transverse atlantal
  transverse carpal
  transverse crural
  transverse genicular
  transverse humeral
  transverse metacarpal
  transverse metatarsal
  transverse perineal
  transverse tibiofibular
  trapezoid
  triangular
  Tuffier inferior
  ulnar collateral
  ulnocarpal
  ulnolunate
  ulnotriquetral
  umbilical
  urachal
  uterine
    broad
    cardinal
    round
  uterosacral
  uterovesical
  venous
  ventral sacrococcygeal
  ventral sacroiliac
  ventricular
  vertebropelvic
  vesicoumbilical
  vesicouterine
  vestibular
  vocal

ligament *(continued)*
  volar
  volar carpal
  Walther oblique
  Weitbrecht
  Winslow
  Wrisberg
  xiphicostal
  xiphoid
  Y-shaped
  Zaglas
  Zinn
ligament of Scarpa
ligament of Struthers
ligament of Testut
ligament of Treitz
ligament shelving edge, Poupart
ligand
ligation, tubal
ligature, elastic
ligature needle
light
  black
  infrared
  polarized
  reflected
  refracted
  Tyndall
  ultraviolet
  white
  Wood
light cell
light cells of thyroid
light-chain proteinuria
light gray stool
light microscope
light microscopy
light scatter gate
ligneous
lilac rash
Lillie allochrome connective tissue
  stain

Lillie azure–eosin stain
Lillie ferrous iron stain
Lillie sulfuric acid Nile blue stain
limb
   afferent
   ampullary
   efferent
   jejunal
   lower
   phantom
   Roux-en-Y jejunal
   sagittal
   upper
limb lead
limb muscle
limb stump
limbus fossae ovalis
limit of resection
limiting membrane
limits, within normal (WNL)
limnemia (chronic malaria)
limp
Limulus amebocyte lysate assay
limulus lysate test
Limulus polyphemus
limulus test
Lindemann test for acetoacetic acid
   in urine
line (pl. lines)
   absorption
   accretion
   alveolonasal
   anocutaneous
   anorectal
   arcuate
   axillary
   azygos venous
   basinasal
   Beau
   Brödel white
   Brücke
   calcification

line *(continued)*
   cell
   cement
   cervical
   Chaussier
   Clapton
   cleavage
   contour
   copper
   Corrigan
   costoclavicular
   costophrenic septal
   dentate
   developmental
   Eberth
   epiphysial
   established cell
   Frommann
   Hunter
   iliopectineal
   incremental
   Langer
   midaxillary
   midclavicular
   midscapular
   milk
   pectinate
   period
   polypropylene
   pubic hair
   pubococcygeal
   Retzius
   Rex-Cantli-Serege
   semilunar
   skin
   suture
   white l. of Toldt
   Z
   Zahn
linea alba
linea nigra
lineae (pl. of linea)

linear cutaneous lesion
linear defect
linear epidermal nevus
linear fraction
linear fracture
linear IgA bullous disease
linear morphea
line of arrested growth
line of Ebner
line of ilium, arcuate
line of Kaes
line of resection
line of Retzius
line of Toldt
line of Zahn
line test for rickets
lingua (tongue)
lingua apex
lingua nigra (black tongue)
lingual aponeurosis
lingual artery, deep
lingual atrophy
lingual bone
lingual frenulum
lingual goiter
lingual muscle
lingual papilla
lingual root
lingual septum
lingual tonsil
lingual vein
lingula (pl. lingulae)
lining cell
lining, ependymal
linitis plastica
lip
   articular
   cleft
   hypoplastic
   lower
   rhombic
   upper

lipase
   pancreatic
   serum
lipase enzyme
lipase test for liver function
lipedematous alopecia
lipemic
lipid-associated sialic acid (LASA)
lipid compound
lipid island
lipid-laden macrophages
lipid material, macrophages stuffed
   with
lipid metabolism, disorders of
lipid-mobilizing hormone
lipidosis
lipid pigment
lipid profile
lipid test on venous blood
liplike projections of cartilage
lipoatrophic diabetes
lipoatrophy
lipoblast
lipocyte
lipodystrophy, familial
lipofuscin
lipogenous diabetes
lipoid, anisotropic
lipoid granuloma
lipoid nephrosis
lipoid pneumonia
lipoid pneumonitis
lipoid proteinosis
lipoid substance
lipoidal degeneration
lipolytic enzyme
lipoma
lipomatosis
lipomatous-like tissue
lipomatous nevus
lipomatous polyp
lipophage

lipophagic granuloma
lipopolysaccharide (LPS)
lipoprotein (LP)
   $alpha_1$-
   beta
   high density (HDL)
   low density (LDL)
   very low density (VLDL)
lipoprotein electrophoresis (LPE)
lilpoproteinemia
lipoprotein metabolism, disorder of
liposarcoma
lipotropic factor
lipotropic hormone
lipping of vertebrae
lips of hilum
Lipschütz body
Lipschütz cell
lipuria
liquefaction degeneration
liquefaction, gas
liquefaction necrosis
liquefaction of debris
liquefying
liquid chromatography
liquid material
liquid nitrogen
liquor folliculi
liquid stool
Lisfranc joint
Lisfranc ligament
Lison-Dunn stain
Listeria monocytogenes
listeriosis
Lister tubercle
liter (L)
lithium-carmine stain
litmus milk test for pancreatic lipase
littoral cell
Littré gland
livedoid dermatitis
livedo, postmortem

liver
   albuminoid
   bare area of
   biliary cirrhotic
   black
   blue
   brimstone
   bronze
   capsule of
   caudate lobe of
   centrilobular region of
   cirrhosis of
   degenerative
   degraded
   diaphragmatic surface of
   dome of
   duodenal impression on
   fatty
   floating
   foamy
   frosted
   green
   hobnail
   icing
   infantile
   iron
   lardaceous
   left lobe of
   metastasis to
   nutmeg
   pigmented
   polycystic
   quadrate lobe of
   renal impression on
   right lobe of
   sago
   stasis
   sugar-icing
   undersurface of
   visceral surface of
   wandering
   waxy

liver adenocarcinoma
liver bed, surface of
liver bile
liver cell
liver cell plate
liver cirrhosis
liver death
liver edge
liver enzyme (glucuronosyltransferase)
liver fluke
liver function test
liver impression
liver iron store
liverlike lung
liver lobule, central vein of
liver panel
liver parenchyma
liver profile
liver segment
liver transplant
liver tumor
livid
lividity
   dependent
   postmortem
livedo reticularis–digital infarct
livedo vasculitis
Livingston triangle
livor mortis
LKS (liver, kidneys, and spleen)
L-L factor (XIII)
LLQ (left lower quadrant)
Loa loa
lobar artery
lobar atrophy
lobar bronchi
lobar consolidation
lobar pneumonia
lobe
   azygos
   caudate (liver)
   cuneiform

lobe *(continued)*
   falciform
   fetal
   flocculonodular
   frontal
   inferior
   left
   occipital
   polyalveolar
   pulmonary
   Riedel
   right
   superior
lobe bronchus
lobectomy
lobed nuclei
Loboa loboi
lobster-claw deformity
lobular architecture
lobular panniculitis
lobular parenchyma
lobular pattern
lobular pneumonia
lobulated
lobulation
lobule
   ansiform
   biventral
   central
   crescentic
   hepatic
   portal
   respiratory
   semilunar
lobule of epididymis
local death
local hormone
localized myeloma
localized nodular synovitis
localized osteitis fibrosa
localized pemphigoid of Brunsting-
   Perry

localized thickenings of Bruch
  membrane
local lesion
locally invasive tumor
local metastasis
locked-in syndrome
locked knee
Lockwood ligament
loculated fluid
Loeffler (Löffler)
Loeffler caustic stain
Loeffler coagulated serum medium
Loeffler methylene blue stain
Loeffler serum
Loeffler stain
Loevit cell
Loewe test for urine glucose
Löffler (Loeffler)
Löhlein-Baehr lesion
loiasis (Calabar swelling)
loin
long-acting thyroid stimulating
  (LATS) hormone test
long axis of spleen
long bone
long chain fatty acid–CoA ligase
long chain triglycerides (LCT)
long ciliary artery
long plantar ligament
long spinous process
long thoracic artery
longitudinal anastomosis
longitudinal arc of skull
longitudinal axis
longitudinal band
longitudinal canals of modiolus
longitudinal cerebral fissure
longitudinal ligament, anterior
longitudinal muscle coat
longitudinal oval pelvis
longitudinal raphe
longitudinal section

loop
  afferent
  bowel
  capillary
  cervical
  closed
  colonic
  duodenal
  efferent
  gamma
  Gerdy interatrial
  Henle
  Hyrtl
  intestinal
  jejunal
  lenticular
  Meyer
  Meyer-Archambault
  open
  peduncular
  pressure-volume
  puborectalis
  sentinel
  sigmoid
  Stoerck
  subclavian
  transverse colon
  ventricular
  Vieussens
loose connective tissue
looseness
loose stool
lordosis
lordotic proteinuria
Lorrain Smith stain
loss of striations
louse (pl. lice)
  body
  hair
  pubic
louse-borne typhus
low birth weight

low density lipoprotein (LDL)
low density lipoprotein receptors
Löwenberg canal
Lowenthal test for glucose not in
urine
lower esophageal sphincter (LES)
lower extremity arteries
lower extremity articulation
lower extremity joint
lower limb
lower lip
lower motor neuron lesion
lower nephron nephrosis
lower respiratory tract smear
lowest splanchnic nerve
low frequency blood group
low-grade dysplasia
low-grade malignancy
low normal test result
low-power field (lpf)
low-viscosity fluid
LP (lumbar puncture)
lpf (low-power field)
LPS (lipopolysaccharide)
LPS-receptor system
L/S (lecithin/sphingomyelin)
L/S ratio in amniotic fluid
lubricant-secreting membrane
lucidum, stratum
Lucio leprosy
Lucio phenomenon
Lucké carcinoma
Lücke test for hippuric acid
Lucké virus
Ludwig angina
Ludwig labyrinth
lues (syphilis) myocarditis
luetic abscess
Luft potassium permanganate fixative
Lugol solution
Lukes-Butler classification of non-
Hodgkin lymphoma

Lukes-Collins classification of non-
Hodgkin lymphoma
lumbar aponeurosis
lumbar artery
lumbar lymph node
lumborum muscle, quadratus
lumbar nerve
lumbar puncture (LP)
lumbar region
lumbar rib
lumbar vein, ascending
lumbar vertebrae (L1 through L5)
lumberman's itch
lumbocostal aponeurosis
lumbocostal arch
lumbocostal ligament
lumbocostoabdominal triangle
lumbosacral arch
lumbosacral articulation
lumbosacral joint
lumbosacral ligament
lumbosacral trunk
lumen (pl. lumens, lumina)
lumiaggregometry
lumina (pl. of lumen)
luminal
lumpectomy
lumpy skin disease
Luna-Ishak stain
Luna modification of Bodian stain
lunate bone
lunate facet
Lundh test for pancreatic function
lung
    airless
    atelectatic
    bird-breeder's
    black
    book
    cardiac
    cheese handler's
    coal-miner's

lung *(continued)*
  drowned
  dull purple
  emphysematous
  farmer's
  fibrinoid
  fissures of
  grain handler's
  hemorrhagic consolidation of
  hilum of
  honeycomb
  humidifier
  hyperlucent
  hypoplastic
  malt worker's
  mason's
  meat wrapper's
  miller's
  miner's
  normal gas exchange in
  pigeon-breeder's
  rudimentary
  shock
  shrunken
  silo-filler's
  silver finisher's
  smoker's
  thresher's
  vanishing
  welder's
  wet
  white
lung abscess
lung adenocarcinoma
lung apex
lung base
lung capacity
lung flukes
lung mass
lung parenchyma
lung plague
lung root

lung tumor
lunotriquetral joint
lunotriquetral ligament
lunula ossicle
lunule
lupoid hepatitis
lupus anticoagulant
lupus band test
lupus erythematosus (LE)
  chilblain
  cutaneous
  discoid (DLE)
  disseminated
  drug-induced
  hypertrophic
  systemic (SLE)
lupus erythematosus cell (LE cell)
lupus erythematosus cell preparation
  test (LE prep)
lupus erythematosus profundus
  (lupus panniculitis)
lupus erythematosus tumidus
lupus hypertrophicus
lupus nephritis
lupus nephrosis
lupus pernio
lupus tumidus
lupus vulgaris
LUQ (left upper quadrant)
Luschka crypt
Luschka gland
Luschka joint
Luschka ligament
Luschka tissue
Lust peroneal nerve phenomenon
luteal cell
luteal phase
luteal phase defect
lutein cell
lutein cyst
luteinization
luteinizing hormone (LH)

luteinizing hormone/follicle-stimulating
 hormone-releasing factor
 (LH/FSH-RF)
luteinizing hormone-releasing
 hormone (LH-RH, LRH)
luteinizing theca cell
Lutembacher syndrome
luteotropic hormone
luteum, corpus
Lutheran blood group
Lutkens sphincter
Luttke test for free hydrochloric acid
 in gastric juice
Luxol fast blue
LVH (left ventricular hypertrophy)
Lyle and Curtman test for blood
Lyme disease
lymph
 aplastic
 chyle
 corpuscular
 croupous
 dental
 euplastic
 inflammatory
 intercellular
 intravascular
"lymphs" (slang for lymphocytes)
lymphadenitis
 caseous
 mesenteric
 necrotizing granulomatous
 nonbacterial regional
 tuberculoid
 tuberculous
lymphadenoid goiter
lymphadenoma cells
lymphadenopathy
lymphadenopathy-associated virus
 (LAV)
lymphangioendothelioma
lymphangioma, cutaneous

lymphangitis
 ascending
 descending
lymphatic abscess
lymphatic, afferent
lymphatic cortex
lymphatic duct
lymphatic edema
lymphatic fluid
lymphatic gland
lymphatic leukemia
lymphatic medulla
lymphatic metastasis
lymphatic network
lymphatic nodules, aggregated
lymphatic obstruction
lymphatic sarcoma
lymphatics of scrotum
lymphatic system
lymphatic tissue
lymphaticum, angioma
lymphatic vessel
lymphatic vessels thickened
lymph capillary
lymph cell
lymph duct
lymphedema
lymph gland
lymph node
 abdominal
 accessory
 anorectal
 aortic
 apical
 appendicular
 auricular
 axillary
 bifurcation
 Bouchard
 brachial
 bronchopulmonary
 buccal

lymph node *(continued)*
  buccinator
  caval
  celiac
  central
  cervical paratracheal
  Cloquet inguinal
  common iliac
  companion
  cubital
  cystic
  Delphian
  deltopectoral
  diaphragmatic
  epicolic
  epigastric
  external iliac
  facial
  fibular
  gastric
  gastroduodenal
  gastroepiploic
  gastro-omental
  gluteal
  hemolymph
  hepatic
  hilar
  ileocolic
  iliac
  iliac circumflex
  infrahyoid
  inguinal
  intercostal
  interiliac
  internal iliac
  interpectoral
  jugular
  jugulodigastric
  jugulo-omohyoid
  lumbar
  malar
  mandibular

lymph node *(continued)*
  mastoid
  mediastinal
  nasolabial
  obturator
  occipital
  palpable regional
  pancreatic
  pancreaticoduodenal
  pancreaticolienal
  pancreaticosplenic
  paracardial
  paracolic
  paramammary
  pararectal
  parasternal
  paratracheal
  parauterine
  paravaginal
  paravesicular
  paratracheal
  parietal
  parotid
  pectoral
  pelvic
  pericardial
  phrenic
  popliteal
  postaortic
  postcaval
  postvesicular
  preaortic
  precaval
  prececal
  prepericardial
  pretracheal
  prevertebral
  prevesicular
  pulmonary
  pyloric
  rectal
  regional

lymph node *(continued)*
  retroaortic
  retroauricular
  retrocecal
  retropharyngeal
  retrorectal
  sacral
  sentinel
  sigmoid
  solitary
  splenic
  submandibular
  submental
  subscapular
  superficial inguinal
  supraclavicular
  supratrochlear
  thyroid
  tracheal
  tracheobronchial
  vesicular
  visceral
lymph node aspiration
lymph node metastasis
lymph node permeability factor
lymph node sinus
lymphoblast
lymphoblastic leukemia
lymphoblastic lymphoma
Lymphocryptovirus
lymphocyte
  atypical
  B
  CD4+
  circulating
  mature
  sinusoidal
  T
  T4
  thymus-dependent
  thymus-independent
lymphocyte-associated virus

lymphocyte-like cell
lymphocyte proliferation test
lymphocyte subset assay
lymphocyte transformation test
lymphocytic choriomeningitis
lymphocytic infiltrate
lymphocytic infiltration of dermis
lymphocytic infiltration of skin
lymphocytic interstitial pneumonitis
lymphocytic leukemia
lymphocytic lymphoma
  plasmacytoid
  poorly differentiated
  well differentiated
lymphocytic myocarditis
lymphocytic thyroiditis
lymphocytopheresis
lymphocytosis, relative
lymphocytotoxic antibody
lymphogenous embolism
lymphogenous metastasis
lymphoglandular body
lymphogranuloma venereum
lymphohistiocytic infiltrate
lymphoid cell
lymphoid follicle
lymphoid hyperplasia
lymphoid interstitial pneumonia
lymphoid leukocyte
lymphoid microabscess
lymphoid polyp
lymphoid tissue, aggregations of
lymphoid tumor
lymphokine-activated killer (LAK) cell
lymphoma
  adult T-cell
  African
  B-cell
  B-cell monocytoid
  Burkitt
  centrocytic
  cleaved cell

lymphoma *(continued)*
  diffuse
  diffuse large cell
  diffuse mixed small and large cell
  diffuse small cleaved cell
  follicular
  follicular center cell
  follicular mixed small cleaved
  follicular predominantly large cell
  follicular predominantly small cell
  giant follicle
  granulomatous
  histiocytic
  Hodgkin
  intermediate lymphocytic
  large cell, immunoblastic
  large cleaved cell
  large noncleaved cell
  Lennert
  lymphoblastic
  lymphocytic plasmacytoid
  lymphocytic poorly differentiated
  lymphocytic well differentiated
  malignant
  mantle zone
  Mediterranean
  mixed lymphocytic-histiocytic
  nodular
  non-Hodgkin
  pleomorphic
  primary of central nervous system
  small B-cell
  small cleaved cell
  small lymphocytic
  small noncleaved cell
  T-cell
    convoluted
    cutaneous
    small lymphocytic
  U-cell
  undefined
  undifferentiated

lymphoma cutis
lymphomatoid papulosis
lymphomatosis
lymphomatous
lymphomyxoma
lymphonodulus (pl. lymphonoduli)
lymphopathy, ataxic
lymphopenia
lymphoplasia
lymphoplasmapheresis
lymphopoiesis
lymphoproliferative
lymphoreticular cell
lymphoreticular tissue
lymphoreticulosis
lymphorrhage
lymphorrhagia
lymphorrhea
lymphorrhoid
lymphosarcoma
lymphostasis
lymphotaxis
lymphotrophy
lymphotropic
lymph plexus
lymph tissue
lymph trunk, bronchomediastinal
lymphvascular
lymph vessel
lysate of blood cells
lyse, lysed
lysing
lysis, euglobulin clot
lysis of cells
lysosomal protease
lysosome
lysozyme
lyssa inclusion body
Lyssavirus
"lytes" (slang for electrolytes)
lytic lesion
lytic virus

M, m

Macalister muscle
Macchiavello stain
MacConkey agar
Macdonald test for liver function
MAC EIA (IgM antibody capture
   enzyme immunoassay)
macerate
macerated fetus
maceration
Machado-Guerreiro test for Chagas
   disease
Machado test for Chagas disease
Mach band
Mackenrodt ligament
Mackenzie point
Maclagan thymol turbidity test
MacLean–de Wesselow urea
   concentration test
MacLean test for lactic acid
   in gastric juice
MacMunn test for indican
MacNeal tetrachrome blood stain
macrocytic anemia
macrocytosis
macroglia cell
macroglobulin
macroglobulinemia, Waldenström

macroglossia
macrognathia
macrolobular cirrhosis
macrometastasis
macrophage
   alveolar
   armed
   fixed
   free
   hemosiderin-laden
   inflammatory
   lipid-laden
   pulmonary
macrophage-activating factor
macrophage colony-stimulating factor
macrophage inflammatory protein
macrophage migration inhibition test
macrophages stuffed with lipid material
macroscopic diagnosis
macroscopic hematuria
macroscopic report
macrosomia
MACS immunomagnetic cell sorter
macula (pl. maculae)
macula, false
macular artery
macular atrophy

macular degeneration
macule
maculopapular exanthem
maculopapular rash
MacWilliam test for albumin
Madayag biopsy needle
Madelung deformity
Madelung neck
Madurella mycetomatis
maduromycosis
Magendie space
magna, lacuna
magnesionitric test for albumin in urine
magnesium (Mg)
Magpie test
mahogany-colored stool
Maier sinus
main artery
main pancreatic duct (MPD)
main stem bronchus
maintenance protein
Maissiat band
Maissiat ligament
Maissiat tract
Majocchi disease
Majocchi granuloma
major branch
major calyx
major duodenal papilla
major, pelvis
major salivary gland
major vessel
majus (pl. majora)
    labium (pl. labia)
    omentum
malabsorption
    congenital lactose
    glucose-galactose
    sucrose-isomaltose, congenital
malabsorption of fats
malabsorption of vitamin B_{12}
malabsorption state

malabsorption syndrome
Malacarne space
malachite green
malar bone
malaria
  acute
  algid
  autochthonous
  avian
  benign tertian
  bilious remittent
  cerebral
  congenital
  double tertian
  dysenteric algid
  falciparum
  gastric algid
  hemolytic
  hemorrhagic
  induced
  intermittent
  malignant tertian
  nonan
  ovale
  pernicious
  quartan
  quotidian
  relapsing
  remittent
  tertian
  therapeutic
  transfusion
  vivax
malarial cachexia
malarial cirrhosis
malarial granuloma
malaria-like illness
malarial knobs
malarial pigment
malarial pneumonitis
malaria smear
malariotherapy

malar rash
malar skin
Malassezia furfur
Malassezia pachydermatis
Malbin-Sternheimer stain
Maldonado–San Jose stain
male pattern alopecia
male pattern baldness
male pelvis
male reproductive system
male sex cell
malformation
   Arnold-Chiari
   cystic adenomatoid
   dancer foot
   Dieulafoy vascular
malignancy
   aggressive
   borderline
   grading of
   hematologic
   hematopoietic
   high-grade
   intraocular
   low-grade
   metastatic
   primary
   prostatic
   staging of
malignant atrophic papulosis
malignant cell
malignant change
malignant degeneration
malignant edema
malignant fibrous histiocytoma
malignant glioma tumor
malignant hyperphenylalaninemia
malignant hypertension
malignant lentigo
malignant lymphoma
malignant melanoma
malignant melanoma in situ

malignant melanoma metastatic
   to heart
malignant mesothelioma
malignant mole
malignant neoplasm
malignant nephrosclerosis
malignant pheochromocytoma
malignant teratoma of heart
malignant tertian malaria
malleolar artery
malleus bone
malleus, ligaments of
Mallory aniline blue stain
Mallory-Azan stain
Mallory body
Mallory collagen stain
Mallory hemofuchsin stain
Mallory hyalin body
Mallory iodine stain
Mallory iron stain
Mallory phloxine stain
Mallory phosphotungstic acid-
   hematoxylin stain
Mallory trichrome stain
Mallory triple stain
Mallory-Weiss lesion
Mallory-Weiss syndrome
Mallory-Weiss tear
malnutrition
malodorous stool
Malot test
malpighian body
malpighian cell
malpighian corpuscle
malpighian follicle
malpighian gland
malpighian layer
malrotation of intestine
Malta fever
maltose test
malunion of fracture fragments
mamillary body

mammary abscess
mammary adenoma
mammary adenosis
mammary artery
mammary atrophy
mammary cyst
mammary duct obstruction
mammary dysplasia
mammary gland
mammotropic factor
mammotropic hormone
Manchurian fever
Mancini iodine technique
mandible
    alveolar border of
    angle of
mandible bone
mandible joint
mandibular arch
mandibular artery
mandibular canal
mandibular disk
mandibular gland
mandibular incisor angle, Frankfort
mandibulofacial dysostosis
manganese (Mn)
manganese pneumonitis
mango dermatitis
Mann methyl blue-eosin stain
Mann-Whitney test
Mann-Whitney-Wilcoxon test
Manson pyosis
mantle, brain
mantle zone lymphoma
Mantoux intracutaneous tuberculin test
Mantoux skin test
manubriosternal articulation
manubriosternal joint
manubrium, inferior border of
manubrium of sternum
many-sided
maple syrup odor in urine

maple syrup urine disease
maprotiline
marantic clot
marasmus
marble bone disease
marble bones
Marburg disease
Marburg virus
Marchand adrenal gland
Marchand wandering cell
Marchi fixative
Marchi method of staining
Maréchal test for bile pigments in urine
Marfan syndrome
margin
margin of pupil
margin of resection
marginal artery
marginal artery of colon
marginal artery of Drummond
marginal osteophyte
marginal sinus
marginatum erythema
Marie-Strümpell (Struempell) disease
marine dermatitis
mark, Unna
marked focal hyperkeratosis
marker (see *tumor marker*)
markings, haustral
maroon-colored stool
Marquis test for morphine
marrow
    bone
    depressed
    erythroid hyperplasia of
    fat
    gelatinized
    hyperplasia of
    red
    spinal
    yellow
marrow aspiration

marrow canal
marrow cell
marrow harvesting, stem cell
Martinotti cell
masculine pelvis
mask, ecchymotic
masked virus
mass
  appendiceal
  apperceptive
  body cell
  brittle
  concentrically laminated
  conical
  cystic
  elongated
  encapsulated
  firm
  fleecy
  friable
  fungating
  glistening
  injection
  inner cell
  irregular
  lean body
  lung
  molar
  molecular
  multilocular
  nodular
  pearly white
  relative molecular
  sex chromatin
  shiny
  slowly enlarging
  stonelike
  tigroid
mass effect
masseteric artery
Masset test for bile pigments in urine
mass infection

massive coagulation
massive deposits of glycogen in muscle
massive embolism
massive hepatic necrosis
massive pneumonia
massive pulmonary hemorrhagic
  edema
mass of congealed blood
Masson argentaffin stain
Masson-Fontana ammoniacal silver
  stain
Masson trichrome stain
mass spectrometry
mast cell
mast cell leukemia
master gland
mast leukocyte
masticate
mastitis
  acute
  chronic
  cystic
  gargantuan
  glandular
  interstitial
  lactational
  parenchymatous
  periductal
  phlegmonous
  plasma cell
  puerperal
  retromammary
  stagnation
  submammary
  suppurative
mastocytosis, diffuse cutaneous
mastoid abscess
mastoid air cells, epithelium-lined
mastoid antrum
mastoid artery
mastoid bone
mastoid cell

mastoid fontanelle
mastoid process
mastoiditis
mater (note: one *t*)
   dura
   pia
material
   amorphous
   base
   breadlike
   calcareous
   coffee-grounds
   colloid
   cross-reacting (CRM)
   cytoplasmic
   dried out
   eosinophilic
   extracellular (ECM)
   fluid
   foamy
   foreign
   functional
   gelatinous
   gel-like
   genetic
   globoid
   gritty
   grumous
   hemorrhagic
   homogeneous
   inspissated
   jelly-like
   liquid
   lumpy
   mucoid
   myxoid
   noncellular
   nonfibrous
   purulent
   refractile
   sandy
   sarcoplasmic

material *(continued)*
   semisolid
   thickened
   tissue equivalent
maternal diabetes
maternal phenylketonuria
Mathews test for lactose and glucose
matrix
   amphophilic
   bone
   cartilage
   cytoplasmic
   extracellular (ECM)
   interterritorial
   mitochondrial
   nail
   sarcoplasmic
   solid
   territorial
matrix band
matrix cell
matrix granule
matrix hyaline
matrix of collagenic fibers
matt or matte
matter
   gray
   white
matting
maturation
maturation index
mature lymphocyte
maturity-onset diabetes
maturity-onset diabetes of youth
   (MODY)
Mauchart ligament
Maumené test for glucose
Maurer dots
Mauthner cell
maxilla (pl. maxillae)
maxillary antrum
maxillary artery

maxillary articulation
maxillary bone
maxillary canal
maxillary nerve
maxilloturbinal bone
Maximow fixative
Maximow solution
Maximow stain
maximum breathing capacity
maximus, gluteus
Mayaro virus
Mayer hematoxylin
Mayer hematoxylin counterstain
Mayer mucicarmine
Mayer stain
Mayerhofer test
Mayer test for alkaloids
May-Grünwald-Giemsa stain
mazoplasia
Mazzotti test for onchocerciasis
M band
MB band
MBC (minimum bactericidal
  concentration)
MB fraction
MB isoenzyme
MBP (myelin basic protein)
MCB Tissue Freeze
McBurney point
McCort sign
McCoy cell
mcg (microgram)
MCH (mean corpuscular hemoglobin)
MCHC (mean corpuscular hemoglobin
  concentration)
McKrae strain of herpesvirus
McLeod blood phenotype
MCV (mean corpuscular volume)
MD (muscular dystrophy)
MDM2 expression
meadow dermatitis
meadow grass dermatitis

meal
  barium
  fatty
  opaque
  retention
  test
mealy
mean corpuscular hemoglobin (MCH)
mean corpuscular hemoglobin concentration (MCHC)
mean corpuscular volume (MCV)
mean platelet volume (MPV)
measles (rubeola)
measles encephalitis
measles-like viruses
measles virus
measurement
  axial extinction
  slit-scan
meatus
  acoustic
  external auditory
meaty appearance
meaty texture
mechanical vector
mechanism
  deglutition
  Frank-Starling
  humeral
  immune
  sphincteric
  swallowing
Meckel band
Meckel diverticulitis
Meckel diverticulum
Meckel ligament
Meckel space
meconium plug
meconium-stained amniotic fluid
meconium-stained membrane
medial antebrachial cutaneous nerve
medial arcuate ligament

medial atlantoaxial joint
medial circumflex artery of thigh
medial collateral ligament of elbow
medial crus (pl. crura)
medial crus of superficial inguinal ring
medial cuneiform bone
medial cutaneous nerve
medial cutaneous nerve of arm
medial cystic necrosis
medial eminence
medial epicondyle
medial frontobasal artery
medial ligament of knee
medial ligament of talocrural joint
medial lumbocostal arch
medial necrosis of large arteries
medial palpebral artery
medial palpebral ligament
medial puboprostatic ligament
medial striate artery
medial surface of lung
medial surface, vertebral part of
medial talocalcaneal ligament
medial tarsal artery
medial umbilical fold
medial umbilical ligament
medial wall of nasal cavity
median antebranchial vein
median aperture
median arcuate ligament
median eminence
median groove
median lobe of prostate
median plane
median raphe
median sacral artery
median umbilical fold
media, otitis
mediastinal artery
mediastinal fibrosis
mediastinal lymph node
mediastinal pleura

mediastinal pleurisy
mediastinitis
   fibrous
   indurative
mediastinodiaphragmatic pleural
   reflection
mediastinum
mediate transfusion
media tunica
medical mycology
medical surveillance
medical technologist
medicolegal autopsy
Mediterranean anemia
Mediterranean lymphoma
medium (pl. media)
   agar
   AimV serum-free
   alkaline
   Apathy mounting
   artificial
   balsam mounting
   Bruns glucose
   Clarite mounting
   clear (or clearing)
   contrast
   culture
   embedding
   HAT (hypoxanthine, aminopterin, thymidine)
   homogeneous
   infiltration
   jelly-like
   Loeffler
   mounting
   nutrient
   Permount mounting
   refractile
   Sabouraud culture
   Spurr
   Stuart
   Thayer-Martin

medium *(continued)*
    transparent
    transport
medium chain fatty acid (MCFA)
medium chain triglycerides (MCT)
medius, scalenus
medulla (pl. medullas, medullae)
    adrenal
    dusky
    lymphatic
    ovarian
    renal
    spinal
medulla oblongata
medulla of bone
medulla of kidney
medulla of lymph node
medulla of thymus
medullary artery
medullary bone
medullary canal
medullary carcinoma
medullary cavity
medullary cord
medullary ray
medullary sarcoma
medullary sinus
medullary sponge kidney
medullary substance
medullary zone
medulloblastoma
medusae, caput
megacolon, congenital
megakaryocyte
megakaryocyte progenitor cell
megakaryopoiesis
megaloblastic anemia
megaloblastic bone marrow
megaspore mother cell
meibomian cyst
meibomian froth
meibomian gland

Meigs syndrome
Meigs test for fat in milk
meiosis
Meirowsky phenomenon
Meissner corpuscle
Meissner plexus in submucosa
melanin-containing cell
melanin deposition
melanin incontinence
melanin synthesis, defect in
melanin test
melanoblasts
melanocyte
melanocyte-stimulating hormone
melanocytic nevus
melanocytoma, dermal
melanocytosis
melanoma
    acral-lentiginous
    amelanotic
    benign juvenile
    benign uveal
    desmoplastic malignant
    halo
    intraocular
    juvenile
    lentigo maligna
    malignant
    malignant lentigo
    minimal deviation
    mucosal
    nodular
    ocular
    staging of malignant
    subungual
    superficial spreading
    uveal
melanomatosis
melanophage
melanosis
melanosis coli
melanosome

melanotic freckle, Hutchinson
melanotic pigment
melanotic prurigo
melanotropic
melanotropin release-inhibiting
   hormone (MIH)
melanotropin-releasing factor
melanotropin-releasing hormone
   (MRH)
melasma
melatonin
melenic stool
mellitus, diabetes
membrane
   allantoid
   alveolodental
   anal
   arachnoid
   arachnoidal
   areolar
   atlanto-occipital
   basement
   basilar
   boundary
   Bowman
   Bruch
   bucconasal
   buccopharyngeal
   cell
   chorioallantoic
   cloacal
   closing
   cricothyroid
   cricotracheal
   cricovocal
   croupous
   deciduous
   Descemet
   diphtheritic
   drum
   dysmenorrheal
   egg

membrane *(continued)*
   elastic
   embryonic
   enamel
   epipapillary
   exocelomic
   external intercostal
   false
   fenestrated
   fertilization
   fetal
   fibrous
   flaccid
   gelatinous otoli sthic
   germ
   germinal
   glomerular capillary
   hyaline
   inner
   innermost intercostal
   intact
   internal elastic
   internal intercostal
   interosseous
   limiting
   localized thickenings of Bruch
   Millipore
   mucous
   nitrocellulose
   nuclear
   obturator
   otolithic
   outer
   perforated tympanic
   perineal
   phrenoesophageal
   placental
   plasma
   pleuroperitoneal
   polyvinylidene difluoride
   serous
   suprapleural

membrane *(continued)*
  synovial
  tympanic
membrane permeability
membranoproliferative glomerulonephritis
membranous deep layer
membranous glomerulonephritis
membranous labyrinth
membranous pneumonocyte
membranous pregnancy
membranous stomatitis
membranous urethra
memory cell
MEN (multiple endocrine neoplasia)
  type I (Wermer syndrome)
  type II (Sipple syndrome)
  type III (mucosal neuroma
    syndrome)
Mendel test
Menghini needle
meningeal adhesion
meningeal artery
meningeal carcinoma
meningeal petechiae
meningeal plague
meningeal tuberculosis
meninges (pl. of meninx)
meningioma
  angioblastic
  cerebellopontine angle
  clival
  convexity
  cystic
  falcine
  falx
  fibroblastic
  fibrous
  malignant
  meningotheliomatous
  parasagittal
  posterior fossa

meningioma *(continued)*
  psammomatous
  suprasellar
  syncytial
  tentorial
  transitional
meningioma of olfactory groove
meningioma of sphenoid ridge
meningitis
  aseptic
  bacterial
  basilar
  benign lymphocytic
  cerebral
  cerebrospinal
  chronic
  coccidioidal
  cryptococcal
  eosinophilic
  epidemic cerebrospinal
  gummatous
  Haemophilus influenzae
  meningococcal
  Mollaret
  mumps
  neoplastic
  occlusive
  otitic
  plague
  pneumococcal
  purulent
  pyogenic
  Quincke
  serous
  spinal
  sterile
  syphilitic
  tuberculous
  viral
meningitis necrotoxica reactiva
meningitis ossificans
meningoarteritis

meningocele
  anterior
  cranial
  sacral
  spinal
  spurious
  traumatic
meningocephalitis (also, meningoencephalitis)
meningocerebritis
meningococcal meningitis
meningococcal myocarditis
meningococcal septicemia
meningococcus
meningoencephalitis
meningoencephalomyelitis
meningomyelocele
meningothelial cell
meningotheliomatous meningioma
meningothelium
meningotyphoid fever
meninx (pl. meninges)
meniscal horn
menisci (pl. of meniscus)
meniscofemoral ligament
meniscus (pl. menisci)
  articular
  diverging
meniscus homologue
menstrual endometrium
menstrual stage
menstruation
mental artery
mental canal
mental deterioration
mental impairment
mental retardation
mental spine of maxilla
mentolabial sulcus
mEq (milliequivalent)
mEq/L (milliequivalents per liter)
M/E (myeloid/erythroid) ratio

mercurial stomatitis
mercuric chloride
mercuric salts
mercury poisoning
mercury test
Merkel-Ranvier cell
Merkel tactile cell
Merkel tactile disk
mermaid deformity
merocrine gland
Mery gland
Merzbacher-Pelizaeus disease
mesangial cell
mesangial cell fibronectin
mesangial cell proliferation
mesangium
mesarteritis, Mönckeberg
mesatipellic pelvis
mesencephalic artery
mesencephalon
mesenchyma
mesenchymal cell
mesenchymal model
mesenchymal tissue
mesenchymoma
  benign
  malignant
mesenteric artery
mesenteric gland
mesenteric plexus
mesenteric pregnancy
mesenteric soft tissue
mesenteric triangle
mesenteric vein
mesentery
  fan-shaped
  leaves of
  root of
  ventral
mesentery of appendix
mesentery of ileum
mesentery of jejunum

meshwork of connective tissue
meshwork of glial fibrils as repair
  material
mesoappendix
mesocardium, arterial
mesocolic band
mesocolic gland
mesocolon
mesocolonic fat tissue
mesoderm
    extraembryonic
    gastral
mesodermal factor
mesogastrium, dorsal
mesoglial cell
mesorectum
mesosalpinx
mesosigmoid colon
mesothelial cell
mesothelial cyst
mesothelioma of pleura
mesothelium
mesothial cell
mesovarium
Mester test for rheumatic disease
metabisulfite test for sickle cell
  hemoglobin
metabolic acidosis
metabolic alkalosis
metabolic cirrhosis
metabolic coma
metabolic disorder
metabolic disturbance of acid-base
  balance
metabolic encephalopathy
metabolic insult
metabolism
    abnormal glucose
    basal
    carbohydrate
    carbon dioxide
    electrolyte

metabolism *(continued)*
    energy
    glucose
    inborn error of
    intermediary
    mucopolysaccharide
    primary
    protein
    respiratory
    secondary
metacarpal artery
metacarpal bone
metacarpophalangeal articulation
metacarpophalangeal joint
metacarpus (pl. metacarpi)
metachromatic leukodystrophy
metachromatic stain
metahypophysial diabetes
metamorphosis
    fatty
    platelet
    retrograde
    tissue
    viscous
metamyelocyte
metanephric diverticulum
metanephrines in urine
metaphyseal artery
metaphyseal dysplasia
metaphysis (pl. metaphyses)
    agnogenic myeloid
    apocrine
    apocrine (of breast)
    autoparenchymatous
    celomic
    columnar
    fundic
    intestinal
    myeloid
    primary myeloid
    secondary myeloid
    squamous

metaplastic squamous cell epithelium
metapneumonic pleurisy
metastasis (pl. metastases)
    calcareous
    drop
    hematogenous
    local
    lymphatic
    lymph node
    pulsating
    satellite
    widespread
metastasis staging
metastasis to bone
metastasis to brain
metastasis to liver
metastasis to lung
metastatic abscess
metastatic calcification
metastatic carcinoma
metastatic disease
metastatic inflammation
metastatic malignancy
metastatic orchitis
metastatic pneumonia
metastatic polyp
metastatic tuberculous abscess
metastatic tumor
metatarsal artery
metatarsal bone
metatarsal plantar artery
metatarsophalangeal articulation
metatarsophalangeal joint
metatarsus (pl. metatarsi)
metazoal myocarditis
methanol (methyl alcohol)
methanol-based polychrome stain
methanol fixative
metHb (methemoglobin)
methemalbumin
methemalbuminemia
methemoglobin (metHb)

methemoglobinemia
    acquired
    congenital
    enterogenous
    hereditary
    primary
    secondary
methemoglobinuria
methicillin-resistant *Staphylococcus aureus* (MRSA)
methionine test
method (staining) (see *solution, stain*)
    ABC peroxidase
    Abell-Kendall
    absorption
    Altmann-Gersh
    AMEX (of processing and embedding)
    Ashby
    Bielschowsky
    Billheimer assay
    capillary gap
    cell separation
    cooled-knife
    copper sulfate
    disk sensitivity
    Filley
    Gallyas
    immunofluorescence
    Jenner
    Klumpp & Bieth
    Kokoskin modified Weber
    Lee-White
    Marshall
    Millipore
    Nuclepore
    PAP
    Parham
    peroxidase/antiperoxidase protein labeling
    phenol/chloroform
    RNAzolB (of RNA extraction)

method *(continued)*
  Sainte-Marie (of alcoholic fixation
    and paraffin embedding)
  strong trichrome staining
  thermodilution
  Torrance and Bothwell
  Towbin (of immunoblotting)
  Warthin-Starry tissue staining
  Weber staining
  Westergren
  Wijsman (of end-labeling)
  Wu
  Ziehl-Neelsen
methyl alcohol
methylene blue stain
  Kühne
  Loeffler
  polychrome
methyl green–pyronin stain
methylphenylhydrazine test for
  fructose
methyl red test
methylumbelliferylglucuronide (MUG)
methyl violet stain
metopic suture
metrotrophic test
Mett test for estimating pepsin
metyrapone test
Mexican hat cell
Mexican spotted fever
Meyenburg complex
Meyer-Archambault loop
Meyer loop
Meynert cell
mg/dl (milligrams per deciliter)
Mg (magnesium)
MHA-TP (microhemagglutinin-
  Treponema pallidum) test
MIC (minimum inhibitory concentra-
  tion)
mice, joint
Michaelis stain

Michailow test for proteins
Michel transport fixative
microabscess
  dermal
  lymphoid
  Munro
  Pautrier
microabscess of lung
microabscess of skin
microaerophilic
microaneurysm of retina, capillary
microangiopathy, diabetic
microbe
microbial
microbiology
microchemotaxis chamber
Micrococcus
microcytosis
microcytotoxicity assay
microfilaria
microfilariae in blood
microfilariae in subcutaneous tissue,
  skin, eye
microfocus
microglandular
microglia
microglial cell
micrognathia
microgram (mcg)
microhemagglutination test for
  Treponema pallidum (MHA-TP)
microhematocrit
microinfarcts of spleen
microinvasion
microinvasive carcinoma
microinvasive carcinoma classification
microkatal
microliter (μL)
microlobular cirrhosis
micrometastasis
micrometer (μm)
micromolar

micromole (μmol)
micromyeloblastic leukemia
micronodular cirrhosis of liver
micronodular fibrotic pattern
microorganism, pathogenic (see
   pathogen)
microprecipitation test
microscope
   BHS-RFC A3 fluorescence
   cervical
   confocal epifluorescence
   darkfield
   electron
   fluorescence
   JEOL 100 CX electron
   light
   Olympus B-Max
   phase-contrast
   Phillips 300 transmission electron
   polarizing
   Sarastro-2000 confocal scanning
   transmission electron
   Vanox fluorescence
   Vanox-T
   Zeiss Axiolab light
microscopic clefts
microscopic diagnosis
microscopic hematuria
microscopy
   confocal laser scanning
   darkfield
   electron
   fluorescent
   intravital
   light
microsomal antibodies, thyroid
microsomal TRC antibody titer
microsomes
microsomia
Microsporum
Microsporum amazonicum
Microsporum audouinii

Microsporum boullardii
Microsporum canis
Microsporum cookei
Microsporum equinum
Microsporum faeni
Microsporum ferrugineum
Microsporum floccosum
Microsporum fulvum
Microsporum gallinae
Microsporum gypseum
Microsporum nanum
Microsporum persicolor
Microsporum praecox
Microsporum racemosum
Microsporum ripariae
Microsporum vanbreuseghemii
Microtainer (B-D Microtainer)
microtome
   freezing
   rocking
   rotary
   sliding
microtubule-associated protein (MAP)
microvesicular fat
microvesiculation
microvillus (pl. microvilli)
midabdominal wall
midaxillary line
midbody
midbrain
midcarpal joint
midcarpal portal
midclavicular line
midcolon
midcycle cervical mucus
middle capsular artery
middle cardiac vein
middle cell
middle cerebral artery
middle collateral artery
middle costotransverse ligament
middle cuneiform bone

middle ear
middle ethmoidal air cell
middle extrahepatic bile duct
middle genicular artery
middle hemorrhoidal artery
middle lobe bronchus
middle meatus
middle mediastinum
middle meningeal artery
middle nasal concha
middle radioulnar joint
middle rectal artery
middle rectal vein
middle sacral artery
middle suprarenal artery
middle temporal artery
middle turbinated bone
middle umbilical ligament
middle vesical artery
midepigastric area
midepigastrium
midesophagus
midface
midfoot
midfrontal
midget bipolar cell
midgut
midgut artery
midinguinal point
midlateral
midline abdominal crease
midline granuloma
midpoint of clavicle
midportion
mid-pretibial
midrectal area
midscapular line
midsection
midsigmoid colon
midstream urine specimen
midtarsal
midtarsal joint

midthigh
midzonal hepatic necrosis
Mielke bleeding time
Mignon eosinophilic granuloma
migrating abscess
migrating neuritis
migration inhibition test
migration inhibitory factor (MIF)
migration inhibitory factor (MIF) test
migration of leukocytes
migration, transepithelial
migratory cell
migratory pneumonia
migratory polyarthritis
Mikulicz cell
Mikulicz syndrome
miliaria
miliary abscess
miliary aneurysm
miliary embolism
miliary fever
miliary granuloma
miliary pattern
miliary tubercles
miliary tuberculosis
milker node virus
milk fever
milk-filled cyst
milk line
milk protein antibody
milk teeth
Millard test for albumin
Miller-Galante knee
Miller-Kurzrok test
milliequivalent (mEq)
milliequivalents per liter (mEq/L)
Milligan trichrome stain
milliliter (mL, ml)
millimeter (mm)
millimole (mmol)
millimoles per liter (mmol/L)
milliosmole (mOsm)

Millipore filter
Millipore membrane
Millipore method
Millonig phosphate-buffered formalin
Millon-Nasse test for protein
Millon test for proteins and
    nitrogenous compounds
Mima polymorpha (now *Acinetobacter
    calcoaceticus,* var. *lwoffi*)
mineralocorticoid
minilaparotomy
minimal deviation melanoma
minimum bactericidal concentration
    (MBC) culture
minimum inhibitory concentration
    (MIC)
minimum lethal concentration (MLC)
minor (pl. minora)
    labia
    pelvis
minor calyx
minor duodenal papilla
mirror image breast biopsy
mirror-image cell
mismatched blood transfusion
missed abortion
mites in cutaneous burrows
mites in skin scrapings
mitochondria
mitochondrial antibody
mitochondrial gene
mitochondrial matrix
mitogen
mitosis (pl. mitoses), multipolar
mitotic activity
mitotic division
mitotic figures, bizarre
mitotic index
mitotic rate
mitral arcade
mitral cell
mitral orifice

mitral stenosis
mitral valve
mitral valvular leaflet
Mitscherlich test for phosphorus
    in stomach
Mittendorf dot
mIU (milli-international unit)
mixed agglutination test
mixed cell sarcoma
mixed flora
mixed gland
mixed infection
mixed leukocyte culture (MLC)
mixed lymphocyte culture (MLC) test
mixed lymphocytic-histiocytic
    lymphoma
mixed phase endometrium
mixed proteinuria
mL, ml (milliliter)
MLC (minimum lethal concentration)
mm (millimeter)
MM band
MM isoenzyme
MM virus
mm^3 (cubic millimeter)
mmol (millimole)
mmol/L (millimoles per liter)
Mn (manganese)
MNS blood group
mobile gallbladder
moderator band
Modic disk abnormality classification
modicum
modifier gene
MODY (maturity-onset diabetes
    of youth)
Mohrenheim space
Mohr test for hydrochloric acid
    in stomach contents
Mohs surgery
moist scaling
Mokola virus

mol (mole)
molar gland
molar mass
molar pregnancy
molar tissue
mold
mold fungus
mole (mol) (measurement)
    blood
    Breus
    cystic
    false
    fleshy
    hairy
    hydatidiform
    invasive
    malignant
    pigmented
    stone
    true
    tubal
    vesicular
molecular death
molecular lesion
molecular mass
molecular weight
Molisch test for urine glucose
Mollaret meningitis
Moll gland
Molluscipoxvirus
molluscum body
molluscum contagiosum
molluscum contagiosum virus
Moloney test
molybdenum
Mönckeberg arteriosclerosis
Mönckeberg calcification
Mönckeberg degeneration
Mönckeberg sclerosis
Mondor disease
mongolian spot-like lesion
mongolism

Monilia (former name of *Candida*)
Monilia sitophila
moniliaceous
moniliasis
monkeypox virus
"mono" (slang for infectious mononu-
    cleosis)
"monos" (slang for monocytes)
monoamino-monocarboxylic acids,
    impaired transport of
monoblast
monoclonal antibody (see *antibody*)
monoclonal gammopathy
monoclonal immunoglobulin
monoclonal immunoglobulin light
    chains in serum
monoclonal light chains
monoclonal peak
monocyte
monocyte chemoattractant protein-1
    (MCP-1)
monocyte derived neutrophil chemo-
    tactic (MDNCF)
monocytic leukemia
monocytoid cell
monocytopenia
monocytosis
Mono-Diff test
monolayer
monoleptic fever
monomorphous oval cell
mononeuritis
mononuclear and neutrophilic exudate
mononuclear cell infiltrate
mononuclear cells in circulating blood
mononuclear infiltrate
mononucleosis
monoptychic gland
monosaccharide
Monoscreen test
monosexual
monosome

monosomic
monosomy
Monospot test (also, MonoSpot)
Monosticon Dri-Dot test
Monsel solution
mons pubis
monstrocellular nuclei
Montenegro test
Montgomery gland
moon face (facies)
Moore test for carbohydrate
Mooser cell
Morax-Axenfeld bacillus
Moraxella atlantae
Moraxella catarrhalis
Moraxella lacunata
Moraxella nonliquefaciens
Moraxella osloensis
Moraxella phenylpyruvica
Moraxella urethralis
morbid obesity
morbilliform
Morbillivirus, morbillivirus
mordant (see *stain*)
mordant solution
Morel ear
Morelli test (exudate v. transudate)
   (*not* Moretti)
Moretti test for typhoid fever
morgagnian cyst
Morgagni appendix
Morgagni crypt
Morgagni gland
Morgagni hydatid
Morgagni nodule
Morgagni ventricle
Morgan bacillus
Morganella
Morganella morganii
morgue
moribund
Morison pouch

Moritz test
Mörner test for tyrosine
morphea (localized scleroderma)
   generalized
   guttate
   linear
morphogenic field
morphologic change
morphologic classification
morphology
Morquio disease
mortar kidney
mortem (see *antemortem* and
   postmortem)
Mortierella wolfii
mortis
   algor
   livor
   rigor
mortise
mortise joint
morula (pl. morulae)
mosaic fungus
mosaic pattern
mosaic wart
Mosenthal test
Mosler diabetes
mOsm (milliosmole)
mosquito
   Culex
   Wyeomyia melanocephala
mosquito-borne febrile exanthem
mosquito-borne virus
mossy cell
moth-eaten alopecia of secondary
   syphilis
mother cell
motile
motile bacillus
motile leukocyte
motile sperm
motility, sperm

motility test
motor cell
motor cortex
motor end plates
motor fiber
motor neuron, cell body of
motor root
motor supply
motor unit
Mott cell
mottled appearance
Motulsky dye reduction test
mound, infraumbilical
mount, KOH (potassium hydroxide)
mounted
mounting medium
mounting of tissue section
mouth, foot, and hand disease
mouth of processus vaginalis
movable articulation
movable joint
movable kidney
movement, ameboid
movers, prime
Mowry colloidal iron stain
moyamoya
Mozart ear
MPD (main pancreatic duct)
MP, MCP (metacarpophalangeal) joint
MP, MTP (metatarsophalangeal) joint
M protein
MPV (mean platelet volume)
MRSA (methicillin-resistant
    Staphylococcus aureus)
MSB trichrome stain
MSTS (Musculoskeletal Tumor
    Society) staging system
M-25 virus
μL (microliter)
μmol (micromole)
Much bacillus
Much granule

mucicarmine
mucilaginous gum
mucin clot formation
mucin clot test
mucin, gastric
mucinoid degeneration
mucinosis
    follicular
    papular
mucinous adenocarcinoma
mucinous carcinoma
mucinous cystadenocarcinoma
mucinous degeneration
mucinous nest
mucin-secreting columnar cell
mucin stain
mucoalbuminous cell
mucocutaneous lymph node syndrome
mucocutaneous pigmentation
mucoid degeneration
mucoid impaction of bronchus
mucoid material
mucoid stool
mucoperichondrium
mucopolysaccharide metabolism
mucopolysaccharides, excessive
    production of
mucopolysaccharides in intima of
    arteries
mucoprotein
mucopurulent exudate in alveoli
mucopus (mucus and pus)
Mucor
Mucor ramosissimus
Mucor rouxianus
mucormycosis
mucorrhea
mucosa (mucous membrane)
    alimentary
    alveolar
    antral
    auditory

mucosa *(continued)*
   bronchial
   buccal
   bulging of
   cardiac m. of stomach
   colorectal
   endocervical
   foveolar gastric
   foveolosulciolar gastric
   gallbladder
   gingival
   intestinal
   oxyntic
   pyloric
   rectal
   sulciolar gastric
   urinary
   vaginal
mucosal bridge
mucosal disease virus
mucosal folds
mucosal hyperemia
mucosal hyperplasia
mucosal injection
mucosal island (on x-ray)
mucosal junction, squamocolumnar
mucosal melanoma
mucosal necrosis
mucosal patch
mucosal pattern
mucosal ring, esophageal
mucosal suspensory ligament
mucosal ulcer
mucosal zone
mucoserous cell
mucous cell
mucous cyst
mucous degeneration
mucous diarrhea
mucous gland
mucous glands of auditory tube
mucous glands of duodenum

mucous glands of eustachian tube
mucous lake of stomach
mucous membrane
mucous neck cell
mucous plug
mucous polyp
mucous salivary gland
mucous shred
mucous stool
mucous strand
mucous surface
mucoviscidosis
mucus (noun)
   cervical
      midcycle cervical
   ovulatory
mucus-secreting cell
mucus-secreting epithelium
mucus-secreting gland
mud, biliary
MUG (methylumbelliferylglucuronide)
mulberry cell
mulberry ovary
mulberry-shaped intracytoplasmic
   inclusion
Mulder test for glucose
Müller (Mueller)
Müller canal
müllerian cyst
müllerian duct
Müller radial cell
Müller solution
Müller trigone
multangular bone
multiaxial articulation
multiaxial joint
multicellular gland
multicellular organism
multicentric osteosarcoma
multi-colony-stimulating factor
   (multi-CSF)
multifaceted

multifocal area
multifocal encephalomalacia
multifocal osteitis fibrosa
multilobular cirrhosis
multilocular cyst
multiloculated cyst
multiloculated pustule
multinodular goiter
multinucleate cell
multinucleate giant cell
multinucleate giant cells with
    cytoplasmic inclusions
multinucleate globoid cell
multinucleated giant cell
multiparity
multipennate muscle
multiple embolism
multiple endocrine neoplasia (MEN)
    type I (Wermer syndrome)
    type II (Sipple syndrome)
    type III (mucosal neuroma
        syndrome)
multiple familial polyposis
multiple idiopathic hemorrhagic
    sarcoma
multiple intestinal polyposis
multiple myeloma
multiple myositis
multiple neuritis
multiple organ failure
multiple osteochondromatosis
multiple pregnancy
multiple-puncture intracutaneous
    tuberculin test
multiple sclerosis
multiple stain
multiple system atrophy
multiple trauma
multipolar cell
multipolar mitosis
multiseptate, brown distorted hyphae
multiseptate gallbladder

multiseptate hyphae
Multistix
multisystem failure
mummification
mumps
mumps encephalitis
mumps meningitis
mumps meningoencephalitis
mumps sensitivity test
mumps virus
Munro abscess
Munro microabscess
Munro point
mural aneurysm
mural cell
mural kidney
mural pregnancy
mural thrombus
muramidase
Murayama test
murine leukemia virus
murine typhus
murmur grades
Murray Valley encephalitis virus
muscle (see Table of Muscles for
    anatomical names)
    abdominal
    accessory
    Aeby
    agonistic
    Albinus
    anterior
    antigravity
    auricular
    axillary
    Bell
    bipennate
    Bochdalek
    Bovero ("sucking")
    Bowman
    Braune
    Brücke

muscle *(continued)*
    bulbocavernosus
    canine
    cardiac
    Casser
    casserian
    cervical
    Crampton
    Chassaignac
    chin
    Coiter
    deep
    detrusor
    digastric
    dorsal
    Dupré
    Duverney
    emergency
    external
    fast (white)
    fixation
    fixator
    Folius
    Gantzer
    Gavard
    greater
    Guthrie
    Hilton
    Horner
    Houston
    iliococcygeal
    iliocostal
    inferior
    internal
    interosseous
    interspinal
    intertransverse
    intra-auricular
    involuntary
    ischiocavernosus
    Jung
    Klein

muscle *(continued)*
    lateral
    lesser
    levator
    longitudinal
    major
    Macalister
    Marcacci
    medial
    Merkel
    middle
    minor
    Müller (Mueller)
    multipennate
    nonstriated
    oblique
    Ochsner
    Oddi
    Oehl
    opposing
    organic
    Phillips
    posterior
    Pozzi
    pubococcygeal
    quadrate
    red (slow)
    Reisseisen
    ribbon
    rider
    Riolan
    Rouget
    round
    Ruysch
    Santorini
    sartorius
    scalp
    Sebileau
    semimembranous
    semispinal
    semitendinous
    short

muscle *(continued)*
  Sibson
  skeletal
  slow (red)
  smaller
  smooth
  Soemmerring
  somatic
  spindle-shaped
  strap
  striated
  "sucking" (Bovero)
  superficial
  synergic
  synergistic
  tailor's
  Theile
  Tod
  Toynbee
  transverse
  Treitz
  triangular
  trigonal
  true back
  two-bellied
  unipennate
  unstriated
  unstriped
  Valsalva
  ventral
  vertical
  visceral
  vocal
  voluntary
  white (fast)
  Wilson
  wrinkler
  yoked
muscle cell
muscle coat
  circular
  longitudinal

muscle contusion
muscle cramp
muscle enzyme
muscle fiber
  cardiac
  skeletal
  sling
muscle rigidity
muscle shortening
muscle tearing
muscle tissue
muscle twitching
muscle wasting
muscular artery
muscular atrophy
muscular degeneration
muscular dystrophy
  Dejerine-Landouzy
  Duchenne
  Erb
  Landouzy-Dejerine
muscular ring, esophageal
muscular spasticity and rigidity
muscular tube
muscular twig
musculature
musculi (pl. of musculus)
musculophrenic artery
musculophrenic vessel
musculoskeletal
musculotendinous
musculotendinous crura
musculotubal canal
musculus (pl. musculi) (see Table of
  Muscles)
musculus uvulae
mushroom cap
mushroom caps of mucus-like
  pseudomembrane
mushroom-like excrescence
mushroom poisoning
mushy stool

mutant gene
mutant protein
mutant tumor suppressor
mutton fat KPs (keratic precipitates)
myalgia
myasthenia gravis
Mycelia sterilia
mycelial fungus
mycelium
MycoAKT latex bead agglutination test
mycobacteria
mycobacterial antibody
Mycobacterium asiaticum
Mycobacterium avium
Mycobacterium avium-intracellulare
   (MAI) complex
Mycobacterium bovis
Mycobacterium celatum
Mycobacterium chelonei (formerly
   Mycobacterium abscessus)
Mycobacterium cookii
Mycobacterium flavescens
Mycobacterium fortuitum
Mycobacterium gastri
Mycobacterium genavense
Mycobacterium gordonae
Mycobacterium haemophilum
Mycobacterium intracellulare
Mycobacterium kansasii
Mycobacterium leprae
Mycobacterium malmoense
Mycobacterium marinum
Mycobacterium microti
Mycobacterium paratuberculosis
Mycobacterium phlei
Mycobacterium scrofulaceum
Mycobacterium shimoidei
Mycobacterium simiae
Mycobacterium smegmatis
Mycobacterium szulgai
Mycobacterium terrae
Mycobacterium triviale

Mycobacterium tuberculosis
Mycobacterium ulcerans
Mycobacterium xenopi
Mycocentrospora acerina
mycologic test for sugar in urine
mycoplasma (pl. mycoplasmata)
Mycoplasma buccale
Mycoplasma faucium
Mycoplasma fermentans
Mycoplasma genitalium
Mycoplasma hominis
mycoplasmal pneumonia
Mycoplasma orale
Mycoplasma pharyngis
Mycoplasma pneumoniae
Mycoplasma salivarium
mycosis (pl. mycoses)
mycosis cell
mycosis cutis chronica
mycosis fungoides
mycosis intestinalis
mycotic aneurysm
mycotic keratitis
mycotic stomatitis
mycotoxicosis
mydriasis
myelination, incomplete (of nerve
   fibers in brain and spinal cord)
myelin basic protein (MBP)
myelin degeneration of peripheral
   nerves
myelinic degeneration
myelin kidney
myelinogenic field
myelin oligodendrocyte glycoprotein
myelin sheath
myelitic
myelitis
   acute
   ascending
   bulbar
   cavitary

myelitis *(continued)*
    central
    chronic
    compression
    concussion
    cornual
    diffuse
    disseminated
    hemorrhagic
    neuro-optic
    periependymal
    postinfectious
    postvaccinal
    subacute
    subacute necrotic
    syphilitic
    transverse
    viral
myeloblast
myeloblastic leukemia
myeloblastic protein
myelocele
myelocytic leukemia
myelofibrosis
myelogenic osteopathy
myelogenic sarcoma
myelogenous leukemia
myeloid cell
myeloid leukocyte
myeloid metaplasia
myeloid sarcoma
myeloid tissue
myeloma
    giant cell
    indolent
    localized
    multiple
    plasma cell
    sclerosing
    solitary
myeloma cell
myeloma kidney

myeloma protein
myelomonocytic leukemia
myelopathic muscular atrophy
myeloperoxidase
myeloproliferative disease
Myers and Fine test for amylolytic
    activity
Mylius test for bile acids
mylohyoid artery
myoblast
myoblastoma
myocardial depressant
myocardial fiber
myocardial hypertrophy
myocardial infarction
myocardial ischemia
myocardial necrosis
myocardial scarring
myocarditis (MC)
    acute bacterial
    acute interstitial
    acute isolated
    acute rheumatic
    aseptic (of newborn)
    bacterial
    chronic
    chronic hypertrophic
    chronic interstitial
    chronic pernicious
    coxsackievirus
    diphtheritic
    eosinophilic
    fibroid
    fibrous
    Fiedler
    fragmentation
    fungal
    giant cell
    granulomatous
    Histoplasma
    hypersensitivity
    idiopathic

myocarditis *(continued)*
  infectious
  infective
  inflammatory
  influenzal
  interstitial
  isolated diffuse
  Löffler (Loeffler)
  lues
  lymphocytic
  meningococcal
  metazoal
  neutrophilic
  nonspecific granulomatous
  parenchymatous
  peripartum
  pernicious
  pneumococcal
  protozoal
  rheumatic
  rickettsial
  senile
  septic
  spirochetal
  staphylococcal
  subepicardial
  syphilitic
  toxic
  toxoplasmotic
  Trichinella
  tuberculoid
  tuberculous
  viral
myocardium
  senile
  stunned
myocellular area
myoclonic encephalopathy
myocyte
myocyte necrosis
myocytic lysosome
myocytolysis, focal

myoendocarditis
  acute
  subacute
myoepithelial cell
myofiber
myofibrillar area
myofilament protein
myoglobin in urine
myoid cell
myoma (pl. myomata)
myomastoid artery
myomatous polyp
myometrial gland
myometrium, uterine
myopathic atrophy
myopericarditis
myosarcoma
myosin
myosin heavy chain
myosin light chain
myositis
  acute disseminated
  acute progressive
  inclusion body
  infectious
  interstitial
  multiple
  parenchymatous
  primary multiple
  progressive ossifying
  proliferative
  rheumatoid
  spontaneous bacterial
  trichinous
myositis fibrosa
myositis ossificans
myositis serosa
myotome
myotubular myopathy
myxedema
myxedema heart
myxoid cyst

myxoid degeneration
myxoid fibroma
myxolipoma
myxoliposarcoma
myxoma (pl. myxomas, myxomata)
myxoma syndrome with facial
    freckling

myxomatous degeneration
myxomatous tumor
myxopapilloma
myxosarcoma
myxovirus

N, n

Naboth gland
nabothian cyst
nabothian follicle
nabothian gland
NADH diaphorase
NADH methemoglobin reductase
nadir
Naegeli monocytic leukemia
Nägele pelvis
Nageotte cells
nail bed
nail fungal infection
nail matrix
Nairovirus
Najjar-Crigler syndrome
Nakanishi stain
Nakayama test for bile pigments
naked virus
Nakiwogo virus
nalidixic acid
nanogram (ng)
nanoliter (nL)
nanometer (nm)
nanomole (nmol)
NAP (neutrophil activating protein)
nape nevus
naphthalene poisoning

naphthol-ASD chloroacetate esterase
naphthol green B stain
naphthol yellow S stain
napkin (diaper) dermatitis
napkin-ring lesion
narcotic abuse
narcotism, intravenous
naris (pl. nares)
narrow-angle glaucoma
nasal ala
nasal aperture
nasal arch
nasal artery
nasal bone
nasal canal
nasal cavity
nasal concha
nasal fossa
nasal gland
nasal part of pharynx
nasal polyp
nasal secretions
nasal septum
nasal smear
nasion
nasobregmatic arc
nasolabial sulcus

nasolacrimal canal
nasolacrimal duct
naso-occipital arc
nasopalatine artery
nasopalatine canal
nasopalatine nerve
nasopharyngeal carcinoma
nasopharyngeal culture
nasopharyngeal flora
nasopharyngeal secretions
nasopharynx
native albumin
native protein
natural body fluid
natural death
natural killer (NK) cell
natural killer cell stimulating factor
  (NKSF)
nausea
Nauta stain
navicular bone of hand
navicular fossa
N-b band
NBT (nitroblue tetrazolium)
NCL-Arp monoclonal antibody
NCL-Cdm
NCL-ER-LHZ monoclonal antibody
NCL-PGR monoclonal antibody
NCL-pS2
Necator americanus
neck
  dental
  femoral
  Madelung
  bladder
  gallbladder
  pancreas
  rib
  surgical
  transverse artery of
  webbed
  wry

necklike
neck of femur
neck of gallbladder
neck of humerus, anatomical
necrobacillosis
necrobiosis
necrobiotic core
necrocytosis
necrocytotoxin
necrogenic
necrolysis
necrophilia
necrophilic
necropneumonia
necropsy
necrosis
  acute tubular
  arteriolar
  aseptic
  avascular
  bacillary
  Balser fatty
  bilateral cortical
  bloodless zone of
  bridging
  caseous
  central
  centrilobular
  cheesy
  coagulation
  colliquative
  contraction band
  cystic medial
  diffuse
  dry
  epiphyseal ischemic
  Erdheim cystic medial
  exanthematous
  fat
  fibrinoid
  focal
  focal hepatic

necrosis *(continued)*
  focal hepatocellular n. with
    hemorrhagic cysts
  frank
  gangrenous
  gangrenous pulp
  hemorrhagic
  hepatic
  hyaline
  indurative
  infectious pancreatic
  ischemic
  liquefaction
  localized
  massive hepatic
  medial cystic
  midzonal
  mucosal
  myocardial
  Paget quiet
  papillary
  peripheral
  peripheral hepatic
  phosphorus
  piecemeal
  postpartum pituitary
  pressure
  progressive emphysematous
  radiation
  renal tubular
  septic
  stromal
  subacute hepatic
  subcutaneous fat
  submassive hepatic
  superficial
  syphilitic
  total
  tracheobronchial mucosal
  Zenker
  zonal
necrosis of bladder epithelium

necrosis of bladder mucosa
necrosis of ductal epithelium
necrosis of hepatocytes
necrosis of muscle
necrosis of muscle cells
necrosis of small bowel mucosa
necrosis of tissue
necrotic "anchovy paste" material in
  hepatic abscess
necrotic bone
necrotic debris
necrotic inflammation
necrotic lesion in retina
necrotic tissue
necrotizing and suppurative
  osteomyelitis of maxilla
  and mandible
necrotizing arteriolitis in kidney
necrotizing arteritis
necrotizing fasciitis
necrotizing gastritis
necrotizing gingivitis
necrotizing glomerulonephritis
necrotizing granulomatous
  lymphadenitis
necrotizing nephrosis
necrotizing papillitis
necrotizing pneumonia
needle
  Abrams
  aneurysm
  aspirating
  Brockenbrough
  cataract
  Chiba aspiration biopsy
  Cook aspiration biopsy
  Cope
  cutting biopsy
  Deschamps
  discission
  double-pointed
  fine

needle *(continued)*
  Franseen
  Greene biopsy
  Hagedorn
  hollow
  hypodermic
  Jamshidi biopsy
  Lee cutting biopsy
  ligature
  Madayag biopsy
  Menghini
  Reverdin
  Rotex cutting biopsy
  Seldinger
  Silverman
  Skinny
  swaged
  transseptal
  Trucut cutting biopsy
  Turner biopsy
  Vim-Silverman
  Westcott cutting biopsy
needle aspiration, fine-
needle biopsy, fine-
needle core biopsy
needle puncture
needle puncture wound
Neer shoulder fractures I, II, III
  classification
negative
  false
  Rh
negative charge
negative control
negative stain
negative strand virus
Negri bodies in neurons
Negri inclusion body
Neisseria
Neisseria catarrhalis
Neisseria cinerea
Neisseria elongata

Neisseria flavescens
Neisseria gonorrhoeae
Neisseria lactamica
Neisseria meningitidis
Neisseria mucosa
Neisseria sicca
Neisseria subflava
Neisser stain
Neisser-Wechsberg leukocidin
Neisser-Wechsberg phenomenon
Nélaton fold
Nélaton sphincter
Nencki test for indole
neonatal diagnosis
neonatal hepatitis
neonatal jaundice
neonatal lupus
neoplasia
  cervical intraepithelial (CIN)
  lobular
  gestational trophoblastic (GTN)
  multiple endocrine (MEN)
    type I (Wermer syndrome)
    type II (Sipple syndrome)
    type III (mucosal neuroma
      syndrome)
  vaginal intraepithelial (VIN)
neoplasm
  benign
  encapsulated
  firm
  functioning
  gonadal
  grading
  hormone-dependent
  lethal
  malignant
  ovarian
  premalignant
  spherical
  staging
  well-circumscribed

neoplastic cell
neoplastic cyst
neoplastic meningitis
neoplastic tissue
Neoprobe cancer detector device
neorectum
Neotestudina rosatii
neovascularization
nephelometry
nephritic factor
nephritis
  acute
  arteriosclerotic
  azotemic
  bacterial
  Balkan
  capsular
  caseous
  cheesy
  chloro-azotemic
  chronic
  congenital
  croupous
  degenerative
  exudative
  fibrolipomatous
  glomerular
  glomerulocapsular
  hemorrhagic
  interstitial
  Lancereaux
  lupus
  parenchymatous
  pneumococcus
  potassium-losing
  productive
  salt-losing
  saturnine
  scarlatinal
  subacute
  suppurative
  syphilitic

nephritis *(continued)*
  transfusion
  tubal
  tuberculous
  vascular
nephritis dolorosa
nephritis gravidarum
nephritogenic strains of betahemolytic
  streptococci
nephroblastoma
nephrocalcinosis
nephrogenic zone
nephrogenous proteinuria
nephropathy, diabetic
nephrosclerosis
  arterial
  arteriolar
  benign
  hyperplastic arteriolar
  malignant
  senile
nephrosis
  acute
  amyloid
  cholemic
  Epstein
  glycogen
  hydropic
  hypokalemic
  infectious avian
  lower nephron
  lupus
  necrotizing
  osmotic
  toxic
  vacuolar
nephrotic syndrome
nerve (see Table of Nerves)
nerve cell
nerve cell degeneration
nerve degeneration
nerve fasciculus

nerve fiber
nerve fibril
nerve growth factor (NGF)
nerve plexus
nerve root
nerve sheath cell
nerve supply, parasympathetic
nerve tissue damage
nerve tissue degeneration
nerve tissue inflammation
nerve tracts, disruption of
nerve trunk
nervous pregnancy
nervous system
   autonomic
   central
nest
   Brunn
   cell
   epithelial
   isogenous
   mucinous
nests and clumps
nests of radially disposed cells
net knot
network
   articular
   cell
   lymphatic
   venous
Neubauer artery
Neufeld capsular swelling
Neukomm test for bile acids
Neumann cell
neural arc
neural factor
neural (neuroid) nevus
neural arch
neural atrophy
neural canal
neuralgic amyotrophy
neural groove

neural tube
neural tube defect
neurenteric canal
neurilemma
neurilemma cell
neurilemmitis
neurilemoma
   acoustic
   Antoni type A
   Antoni type B
neurinoma, acoustic
neuritic muscular atrophy
neuritic pain
neuritic plaque
neuritis (pl. neuritides)
   adventitial
   ascending
   brachial
   descending
   dietetic
   Eichhorst
   fallopian
   Gombault
   hereditary optic
   interstitial hypertrophic
   intraocular
   Leyden
   migrating
   multiple
   optic
   orbital optic
   parenchymatous
   periaxial
   peripheral
   postfebrile
   postocular optic
   radiation
   radicular
   retrobulbar optic
   sciatic
   segmental
   serum

neuritis *(continued)*
    shoulder-girdle
    syphilitic
    toxic
    traumatic
    vestibular
neuritis migrans
neuroastrocytoma
neuroblastoma
neurocentral joint
neurocentral junction
neurodegenerative disease
neuroendocrine cell
neuroendocrine transducer cell
neuroepithelial cell
neurofibril
neurofibrillary tangle
neurofibroma
neurofibromatosis
neurofibrosarcoma
neurofilament
neurofilament triplet protein
neurogenic bladder
neurogenic diabetes
neurogenic sarcoma
neuroglia
neuroglial cell
neurohypophyseal tract of hypo-
    thalamus
neurohypophysis
neuroma, acoustic
neuromuscular cell
neuromuscular excitability
neuromuscular junction
neuromyelitis, optic
neuron
    autonomic motor
    commissural
    degenerating
    gamma motor
    motor
    spinal

neuronal degeneration
neuronitis
neuronophagia of anterior horn cells
    of spinal cord
neuron-specific enolase
neuro-optic myelitis
neuropathic atrophy
neuropathic joint
neuropathy
    diabetic
    peripheral
    segmental (demyelination)
neuropore, caudal
neurosecretory cell
neurosyphilis
neurotonic congestion
neurotrophic atrophy
neurotropic hormone
neurotropic virus
neurovascular bundle
Neusser granule
neutral (buffered) formalin
neutralization test
neutral red stain
neutral zone
neutropenia
neutrophil
    band
    filamented
    giant
    immature
    juvenile
    nonfilamented
    rod
    segmented
    stab
    unsegmented
neutrophil activating protein (NAP)
neutrophil alkaline phosphatase
neutrophil chemotactant factor
neutrophilia
neutrophilic exudate

neutrophilic infiltrate
neutrophilic leukocyte
neutrophilic myocarditis
nevocyte
nevocytic nevus
nevoid lentigo
nevolipoma
nevus (pl. nevi)
  achromic
  acquired
  amelanotic
  anemic
  balloon cell
  basal cell
  bathing trunk
  Becker
  benign pigmented
  blue
  blue rubber-bleb
  capillary
  cellular blue
  choroidal
  comedo
  compound
  congenital
  connective tissue
  dermal
  dysplastic
  fatty
  flame
  giant hairy
  giant pigmented
  hairy
  halo
  intradermal
  Ito
  Jadassohn
  Jadassohn-Tièche
  junction
  juvenile
  linear epidermal
  melanocytic

nevus *(continued)*
  nape
  neural (neuroid)
  nevocytic
  oral epithelial
  organoid
  Ota
  pigmented
  pigmented hairy
  pigmented hairy epidermal
  port-wine
  sebaceous
  spider
  spindle and epithelioid cell
  spindle cell
  Spitz
  stellar
  strawberry
  Sutton
  systematized
  Unna
  uveal
  vascular
  verrucous
  white sponge
  woolly-hair
nevus cell
  A-type
  B-type
  C-type
nevus-type giant cell
new bone formation
newborn
    gonococcal ophthalmia of the
    hemolytic disease of the
newborn pneumonitis virus
Newcastle disease virus
Newcastle-Manchester bacillus
newly woven bone
NF (neurofibromatosis)
NF1 tumor suppressor gene
NF2 tumor suppressor gene

ng (nanogram)
niacin (nicotinic acid)
niacin test for *Mycobacterium*
    tuberculosis
niche, Barclay
niche en plateau
nickel dermatitis
nickel grid
Nickerson-Kveim test
nicking
Nicolle stain
nidus
nidus of inflamed tissue
nidus of necrotic tissue
nidus of stone formation
Niemann-Pick cell
Niemann-Pick disease
nigra
    linea
    substantia
    tinea
Nikolsky sign
Nile blue fat stain
ninhydrin reagent
ninhydrin-Schiff stain
ninhydrin test
Nippe test for blood
nipple
    accessory
    supernumerary
nipple-areola complex
nipple inversion
nipplelike projections
Nissl body
Nissl degeneration
Nissl granule
Nissl method of staining
Nissl stain
Nissl substance
nitrate reduction test
Nitrazine positive test
Nitrazine test

nitric acid
nitric acid–magnesium sulfate test
nitric acid test for albumin
nitrites test in saliva
nitroblue tetrazolium (NBT) test
nitrocellulose membrane
nitrogen
    alpha amino
    blood urea (BUN)
    liquid
    total
nitrogen gas
nitrogenous compounds test
nitrogenous waste
nitrogen oxide poisoning
nitrogen waste
nitropropiol test for urine glucose
nitroprusside reaction
nitroprusside test for cysteine
nitroso-indole-nitrate test
NK (natural killer) cell
nL (nanoliter)
nm (nanometer)
nmol (nanomole)
N-Multistix
N-myc oncogene
Nobel agar
Nobel stain
Nobel test for acetoacetic acid and
    acetone
Nocardia
Nocardia asteroides
Nocardia brasiliensis
Nocardia caviae
nocardiosis
nodal artery
nodal fever
nodal tissue
node (see also *lymph node*)
    abdominal lymph
    accessory lymph
    anorectal lymph

node *(continued)*
 aortic lymph
 apical lymph
 appendicular lymph
 Aschoff AV (atrioventricular)
 atrioventricular
 auricular lymph
 AV (atrioventricular)
 axillary lymph
 bifurcation lymph
 Bouchard
 brachial lymph
 bronchopulmonary lymph
 buccal lymph
 buccinator lymph
 caval lymph
 celiac lymph
 central lymph
 cervical paratracheal lymph
 Cloquet inguinal lymph
 common iliac lymph
 companion lymph
 coronary
 cubital lymph
 cystic lymph
 Delphian lymph
 deltopectoral lymph
 diaphragmatic lymph
 Dürck
 epicolic lymph
 epigastric lymph
 epitrochlear
 Ewald
 external iliac lymph
 facial lymph
 fibular lymph
 Flack
 foraminal
 gastric lymph
 gastroduodenal lymph
 gastroepiploic lymph
 gastro-omental lymph

node *(continued)*
 gluteal lymph
 gouty
 Haygarth
 Heberden
 hemal
 hemolymph
 Hensen
 hepatic lymph
 hilar lymph
 ileocolic lymph
 iliac circumflex lymph
 iliac lymph
 infraclavicular
 infrahyoid lymph
 inguinal lymph
 intercostal lymph
 interiliac lymph
 interpectoral lymph
 jugular lymph
 jugulodigastric lymph
 jugulo-omohyoid lymph
 juxtaintestinal
 Keith
 Keith-Flack
 lacunar
 lumbar lymph
 lymph
 malar lymph
 mandibular lymph
 mastoid lymph
 Meynet
 nasolabial lymph
 obturator lymph
 occipital lymph
 Osler
 pancreatic lymph
 pancreaticoduodenal lymph
 pancreaticolienal lymph
 paracardial lymph
 paracolic lymph
 paramammary lymph

node *(continued)*
  pararectal lymph
  parasternal lymph
  paratracheal lymph
  parauterine lymph
  paravaginal lymph
  paravesicular lymph
  parietal lymph
  parotid lymph
  Parrot
  pectoral lymph
  pelvic lymph
  pericardial lymph
  peroneal
  phrenic lymph
  popliteal lymph
  postaortic lymph
  postcaval lymph
  postvesicular lymph
  preaortic lymph
  precaval lymph
  prececal lymph
  prelaryngeal
  prepericardial lymph
  pretracheal
  pretracheal lymph
  prevertebral lymph
  prevesicular lymph
  pulmonary juxtaesophageal lymph
  pulmonary lymph
  pyloric lymph
  Ranvier
  rectal lymph
  retroaortic lymph
  retroauricular lymph
  retrocecal lymph
  retropharyngeal lymph
  retropyloric
  retrorectal lymph node
  Rosenmüller
  Rotter
  SA (sinoatrial)

node *(continued)*
  sacral lymph
  Schmorl
  sentinel
  sigmoid lymph
  signal
  singer
  sinoatrial
  sinus
  splenic lymph
  subcarinal
  submandibular lymph
  submental lymph
  subpyloric
  subscapular lymph
  supraclavicular lymph
  suprapyloric
  supratrochlear lymph
  syphilitic
  teacher
  thyroid lymph
  tibial
  tracheal lymph
  tracheobronchial lymph
  Troisier
  vesicular lymph
  Virchow
  visceral lymph
node of epiploic foramen
node of His, atrioventricular
node of neck of gallbladder
node of Tawara
nodosum (pl. nodosa)
  erythema
  periarteritis
  polyarteritis (PAN)
nodular aneurysm
nodular deposit in cartilage
nodular embryo
nodular excrescence
nodular fibrotic reaction
nodular goiter

nodularity
nodular lymphoma
nodular melanoma
nodular nonsuppurative panniculitis
nodular proliferation
nodular subepidermal fibrosis
nodular texture
nodular thickening of alveolar septa
nodule
  aggregated lymphatic
  Arantius
  cold
  cortical
  cutaneous
  Dalen-Fuchs
  discrete
  easily compressible
  erectile
  fibrous
  Fraenkel typhus
  Gandy-Gamma
  hard
  hemangiomatous
  Hoboken
  hot
  indiscrete
  Koeppe
  laryngeal
  lymphatic
  Morgagni
  myometrial
  nondiscrete
  Picker
  red
  respiratory
  rheumatoid
  rubbery
  Schmorl
  singer's
  Sister Joseph
  soapy
  solitary

nodule *(continued)*
  surfer's
  teacher's
  thin-walled hemangiomatous
  tobacco
  tuberculous
  typhoid
  typhus
  warm
  waxy
Noguchi test for globulin
nomogram
non-A, non-B hepatitis
non-A, non-B hepatitis virus
non-alpha, non-beta pancreatic islet
  cell
nonan malaria
nonbacterial pneumonia
non-beta cell
nonbloody stool
noncaseating
noncellular material
nonclonogenic cell
noncondylomatous
noncoronary cusp
nondeciduate placenta
nondiscrete nodule
nonenveloped virus
nonfibrous material
nonfilamented neutrophil
nonfunctioning tissue
nongerminal tissue
nonglandular cell
nongonococcal urethritis
nongranular leukocyte
non-heme iron protein
non-Hodgkin's lymphoma
non-hormone-producing neoplasms
  of pituitary
Nonidet P40
noninfectious conjunctivitis
noninfectivity

noninvasive
nonisolated proteinuria
nonkeratinizing epithelium
nonlamellar bone
nonlamellated bone
nonlipid histiocytosis
nonlymphocytic leukemia
nonmalignant cell
nonmeconium-stained membrane
nonmotile leukocyte
nonmyelinated axons of nerve cells
non-necrotizing granuloma
non-necrotizing granulomatous
   inflammation
non-neoplastic cyst
non-nerve cell
non-nodular
nonobese population
nonoccluded virus
non-oncogenic virus
nonpathogenic organisms
nonpenetrating wound
nonrachitic bowleg
non-small cell lung carcinoma
   (NSCLC)
nonspecialized cell
nonspecific antigen
nonspecific granulomatous myocarditis
nonspecific protein
nonspecific stomatitis
nonspecific vaginitis
nonstriated muscle
nonthrombocytopenic purpura
nontoxic goiter
nontreponemal antigen test
nonunion of bone fragments
nonunion of fracture
nonvenereal skin disease
nonviable fetus
nonviable tissue
noradrenaline
no-reflow phenomenon

norepinephrine
normal
   borderline
   high
   low
normal calcification
normal flora
normal gas exchange in lungs
normal human plasma
normal range
normal solution
normal test result
normetanephrine, total
normoblast, polychromatophilic
normoblastic
normoblastosis
normocalcemia
normocapnia
normocephalic
normocholesterolemia
normochromasia
normochromia
normochromic anemia
normocrinic
normocyte
normocytic anemia
normocytosis
normoerythrocyte
normoglycemia
normokalemia
normolipidemic
normoorthocytosis
normoskeocytosis
normospermic
normosthenuria
normotest
normotrophic
normouricemia
normouricuria
normovolemia
Norris corpuscle
North American blastomycosis

Northern blot (NB)
Northern blot analysis
Northern blot procedure
Northern blot test
Northern blotting
Northern hybridization
Norwalk disease
Norwalk gastroenteritis
Norwalk virus
nose, alar cartilages of
nosebleed
nosocomial infection
nosocomial pneumonia
nosomycosis
nosoparasite
nosopoietic
nosotoxic
nosotoxicity
nosotoxicosis
notch
   acetabular
   angular
   antegonial
   aortic
   auricular
   cardiac
   cerebellar
   clavicular
   costal
   cotyloid
   craniofacial
   dicrotic
   digastric
   ethmoidal
   fibular
   frontal
   radial sigmoid
   sciatic
   sigmoid
notched incisor teeth
notching of rib
notch of spleen

notochordal canal
novobiocin resistance
NSCLC (non-small cell lung
   carcinoma)
N-terminus
nuchal ligament
nuchal line
nuchal rigidity
Nuck, canal of
nuclear/cytoplasmic ratio
nuclear disintegration
nuclear dust
nuclear fast red
nuclear membrane
nuclear morphometry
nuclear outline
nuclear polarity
nuclear rim fluorescence
nuclear:cytoplasmic ratio
nucleated cell
nucleated erythrocyte
nucleated red blood cell (RBC)
nucleocytoplasmic
nucleolar fluorescence
nucleolus (pl. nucleoli)
nucleoplasmic index
nucleoprotein
Nuclepore filter
Nuclepore method
Nuclepore prep
nucleus (pl. nuclei)
   abducens
   accessory cuneate
   accessory olivary
   almond
   amygdaloid
   arcuate
   atypical
   auditory
   band-shaped
   benzene
   bizarre

nucleus *(continued)*
  branchimotor
  caudate
  centrally located
  centromedian
  chromatin
  cochlear
  cuneate
  dentate
  descending
  diploid
  dorsomedial
  dorsomedial hypothalamic
  droplet
  eccentrically located
  emboliform
  germ
  horseshoe-shaped
  hyperchromatic
  monstrocellular
  oval
  pleomorphic
  plump
  prominent
  pseudostratified
  pulposus
  pyknotic
  vesicular

nucleus of Perlia
Nuel space
Nuhn gland
null cell
null cell lymphoblastic leukemia
null type non-Hodgkin lymphoma
number, accession
numeric atrophy
nummular eczematous dermatitis
nurse cell
nutmeg appearance
nutmeg liver
nutmeg pattern
nutrient artery
nutrient broth
nutrient canal
nutrient medium
nutritional cirrhosis
nutritional deficiency
nutritional deficiency syndrome
nutritional disorders
NYHA (New York Heart Association)
  classification of congestive heart
  failure
Nyiri test

O, o

O (oxygen)
oat cell
oat cell carcinoma
O-banding
O'Beirne sphincter
Obermayer test for indican in urine
Obermueller test for cholesterol
obesity
    adult-onset
    alimentary
    endogenous
    exogenous
    hyperinsulinar
    hyperinterrenal
    hyperplasmic
    hyperplastic-hypertrophic
    hypertrophic
    hypogonad
    hypoplasmic
    hypothyroid
    lifelong
    morbid
    simple
obesity-associated diabetes
oblique abdominis muscle
oblique fasciculus of pons
oblique fissure of lung

oblique ligament of elbow joint
oblique muscle
oblique pericardial sinus
oblique popliteal ligament
oblique vein
obliterans, thromboangiitis
obliterated hypogastric artery
obliterated umbilical artery
obliterating pericarditis
obliteration, fibrous
obliteration of blood vessels
obliteration of cavity
obliteration of passage
obliteration of structure
obliterative bronchiolitis
obliterative endarteritis
obliterative inflammation
obliterative vasculitis
obstetric canal
obstruction
    arterial
    biliary
    cardiac
    closed-loop
    false colonic
    gastric
    hepatic

obstruction *(continued)*
  intestinal
  lymphatic
  mammary duct
  mechanical
  otic
  pancreatic duct
  renal
  respiratory
  urinary
  venous
obstructive jaundice
obstructive pneumonia
obstructive uropathy
obturating embolism
obturator artery
obturator canal
obturator fascia
obturator foramen
obturator membrane
obturator nerve
occipital artery
occipital belly
occipital bone
occipital eminence
occipital fontantelle
occipital lobe
occipital myotome
occipital node
occipital pole
occipital sinus
occipitoatloid
occipitoaxial ligament
occipitofrontal
occiput
occluding spring embolism
occlusal surface
occlusal zone
occlusion, buccal
occlusive meningitis
occult blood in stool
occult blood in urine

occult blood, positive test for
occupational dermatitis
occupational leukoderma
ochronosis
Ochsner muscle
Ochsner ring
O.C.T. compound
OCT (oxytocin challenge) test
ocular hypertension
ocular melanoma
ocular pemphigoid
ocular sclera
Oddi, sphincter of
odontoid bone
odontoid ligament
odontoma
  ameloblastic
  composite
  fibrous
  radicular
odorant binding protein
odoriferous glands of prepuce
odorless gas
OI (osteogenesis imperfecta)
oil-aspiration pneumonia
oil embolism
oil gland
oil red O
oily stool
Oken, canal of
OKT (Ortho-Kung T)
OKT antibody
OKT cell
OKT4 monoclonal antibody
OKT8 monoclonal antibody
olecranon bursa
olecranon bursitis
olecranon fossa
oleic acid–^{131}I absorption test
Olerud and Molander fracture
  classification
olfactory area of nose

olfactory bulb
olfactory canal
olfactory cell
olfactory nerve
olfactory receptor cell
olfactory sulcus
olfactory tract
oligakisuria
oligemia
oligochromemia
oligoclonal band
oligocystic
oligodendrocyte
oligodendroglia cell
oligodendroglioma
oligodynamic
oligohydruria
oligohypermenorrhea
oligohypomenorrhea
oligomeganephronia
oligomenorrhea
oligomeric plasmid
oligonucleotide probe
oligophosphaturia
oligotrophia
oliguria
olivary nuclei, accessory
olive (also, oliva)
Oliver test for albumin
Olympus B-Max microscope
omega-3 fatty acid
Omenn syndrome
omental artery
omental band
omental bursa
omental tuberosity
omentum
    colic
    gastric
    gastrocolic
    gastrohepatic
    gastrosplenic

omentum *(continued)*
    greater (omentum majus)
    lesser (omentum minus)
    pancreaticosplenic
    splenogastric
omphalomesenteric artery
Omsk hemorrhagic fever
Omsk hemorrhagic fever virus
Onchocerca volvulus
onchocerciasis
oncocyte
oncocytoma
oncofetal antigen, pancreatic (POA)
oncogene (gene)
    bcl-2
    N-myc
    nm23-H1
    p53
    Philadelphia chromosome
    ras
oncogene code
oncogenesis
oncogenic virus
oncogenous osteomalacia
oncotropic
oncovirus
one-stage prothrombin time
onion mite dermatitis
onion scale lesion
onionskin appearance of new bone
    formation
onionskin lesion
Onodi cell
onychomycosis
O'nyong-nyong virus
oocyte
oophorocystosis
oozing from vessel
oozing of fluid
opacification
opacified
opacify

opacifying
opacities
   cloudy "snowflake"
   diffuse
   lenticular
opacity of lens
opalescent
Opalski cell
opaque cornea
OPD4 monoclonal antibody
open-angle glaucoma
open biopsy
open comedo
opening
  aortic
  cardiac
opening cell block
  esophageal
  external urethral
  femoral
  internal urethral
  saphenous
  ureteral
  vaginal
opening of His, atrioventricular
opening of superior vena cava
open loop
open wound
operative diagnosis
operator gene
ophthalmia neonatorum
ophthalmia of the newborn, gonococcal
ophthalmia, sympathetic
ophthalmic artery
Opisthorchis sinensis
opportunistic infection
opportunistic infection in immunodeficiency
opportunistic microorganism
opsonic index
opsonizing antibody
optic atrophy

optic canal
optic chiasm
optic chiasma
optic cup
optic degeneration
optic disk (or disc)
optic fundus
optic nerve
optic neuritis
optic neuromyelitis
optic radiation
optic tract
optic vesicle
Optilyse one-step staining system
optochin disk
optochin sensitivity test
ora serrata retinae
oral administration of medication
oral cavity
oral cavity proper
oral enanthem
oral epithelial nevus
oral fissure
Oral Fluid Vironostika HIV-1
  Microelisa System
oral lactose tolerance test
oral mucosa
oral orifice
oral papilloma
oral part of pharynx
oral smear
oral ulcers
oral vestibule
"oramine"—see *auramine*
orange G
orange, gentian
orange stick
OraSure HIV-1 oral specimen
  collection device
orbicular bone
orbicular ligament
orbit

orbital artery
orbital canal
orbital fissure
orbital gyri
orbital optic neuritis
orbital plate
orbitosphenoidal bone
Orbivirus, orbivirus
orcein
orchitis
   metastatic
   spermatogenic granulomatous
   traumatic
orchitis variolosa
orf (contagious pustular dermatitis)
orf virus
organ
   accessory
   annulospiral
   cell
   circumventricular
   Corti
   critical
   donor
   enamel
   end
   extraperitoneal
   floating
   genital
   poles of
   reticuloendothelial
   retroperitoneal
   vestigial
organ capsule
organelle, cellular
organic acid
organic lesion
organism (see *pathogen* for list)
   acid-fast
   blood-borne
   intracellular
   multicellular

organism *(continued)*
   nonpathogenic
   pathogenic
      bacterium
      fungus
      parasite
      rickettsia
      virus
   pleuropneumonia-like (PPLO)
   pyogenic
   unicellular
   urease-producing
   virulent
organized clot
organized thrombus
organogenesis
organoid array
organoid nevus
organophosphate pesticides
organophosphate poisoning
organosilane-coated glass slide
Oriental sore
orienting reflex
orifice
   anal
   aortic
   atrioventricular
   cardiac
   esophagogastric
   external urethral
   gastroduodenal
   golf-hole ureteral
   ileocecal
   internal urethral
   mitral
   pharyngeal
   pulmonary
   pyloric
   tricuspid
   ureteral or ureteric
   urethral
   vaginal

orofacial fistula
orofacial herpes
"oromine"—see *auramine*
oropharynx
Oropouche virus
orosomucoid test
Oroya fever
orphan virus
Orth fixative
orthochromatic
orthodontic device
orthomyxovirus
orthostatic proteinuria
Orth solution
Orth stain
Orungo virus
os (pl. ossa), cervical
    external
    internal
os coxae (hip bone)
Osgood-Haskins test for albumin
Osgood-Schlatter disease
Osler-Weber-Rendu disease
Osm (osmole)
osmic acid
osmium tetroxide
osmium tetroxide phosphate
osmolality
    serum
    urinary
    urine
osmolality ratio, urine/serum
osmolarity
osmole (Osm)
osmosis
osmotic activity of total solute content
osmotic edema
osmotic fragility test (RBC fragility)
osmotic fragility test for spherocytosis
osmotic nephrosis
osmotic pressure
os pubis, ascending ramus of

ossa (pl. of os)
osseocartilaginous thoracic cage
osseous cell
osseous labyrinth
osseous polyp
osseous portion of auditory tube
ossicle
    auditory
    epactal
    lunula
ossicles of ear
ossificans, myositis
ossification
    abnormal
    enchondral
    intracartilaginous
    intramembranous
    irregular enchondral
    primary center of
    secondary center of
ossification center
osteitis
    acute
    alveolar
    chronic
    condensing
    cortical
    hematogenous
    sclerosing
    vascular
osteitis deformans
osteitis fibrosa cystica
osteitis pubis
osteitis tuberculosa multiplex cystica
osteoaneurysm
osteoarthritis
osteoarthritis grading
osteoarthropathy
    hypertrophic pulmonary
    idiopathic hypertrophic
osteoblast
osteoblastic osteosarcoma

osteoblastoma
osteocachexia
osteocalcin
osteocampsia
osteocele
osteochondral
osteochondritis dissecans
osteochondritis
    juvenile deforming metatarso-
      phalangeal
    syphilitic
osteochondritis necroticans
osteochondrodysplasia
osteochondrodystrophia deformans
osteochondrodystrophy
osteochondrofibroma
osteochondrogenic cell
osteochondrolysis
osteochondroma, fibrosing
osteochondromatosis
    multiple
    synovial
osteochondromyxoma
osteochondrosarcoma
osteochondrosis deformans tibiae
osteoclast
osteoclast activating factor
osteoclastoma
osteocystoma
osteocyte
osteodermia
osteodysplasty
osteodystrophy, renal
osteogenesis imperfecta (OI)
osteogenic cell
osteogenic sarcoma
osteohemachromatosis
osteoid osteoma
osteoid tissue
osteoid trabeculae
osteolipochondroma
osteolysis, focal

osteolytic
osteoma
    cavalryman's
    compact
    giant osteoid
    ivory
    osteoid
    spongy
osteoma cutis
osteomalacia
    antacid-induced
    anticonvulsant
    familial hypophosphatemic
    hepatic
    oncogenous
    puerperal
    renal tubular
    senile
osteomalacic pelvis
osteomyelitis
    chronic diffuse sclerosing
    chronic focal sclerosing
    conchiolin
    focal sclerosing
    Garré
    hematogenous
    salmonella
    sclerosing nonsuppurative
    typhoid
osteomyelitis variolosa
osteomyelodysplasia
osteomyxochondroma
osteon
osteonecrosis
osteopathia striata
osteopathy
    disseminated condensing
    hunger
    myelogenic
osteopenia
osteoperiostitis
osteopetrosis

osteophlebitis
osteophyma
osteophyte, marginal
osteophytosis
osteoporosis
   disuse
   juvenile
   postmenopausal
   post-traumatic
   senile
osteoporosis of bone
osteoporotic bone
osteoprogenitor cell
osteopulmonary arthropathy
osteoradionecrosis
osteorrhagia
osteosarcoma
   chondroblastic
   classical
   extraosseous
   fibroblastic
   high-grade surface
   intracortical
   intraosseous low-grade
   jaw
   juxtacortical
   multicentric
   osteoblastic
   parosteal
   periosteal
   small cell
   synchronous multicentric
   telangiectatic
osteosarcomatosis
osteosclerosis
osteosclerotic anemia
osteosis cutis
osteosis, parathyroid
osteosynovitis
osteothrombophlebitis
osteothrombosis
Osterberg test

ostium (pl. ostia)
   abdominal
   aortic
   auditory tube of pharyngeal
   uterine
Ota nevus
otic abscess
otic atrophy
otic degeneration
otic dystrophy
otic ganglion
otic labyrinth
otic obstruction
otitic meningitis
otitis externa
otitis interna
otitis media, purulent
otitis, serous
otocyst
otogenous abscess
otolithic membrane
otomycosis
otorrhea, cerebrospinal fluid
otosclerosis
ototoxic
Ouchterlony double diffusion method
Ouchterlony test
outer lipoprotein bilayer
outer membrane
outer pigment cell layer
outflow, sacral parasympathetic
outlet
   pelvic
   pyloric
   thoracic
outpouching of joint capsule
outpouching of tendon sheath
outpouring of fluid
output, cardiac
ova and parasites (O&P) test
oval cell
ovale malaria

oval foramen
oval-form colonic groove
ovalis
   annulus
   fossa (saphenous opening)
   limbus fossae
oval nucleus
ovalocyte
ovalocytosis
oval shape
oval-shaped
oval window
ovarian abscess
ovarian adenocarcinoma
ovarian artery
ovarian cortex
ovarian cyst
ovarian fibroma
ovarian fimbria
ovarian follicle
ovarian follicle atresia
ovarian fossa
ovarian hormone
ovarian ligament
ovarian medulla
ovarian nerve
ovarian plexus of nerves
ovarian pregnancy
ovarian tumor
ovario-abdominal pregnancy
ovariocentesis
ovary (pl. ovaries)
   atrophied
   atrophy of
   cyst of
   embryonic
   ligament of
   mulberry
   polycystic
   suspensory ligament of
ovary teratocarcinoma
ovary teratoma

overdevelopment, genetically induced
overdevelopment of bone tissue
overflow proteinuria
overgrowth of poorly mineralized
   osteoid
overhydration
overnutrition
overriding aorta
overt diabetes
oviduct
oviductal pregnancy
ovoid articulation
ovotestis
ovulatory mucus
ovum (pl. ova)
   blighted
   fertilized
OvuQUICK test
oxalate plasma
oxalic acid
ox cell hemolysin test
oxidase test
oxide nitrogen
oxygen (O)
   arterial
   partial pressure of (PO_2)
oxygenated blood
oxygenated hemoglobin
oxygen capacity
oxygen-carrying capacity of blood
oxygen-carrying material of red blood
   cells
oxygen deficiency
oxygen saturation
oxygen tension (hypoxemia)
oxyhemoglobin
oxyntic cell
oxyntic gland
oxyntic mucosa
oxyphil cell
oxyphilic
oxytocin challenge test (OCT)

P, p

P (phosphorus)
Pab 1801 immunostain
pacemaker cell
pacemaker region, gastric
pachyderma of vocal cord
pachymeninges
packed cells, volume of
packed human blood cells
packed red blood cells
pad
    abdominal
    antimesenteric fat
    electrode
    fat
    fibrocartilaginous
pad of fat, ischiorectal
Padykula-Herman stain
Paecilomyces javanicus
Paecilomyces lilacinus
Paecilomyces variotii
Paecilomyces viridis
Paget cell
Paget disease, extramammary
Paget disease of bone
Paget disease of breast
Paget-Eccleston stain
Paget quiet necrosis

pagetoid cell
pagetoid fashion
PAI (plasminogen activator inhibitor)
pain fiber
painful hematuria
painless hematuria
painless indurated ulcer
paired parietal branches
paired visceral branches
palatal abscess
palatal arch
palate
    bony
    Byzantine arch
    cleft
    hard
    smoker's
    soft
palatine aponeurosis
palatine artery
palatine bone
palatine canal
palatine foramen
palatine gland
palatine nerve
palatine process
palatine raphe

palatine root
palatine shelf
palatine tonsil
palatoglossal arch
palatoglossus muscle
palatomaxillary canal
palatopharyngeal arch
palatopharyngeal fold
palatopharyngeus muscle
palatovaginal canal
pale cytoplasm
pale myocardium
pale stool
palisade cell
palisade formation
palisades of proliferating cells
palisading, peripheral
palmar aponeurosis
palmar arch artery
palmar carpal ligament
palmar carpometacarpal ligament
palmar crease
palmar interosseous artery
palmar ligament
palmar metacarpal ligament
palmar radiocarpal ligament
palmar ulnocarpal ligament
Palmer acid test for peptic ulcer
palmin test for pancreatic efficiency
palpable
palpate
palpatory proteinuria
palpebra (pl. palpebrae)
palpebral arch
palpebral artery
palpebral conjunctiva
palpebral fascia
palpebral fissure
palpebral gland
palpebral raphe
pampiniform
pampiniform plexus

PAN (polyarteritis nodosa)
pancake kidney
pancervical smear
pancreas
  aberrant
  accessory
  annular
  anterior surface of
  Aselli
  beta-cells of the
  biopsy of
  degeneration of
  dorsal
  head of
  heterotopic
  inferior surface of
  lesser
  neck of
  posterior surface of
  tail of
  uncinate process of
  ventral
  Willis
  Winslow
pancreas divisum
pancreas transplant
pancreatic abscess
pancreatic acini atrophy
pancreatic bud
pancreatic calculus
pancreatic carcinoma
pancreatic cyst
pancreatic diabetes
pancreatic duct
  accessory
  duodenal end of dorsal
  duodenal end of main
  main
  obstruction of
  proximal part of dorsal
pancreatic duct sphincter
pancreatic enzyme

pancreatic function test
pancreatic hormone
pancreatic islet
pancreatic islet cell
pancreatic juice
pancreatic lipase
pancreaticobiliary common channel
pancreaticobiliary ductal junction
pancreaticobiliary sphincter
pancreaticobiliary tract
pancreatic obstruction
pancreaticoduodenal artery
pancreaticolienal lymph nodes
pancreatic oncofetal antigen (POA)
pancreaticosplenic gland
pancreaticosplenic lymph nodes
pancreaticosplenic omentum
pancreatic phlegmon
pancreatic polypeptide (PP)
pancreatic pseudocyst
pancreatic tumor
pancreatic vein
pancreatin
pancreatitis
     acute
     acute hemorrhagic
     acute interstitial
     calcareous
     centrilobar
     chronic
     chronic relapsing
     interstitial
     necrotizing
     perilobar
     purulent
pancreatoblastoma
pancrelipase
pancreozymin-secretin test
panculture
pancystitis
pancytopenia
panduriform placenta

panel
     arthritis
     chemistry
     electrolyte
     enzyme
     fasting chemistry
     febrile agglutinin
     liver
     rheumatoid (rheumatology)
     rheumatology
     test
     thyroid
panel cell
panel coagulation
panencephalitis
     Pette-Döring
     subacute sclerosing (SSPE)
Paneth granular cell
panhypopituitarism
panic level
panlobular emphysema
Panner disease
panniculitis
     LE (lupus erythematosus)
     lobular
     nodular nonsuppurative
     relapsing febrile nodular
         nonsuppurative
     septal
     subacute nodular migratory
     Weber-Christian
panniculus
panniculus adiposus
panniculus carnosus
pannus formation
pannus of eye
pannus of joint
pannus subcutaneous
panophthalmitis
panoptic stain
panosteitis
pantaloon embolism

Panton-Valentine leukocidin
PAP (Papanicolaou)
PAP smear
PAP stain (or test)
PAP (peroxidase-antiperoxidase) technique for detecting antigen or antibody in tissue sections
PAP (prostatic acid phosphatase)
paper chromatography
paper electrophoresis
papilla (pl. papillae)
   acoustic
   bile
   circumvallate
   clavate
   conical
   dentinal
   dermal
   filiform
   foliate
   fungiform
   lingual
   major duodenal
   minor duodenal
   renal
   urethral
papilla of Vater
papillary adenocarcinoma
papillary carcinoma
papillary cluster of cells
papillary cystadenocarcinoma
papillary cystic adenoma
papillary dermis
papillary hyperplasia of follicles
papillary hypertrophy of conjunctiva
papillary layer of dermis
papillary lesion
papillary muscle
papillary necrosis
papillary proliferation
papillary tumor
papillated surface

papillation
papillitis
   necrotizing
   necrotizing renal
papilloadenocystoma
papillocarcinoma
papilloma
   basal cell
   benign squamous
   choroid plexus
   cockscomb (also coxcomb)
   cutaneous
   duct
   fibroepithelial
   friable
   Hopmann
   intracanalicular
   intracystic
   intraductal
   inverted
   inverted ductal
   oral
   soft
   squamous
   transitional cell
   villous
   warty
papilloma of bladder
papilloma of vocal cord
papillomatosis, confluent reticulated
papillomatosis/epitheliosis, intraductal
papillomatous benign tumor
papilloma virus (also, papillomavirus)
Papnet test
papovavirus
pappataci fever virus
Pappenheimer body
Pappenheim stain
papular dermatitis of pregnancy
papular eruption
papular erythema and scaling
papular fever

papular lesion
papule
    fluid-filled
    lichenoid
    minute
    pedunculated
    pruritic urticarial (of pregnancy)
    rust-colored
    sessile
    transitory
papulonecrotic lesion
papulosis
    bowenoid
    lymphomatoid
    malignant atrophic
papulosquamous
papulovesicular dermatitis
papulovesicular eruption
para 1 (primipara)
para 2 (secundipara)
para-aortic region
paracarmine stain
paracecal appendix
paracentesis
paracentric inversion
parachute deformity
Paracoccidioides brasiliensis
paracoccidioidomycosis
paracolic gutter
paracolic lymph nodes
paracolon bacilli
paracystic
paracystic pouch
paracytic
paradidymis
paradoxical embolism
paraduodenal fold
paraduodenal recess
paradysentery bacillus
parafascicular (PF) nucleus
paraffin
paraffin block

paraffin section
paraffin tumor
paraffin wax
paraffinoma
parafollicular cell
paraformaldehyde
parafrenal abscess
parafrenal gland
paraganglioma
paraganglion (pl. paraganglia)
paraganglionic cell
Paragon stain
paragonimiasis
Paragonimus westermani
parainfluenza 2 virus
parainfluenza 3 virus
parainfluenza 4 virus
parainfluenza virus (PIV)
parakeratosis
parallel pelvic plane
paraluteal cell
paralutein cell
paralysis
paralysis agitans
paramedial
paramedian
paramesonephric duct
parameter
parametrial abscess
parametric abscess
parametrium
Paramyxovirus, paramyxovirus
paranasal sinus
paraneoplasia
paraneoplastic pemphigus
paraneoplastic syndrome
paranephric abscess
paraneural infiltration
paraphimosis
Paraplast embedding medium
Parapoxvirus
paraproctitis

paraproteinemia
parapsoriasis en plaque
pararectal fossa
pararectal lymph node
pararectal pouch
parasagittal meningioma
parasite (see *pathogen* for list)
parasite, bloodsucking intestinal
parasite cyst
parasites in crypts of Lieberkühn
parasitic infiltration
parasitic worms
parasitism, intestinal
parasitize
parasitology
parasternal lymph node
parasympathetic cardiac nerve
parasympathetic ganglion
parasympathetic nerve supply
parasympathetic secretomotor fiber
parasympathetic system
parathormone hormone
parathyroid adenoma
parathyroid gland
parathyroid hormone (PTH, parathormone)
parathyroid hormonelike protein
parathyroid hyperplasia of
parathyroid-like polypeptide
parathyroid osteosis
parathyroid tumor
paratubal cyst
paratyphoid bacillus
paratyphoid fever
paraumbilical region
paraumbilical vein
paraurethral canal
paraurethral duct
paraurethral gland
paravaccinia virus
paravertebral body
paravertebral ganglion

paravertebral groove
paravertebral nerve plexus
paravesical fossa
paravesical pouch
parchment induration
parenchyma
parenchymal cell
parenchymal hemorrhage
parenchymal tissue
parenchymatous degeneration
parenchymatous goiter
parenchymatous inflammation
parenchymatous mastitis
parenchymatous myocarditis
parenchymatous nephritis
parenchymatous neuritis
parenchymatous pneumonia
parent cell
parenteric fever
paresthesia
Parham method of Fab fragment
   preparation
parietal bone
parietal branches
   paired
   unpaired
parietal cell
parietal cell antibody
parietal convolution, ascending
parietal eye
parietal layer
parietal parenchyma
parietal pelvic fascia
parietal pericardium
parietal peritoneum
parietal pleura
parietal pregnancy
parietal tuber
parieto-occipital artery
parieto-occipital sulcus
parieto-temporal artery
Park aneurysm

Parkinson disease
parkinsonism
Park-Williams bacillus
Park-Williams fixative
Parlodion embedding medium
Parona space
parosteal osteosarcoma
parotid abscess
parotid bed
parotid gland
parotid lymph node
parotidoscirrhus
parotid sheath
parotitis
   acute suppurative
   epidemic
parovarian cyst
paroxysmal cold hemoglobinuria
paroxysmal cough
paroxysmal hemoglobinuria
paroxysmal nocturnal hemoglobinuria
paroxysmal proteinuria
parrot fever
part (portion) (see *pars* in reference
   books for anatomical structures)
partial lesion
partial pressure of carbon dioxide
   (PCO_2)
partial pressure of oxygen in arterial
   blood (PO_2)
partial protein
partial-thickness tear
partial thromboplastin time (PTT) test
particle
   beta
   chromatin
   Dane
   elementary
   ribonucleoprotein
particulate matter
partition, gastric
parturient canal

parturition
Parvovirus
parvovirus B19, human
parvum
PAS (periodic acid-Schiff) stain
PAS III flow cytometer
passage, biliary
passive clot
passive congestion
passive cutaneous anaphylaxis
passive hyperemia
passive pneumonia
passive protection test
Pasteur pipette
Pasteurella haemolytica
Pasteurella multocida
Pasteurella pestis
Pasteurella pneumotropica
Pasteurella pseudotuberculosis
Pasteurella ureae
pasteurellosis
patch (pl. patches)
   cotton-wool
   fibrotic
   Peyer
   transdermal (for glucose
     monitoring)
   yellow crusted
patches of vascularization
patch test
patchy intercellular edema
patella
   bipartite
   floating
patellar bone
patellar ligament
patellofemoral articulation
patent
patent ductus arteriosus
patent foramen ovale
paternity test
path, condyle

pathogen (including bacteria, fungi,
      parasites, and viruses)
  Abel bacillus
  Abelson murine leukemia virus
  abortus bacillus
  Absidia corymbifera
  Acanthamoeba
  Achromobacter xylosoxidans
  acid-fast bacillus (AFB)
  Acinetobacter calcoaceticus var.
      anitratus (formerly *Herellea
      vaginicola*)
  Acinetobacter calcoaceticus var.
      lwoffi (formerly *Mima poly-
      morpha*)
  Acremonium
  Acremonium falciforme
  Acremonium kiliense
  Acremonium recifei
  Acremonium restrictum
  Acrodermatitis enteropathica
  *Actinobacillus actinomycetem
      comitans*
  Actinobacillus equuli
  Actinobacillus hominis
  Actinobacillus lignieresii
  Actinobacillus suis
  Actinomadura
  Actinomyces
  Actinomyces gonidiaformis
  Actinomyces israelii
  Actinomyces meyeri
  Actinomyces naeslundii
  Actinomyces odontolyticus
  Actinomyces viscosus
  adenovirus
  Aerobacter (old name for
      Enterobacter)
  Aerobacter aerogenes
  Aerobacter cloacae
  Aerobacter liquefaciens
  Aerococcus

pathogen *(continued)*
  Aeromonas caviae
  Aeromonas hydrophila
  Aeromonas salmonicida
  Aeromonas shigelloides (see
      Plesiomonas shigelloides)
  Aeromonas sobria
  Afipia felis
  Agaricus
  Agrimonia eupatoria
  Ajellomyces capsulatus
  Ajellomyces dermatitidis
  Alcaligenes denitrificans
  Alcaligenes faecalis
  Alcaligenes odorans
  Alphavirus
  Alternaria
  Alternaria alternata
  Alteromonas putrefaciens
  Amanita
  Amanita bisporigera
  Amanita muscaria
  Amanita ocreata
  Amanita phalloides
  Amanita verna
  Amanita virosa
  Amoeba
  *Anaerobiospirillum succinici-
      producens*
  Ancylostoma
  Ancylostoma americanum
  Ancylostoma brasiliense
  Ancylostoma braziliense
  Ancylostoma caninum
  Ancylostoma dermatitis
  Ancylostoma duodenale
  Anisakis marina
  Arachnia
  Arachnia propionica
  arbovirus
  arenavirus
  Argentine hemorrhagic fever virus

pathogen *(continued)*
 Arizona hinshawii
 anthrax bacillus
 arterivirus
 Arthrinium
 Arthroderma
 Arthropoda
 arthropod-borne virus
 Ascaris lumbricoides
 Aspergillus
 Aspergillus flavus
 Aspergillus fumigatus
 Aspergillus glaucus
 Aspergillus niger
 Aspergillus terreus
 Aureobasidium pullulans
 avian leukosis virus
 Avipoxvirus
 Babesia
 Babesia bigemina
 Babesia microti
 Bacillus anthracis
 Bacillus cereus
 Bacillus megaterium
 Bacillus subtilis
 Bacteroides
 Bacteroides asaccharolyticus
 Bacteroides bivius
 Bacteroides buccae
 Bacteroides corporis
 Bacteroides corrodens
  (Bacteroides ureolyticus)
 Bacteroides denticola
 Bacteroides disiens
 Bacteroides distasonis
 Bacteroides eggerthii
 Bacteroides fragilis
 Bacteroides gingivalis
 Bacteroides intermedius
 Bacteroides loescheii
 Bacteroides melaninogenicus
 Bacteroides oralis

pathogen *(continued)*
 Bacteroides oris
 Bacteroides ovatus
 Bacteroides ruminicola
 Bacteroides thetaiotaomicron
 Bacteroides uniformis
 Bacteroides ureolyticus
 Bacteroides vulgatus
 Balantidium coli
 Bang bacillus
 Barr-Epstein virus
 Bartonella bacilliformis
 Basidiobolus ranarum
 Battey bacillus
 beta-hemolytic streptococci
 Bifidobacterium
 Bipolaris australiensis
 Bipolaris hawaiiensis
 Bipolaris spicifera
 BK DNA virus
 Blastomyces dermatitidis
 Blastoschizomyces pseudotricho-
  sporon
 blue pus bacillus
 bluetongue virus
 Boas-Oppler bacillus
 Bolivian hemorrhagic fever virus
 Bordet-Gengou bacillus
 Bordetella bronchiseptica
 Bordetella parapertussis
 Bordetella pertussis
 Bornholm disease
 Borrelia burgdorferi
 Borrelia hermsii
 Borrelia kochii
 Borrelia mazzottii
 Borrelia parkeri
 Borrelia recurrentis
 Borrelia turicatae
 Botryodiplodia theobromae
 Branhamella catarrhalis (formerly
  Neisseria catarrhalis)

pathogen *(continued)*
  Brucella abortus
  Brucella canis
  Brucella melitensis
  Brucella suis
  Bunyavirus, bunyavirus
  butter bacillus
  Calicivirus, calicivirus
  California encephalitis virus
  Calmette-Guérin bacillus
  Calymmatobacterium granulomatis
    (formerly *Donovania granulo-*
    matis)
  Campylobacter cinaedi
  Campylobacter coli
  Campylobacter fennelliae
  Campylobacter fetus (formerly
    Vibrio fetus)
  Campylobacter jejuni
  Campylobacter laridis
  Campylobacter parahaemolyticus
  Campylobacter vulnificus
  Candida
  Candida albicans
  Candida guilliermondii
  Candida krusei
  Candida lusitaniae
  Candida parapsilosis
  Candida pseudotropicalis
  Candida pulcherrima
  Candida ravautii
  Candida rugosa
  Candida stellatoidea
  Candida tropicalis
  Candida viswanathii
  Capnocytophaga canimorsus
  Capnocytophaga ochracea
  Capripoxvirus
  Cardiobacterium hominis
  Cedecea
  Cedecea davisae
  Cedecea lapagei

pathogen *(continued)*
  Cedecea neteri
  Chaetoconidium
  chikungunya virus
  Chlamydia pneumoniae
  Chlamydia psittaci
  Chlamydia trachomatis
  Chromobacterium violaceum
  Chrysosporium
  Chrysosporium parvum
  Citrobacter
  Citrobacter amalonaticus
  Citrobacter diversus
  Citrobacter freundii
  Cladosporium
  Cladosporium bantianum
  Cladosporium carrionii
  Cladosporium cladosporioides
  Cladosporium trichoides
  Cladosporium werneckii
  Clonorchis sinensis
  Clostridium
  Clostridium bifermentans
  Clostridium botulinum
  Clostridium butyricum
  Clostridium cadaveris
  Clostridium difficile
  Clostridium histolyticum
  Clostridium innocuum
  Clostridium novyi
  Clostridium paraputrificum
  Clostridium perfringens
  Clostridium putrificum
  Clostridium ramosum
  Clostridium septicum
  Clostridium sordellii
  Clostridium sphenoides
  Clostridium subterminale
  Clostridium tertium
  Clostridium tetani
  Clostridium welchii
  club-shaped bacillus

pathogen *(continued)*
  Coccidioides immitis
  coliform bacillus
  Colorado tick fever virus
  Comamonas terrigena
  common cold virus
  Conidiobolus coronatus
  Conidiobolus incongruus
  Coprinus cinereus
  corkscrew-shaped bacteria
  Coronavirus, coronavirus
  Corynebacterium acnes
  Corynebacterium bovis
  Corynebacterium diphtheriae
  Corynebacterium equi
  Corynebacterium haemolyticum
  Corynebacterium minutissimum
  Corynebacterium pseudo-
    diphtheriticum
  Corynebacterium pseudotubercu-
    losis
  Corynebacterium ulcerans
  Corynebacterium xerosis
  Coxiella burnetii
  Coxsackie virus
  Crimean-Congo hemorrhagic
    fever virus
  Crithidia luciliae
  croup-associated virus (CA v.)
  Cryptococcus
  Cryptococcus albidus
  Cryptococcus laurentii
  Cryptococcus luteolus
  Cryptococcus neoformans
  Cryptosporidium
  Curvularia geniculata
  Curvularia lunata
  Curvularia pallescens
  Curvularia senegalensis
  Curvularia verruculosa
  cytomegalovirus
  Dactylaria

pathogen *(continued)*
  dengue virus
  Dermatophilus
  Dermatophilus congolensis
  dermatophytic fungi
  dermotropic virus
  DF-2 bacillus
  Dibothriocephalus latus
  Dientamoeba fragilis
  diphtheria bacillus
  Diplococcus pneumoniae
  DNA virus
  DNA tumor virus
  Döderlein bacillus
  Donovania granulomatis
  Dracunculus medinensis
  Ducrey bacillus
  dysentery bacillus
  Eaton agent
  Eberth bacillus
  Ebola virus
  Echinococcus granulosus
  ECHO (enterocytopathogenic
    human orphan) virus
  Edwardsiella
  Edwardsiella tarda
  Ehrlichia canis
  Ehrlichia chaffeensis
  Ehrlichia sennetsu
  Eikenella corrodens
  Eikenella corrodens (formerly
    Bacteroides corrodens, HB-1)
  encephalomyocarditis virus
  Entamoeba histolytica
  enteric bacillus
  enteric orphan viruses
  Enterobacter (formerly
    Aerobacter)
  Enterobacter aerogenes
  Enterobacter agglomerans
  Enterobacter cloacae
  Enterobacter gergoviae

pathogen *(continued)*
    Enterobacter hafniae
    Enterobacter liquefaciens
    Enterobacter sakazakii
    Enterobacteriaceae
    Enterobius vermicularis
    Enterococcus (pl. *Enterococci*)
    Enterococcus avium
    Enterococcus faecalis
    Enterococcus faecium
    enterocytopathogenic human
       orphan (ECHO) virus
    Enterovirus, enterovirus
    epidemic keratoconjunctivitis
       virus
    Epidermophyton
    Epidermophyton floccosum
    Epidermophyton stockdaleae
    Epstein-Barr virus (EBV)
    Erysipelothrix rhusiopathiae
    Escherich bacillus
    Escherichia coli (E. coli)
    Escherichia fergusonii
    Escherichia hermannii
    Escherichia vulneris
    Eubacterium alactolyticum
    Eubacterium lentum
    Eubacterium limosum
    Ewingella
    Exophiala dermatitidis
    Exophiala heteromorpha
    Exophiala jeanselmei
    Exophiala spinifera
    Exserohilum rostratum
    Fasciola gigantica
    Fasciola hepatica
    Fasciolopsis buski
    fibrillary bacteria
    Filobasidiella neoformans
    filament-forming bacillus
    Filovirus
    Fissuricella filamenta

pathogen *(continued)*
    flavivirus
    Flavobacterium meningosepticum
    Flexner bacillus
    Fonsecaea compacta
    Fonsecaea dermatitidis
    Fonsecaea pedrosoi
    Francisella tularensis (formerly
       Pasteurella tularensis)
    Friedländer bacillus
    Frisch bacillus
    funguslike bacteria
    Fusarium moniliforme
    Fusarium oxysporum
    Fusarium solani
    fusiform bacillus
    Fusobacterium
    Fusobacterium mortiferum
    Fusobacterium necrophorum
    Fusobacterium nucleatum
    Fusobacterium russii
    Fusobacterium varium
    Gardnerella vaginitis (formerly
       Haemophilus vaginalis or
       Corynebacterium vaginale)
    Gärtner bacillus
    Gemella morbillorum
    Geotrichum capitatum
    Geotrichum fermentans
    Geotrichum penicillatum
    Ghon-Sachs bacillus
    Giardia lamblia
    Gibberella fujikuroi
    glanders bacillus
    gram-negative diplococci
    gram-negative bacillus
    gram-positive bacillus
    grass bacillus
    Guama virus
    Guaroa virus
    Haemophilus
    Haemophilus aegyptius

pathogen *(continued)*
   Haemophilus aphrophilus
   Haemophilus ducreyi
   Haemophilus haemolyticus
   Haemophilus influenzae
   Haemophilus parahaemolyticus
   Haemophilus parainfluenzae
   Haemophilus paraphrophilus
   Haemophilus segnis
   Haemophilus vaginalis
   Hafnia
   Hafnia alvei (formerly
     Enterobacter hafniae)
   Hansen bacillus
   Hantavirus
   helical bacteria
   Helicobacter pylori
   hepatitis A virus (HAV)
   hepatitis B virus (HBV)
   hepatitis C virus
   hepatitis D (delta) virus
   hepatitis E virus
   Herellea vaginicola (now
     Acinetobacter calcoaceticus)
   herpes simplex virus (HSV)
   herpesvirus
   herpes type 5 virus (cytomegalo-
     virus)
   herpes zoster virus (HZV)
   Histoplasma capsulatum
   Hofmann bacillus
   Hormiscium dermatitidis
   Hormodendrum dermatitidis
   human herpesvirus 3
   human herpesvirus 4
   human immunodeficiency virus
     (HIV)
   human T-cell leukemia virus
   human T-cell lymphoma virus
     (HTLV I and II)
   human T-cell lymphotropic virus
     type I (HTLV-I)

pathogen *(continued)*
   Hymenolepis nana
   intracellular bacteria
   Isospora belli
   Ixodes dammini
   Ixodes pacificus
   Jamestown Canyon virus
   Japanese encephalitis virus
   JC DNA virus
   Johne bacillus
   Kemerovo virus
   Kingella denitrificans
   Kingella indologenes
   Kingella kingae
   Kitasato bacillus
   Klebsiella
   Klebsiella oxytoca
   Klebsiella ozaenae
   Klebsiella planticola
   Klebsiella pneumoniae
   Klebsiella rhinoscleromatis
   Klebs-Loeffler bacillus
   Kluyvera
   Kluyvera ascorbata
   Kluyvera cryocrescens
   Koch bacillus
   Koch-Weeks bacillus
   Korean hemorrhagic fever virus
   Koserella trabulsii
   Kyasanur Forest hemorrhagic
     fever virus
   lactic acid bacillus
   La Crosse virus
   Lactobacillus
   Lecythophora hoffmannii
   Lecythophora mutabilis
   legionnaire's bacillus
   Legionella anisa
   Legionella bozemanii
   Legionella dumoffii
   Legionella feelei
   Legionella gormanii

pathogen *(continued)*
  Legionella jordanis
  Legionella longbeachae
  Legionella micdadei
  Legionella oakridgensis
  Legionella pneumonia
  Legionella pneumophila
  Legionella sainthelensis
  Legionella wadsworthii
  Leishmania brasiliensis
  Leishmania donovani
  Leishmania tropica
  leprosy bacillus
  Leptospira biflexa
  Leptospira icterohemorrhagiae
  Leptospira interrogans
  Leptotrichia
  Listeria monocytogenes
  Loa loa
  Loboa loboi
  Lymphocryptovirus
  Lyssavirus
  lytic virus
  M-25 virus
  Madurella mycetomatis
  Malassezia furfur
  Malassezia pachydermatis
  Marburg virus
  Mayaro virus
  measles virus
  Micrococcus
  Microsporum
  Microsporum amazonicum
  Microsporum audouinii
  Microsporum boullardii
  Microsporum canis
  Microsporum cookei
  Microsporum equinum
  Microsporum faeni
  Microsporum ferrugineum
  Microsporum floccosum
  Microsporum fulvum

pathogen *(continued)*
  Microsporum gallinae
  Microsporum gypseum
  Microsporum nanum
  Microsporum persicolor
  Microsporum praecox
  Microsporum racemosum
  Microsporum ripariae
  Microsporum vanbreuseghemii
  Mima polymorpha (now
    Acinetobacter calcoaceticus
    var. *lwoffi)*
  MM virus
  Mokola virus
  Molluscipoxvirus
  molluscum contagiosum virus
  Monilia sitophila
  Morax-Axenfeld bacillus
  Moraxella atlantae
  Moraxella catarrhalis
  Moraxella lacunata
  Moraxella nonliquefaciens
  Moraxella osloensis
  Moraxella phenylpyruvica
  Moraxella urethralis
  Morbillivirus, morbillivirus
  Morgan bacillus
  Morganella
  Morganella morganii
  Mortierella wolfii
  mosquito-borne virus
  Much bacillus
  Mucor
  Mucor ramosissimus
  Mucor rouxianus
  mumps virus
  murine leukemia virus
  Murray Valley encephalitis virus
  Mycobacterium asiaticum
  Mycobacterium avium
  Mycobacterium avium-intracellu-
    lare (MAI) complex

pathogen *(continued)*
  Mycobacterium bovis
  Mycobacterium celatum
  Mycobacterium chelonei (formerly
    Mycobacterium abscessus)
  Mycobacterium flavescens
  Mycobacterium fortuitum
  Mycobacterium gastri
  Mycobacterium genavense
  Mycobacterium gordonae
  Mycobacterium haemophilum
  Mycobacterium intracellulare
  Mycobacterium kansasii
  Mycobacterium leprae
  Mycobacterium malmoense
  Mycobacterium marinum
  Mycobacterium microti
  Mycobacterium paratuberculosis
  Mycobacterium phlei
  Mycobacterium scrofulaceum
  Mycobacterium shimoidei
  Mycobacterium simiae
  Mycobacterium smegmatis
  Mycobacterium szulgai
  Mycobacterium terrae
  Mycobacterium triviale
  Mycobacterium tuberculosis
  Mycobacterium ulcerans
  Mycobacterium xenopi
  Mycocentrospora acerina
  Mycoplasma
  Mycoplasma buccale
  Mycoplasma fauciuim
  Mycoplasma fermentans
  Mycoplasma genitalium
  Mycoplasma hominis
  Mycoplasma orale
  Mycoplasma pharyngis
  Mycoplasma pneumoniae
  Mycoplasma salivarium
  myxovirus
  Nairovirus

pathogen *(continued)*
  Nakiwogo virus
  Necator
  Necator americanus
  Neisseria
  Neisseria catarrhalis
  Neisseria cinerea
  Neisseria elongata
  Neisseria flavescens
  Neisseria gonorrhoeae
  Neisseria lactamica
  Neisseria meningitidis
  Neisseria mucosa
  Neisseria sicca
  Neisseria subflava
  Neotestudina rosatii
  newborn pneumonitis virus
  Newcastle disease virus
  Newcastle-Manchester bacillus
  Nocardia
  Nocardia asteroides
  Nocardia brasiliensis
  Nocardia caviae
  Norwalk virus
  Omsk hemorrhagic fever virus
  Onchocerca volvulus
  oncogenic virus
  oncovirus
  O'nyong nyong virus
  Opisthorchis sinensis
  Orbivirus, orbivirus
  orf virus
  Oropouche virus
  orphan virus
  Orthomyxovirus, orthomyxovirus
  Orungo virus
  Paecilomyces javanicus
  Paecilomyces lilacinus
  Paecilomyces variotii
  Paecilomyces viridis
  papilloma virus (also, papilloma
    virus)

pathogen *(continued)*
 papovavirus
 pappataci fever virus
 Paracoccidioides brasiliensis
 Paragonimus westermanni
 parainfluenza 2 virus
 parainfluenza 3 virus
 parainfluenza 4 virus
 Paramyxovirus, paramyxovirus
 Parapoxvirus
 paravaccinia virus
 Park-Williams bacillus
 Parvovirus, parvovirus
 parvovirus B19, human
 Pasteurella haemolytica
 Pasteurella multocida
 Pasteurella pestis
 Pasteurella pneumotropica
 Pasteurella pseudotuberculosis
 Pasteurella ureae
 Pediculus
 Pediculus capitis
 Pediculus corporis
 Pediculus humanus
 Pediculus humanus capitis
 Pediculus humanus corporis
 Pediculus humanus humanus (yes)
 Pediculus pubis
 Penicillium chrysogenum
 Penicillium citrinum
 Penicillium commune
 Penicillium expansum
 Penicillium lilacinum
 Penicillium marneffei
 Penicillium spinulosum
 Peptococcus
 Peptococcus niger
 Peptostreptococcus
 Peptostreptococcus anaerobius
 Peptostreptococcus asaccharolyticus
 Peptostreptococcus indolicus
 Peptostreptococcus lanceolatus

pathogen *(continued)*
 Peptostreptococcus magnus
 Peptostreptococcus micros
 Peptostreptococcus parvulus
 Peptostreptococcus prevotii
 Peptostreptococcus productus
 Pestivirus
 Pfeiffer bacillus
 Phaeoannellomyces
 Phaeoannellomyces elegans
 Phaeoannellomyces werneckii
 Phaeococcomyces
 pharyngoconjunctival fever virus
 Phaseolus vulgaris
 Phialophora bubakii
 Phialophora dermatitidis
 Phialophora parasitica
 Phialophora pedrosoi
 Phialophora repens
 Phialophora richardsiae
 Phialophora verrucosa
 Phlebovirus
 Phoma cruris-hominis
 Phoma eupyrena
 Phoma glomerata
 Phoma herbarum
 Phoma hibernica
 Phoma oculo-hominis
 Phthirus pubis
 Phycomycetes
 Pichinde virus
 picornavirus
 Piedraia hortae
 Piry virus
 Pityrosporum
 Pityrosporum orbiculare
 Plasmodium
 Plasmodium falciparum
 Plasmodium malariae
 Plasmodium ovale
 Plasmodium vivax
 Plaut bacillus

pathogen *(continued)*
Plesiomonas shigelloides (formerly
   Aeromonas shigelloides)
pleuropneumonia-like organism
Plotz bacillus
Pneumococcus
Pneumocystis carinii (PCP)
Pneumovirus
poliomyelitis virus
poliovirus
polymorphic fungi
polyoma virus
Polyomavirus, polyomavirus
Pongola virus
Porphyromonas asaccharolytica
Powassan virus
pox virus (also, poxvirus)
Preisz-Nocard bacillus
Prevotella bivia
Prevotella disiens
Prevotella intermedia
Prevotella loeschii
Prevotella melaninogenica
Prevotella oralis
Prevotella oris
Propionibacterium
Propionibacterium acnes (formerly
   Corynebacterium acnes)
Propionibacterium avidum
Propionibacterium freudenreichii
Propionibacterium granulosum
Propionibacterium jensenii
Proteus
Proteus hydrophilus
Proteus inconstans subgroup B
Proteus mirabilis
Proteus morganii
Proteus penneri
Proteus rettgeri
Proteus vulgaris
Proteus zenkeri
Providencia

pathogen *(continued)*
Providencia alcalifaciens
Providencia rettgeri
Providencia stuartii
Pseudallescheria boydii
*Pseudochaetosphaeronema
   larense*
Pseudomonas
Pseudomonas acidovorans (for-
   merly *Comamonas terrigena)*
Pseudomonas aeruginosa
Pseudomonas alcaligenes
Pseudomonas cepacia
Pseudomonas diminuta
Pseudomonas fluorescens
Pseudomonas mallei
Pseudomonas maltophilia
Pseudomonas paucimobilis
Pseudomonas pickettii
Pseudomonas pseudoalcaligenes
Pseudomonas pseudomallei
Pseudomonas putida
Pseudomonas putrefaciens
Pseudomonas stutzeri
Pseudomonas testosteroni
Pseudomonas-like bacteria
pseudorabies virus
pus-forming bacteria
Puumala virus
Quaranfil virus
rabies virus
Ramularia
REO (respiratory enteric orphan)
   virus
reovirus
respiratory syncytial virus (RSV)
respiratory virus
retrovirus
rhabdovirus
Rhinocladiella aquaspersa
rhinoscleroma bacillus
Rhinosporidium seeberi

pathogen *(continued)*
Rhinovirus, rhinovirus
Rhizoctonia
Rhizoctonia solani
Rhizomucor pusillus
Rhizopus
Rhizopus arrhizus
Rhizopus microsporus
Rhizopus nigricans
Rhizopus rhizopodiformis
Rhizopus stolonifer
Rhodotorula
Rhodotorula rubra
ribovirus
Rickettsia
Rickettsia akari
Rickettsia australis
Rickettsia conorii
Rickettsia mooseri
Rickettsia prowazekii
Rickettsia rickettsii
Rickettsia sibirica
Rickettsia tsutsugamushi
Rickettsia typhi
Rift Valley fever virus
RNA tumor virus
RNA virus (ribovirus)
Rochalimaea
Rochalimaea henselae
Rochalimaea quintana
Rocio virus
Roseola infantum
Ross River virus
rotavirus
rotavirus antigen
rotavirus DNA virus
Rous-associated virus (RAV)
Rous sarcoma virus (RSV)
Rous virus
rubella virus
Rubivirus

pathogen *(continued)*
Russian autumn encephalitis virus
Russian spring-summer encephalitis virus
SA virus (simian virus SV5)
Saccharomyces cerevisiae
Sachs bacillus
Saksenaea vasiformis
Salisbury common cold virus
salivary gland virus
Salmonella
Salmonella arizonae
Salmonella choleraesuis
Salmonella enteritidis
Salmonella typhi
sandfly fever–Naples virus
sandfly fever–Sicilian virus
Sarcoptes scabiei
satellite virus
Scedosporium apiospermum
Schistosoma
Schistosoma haematobium
Schistosoma japonicum
Schistosoma mansoni
Schmitz bacillus
Schmorl bacillus
Scopulariopsis brevicaulis
Semliki Forest virus
Semunya virus
Sendai virus
Seoul virus
Serratia
Serratia liquefaciens
Serratia marcescens
Serratia rubidaea
Shiga bacillus
Shigella
Shigella boydii
Shigella dysenteriae
Shigella flexneri
Shigella sonnei

pathogen *(continued)*
  Simbu virus
  simian immunodeficiency virus
    (SIV)
  simian virus 40 (SV40)
  simian virus SV5
  Simplexvirus
  Sindbis virus
  slow virus
  smegma bacillus
  Sonne-Duval bacillus
  spiral-shaped bacteria
  Spirillum
  Spirillum minus
  Spondweni virus
  Sporothrix schenckii
  Sporotrichum schenckii
  Stanley bacillus
  Staphylococcus
  Staphylococcus albus
  Staphylococcus aureus
  Staphylococcus auricularis
  Staphylococcus capitis
  Staphylococcus cohnii
  Staphylococcus epidermidis
  Staphylococcus haemolyticus
  Staphylococcus hominis
  Staphylococcus pyogenes
  Staphylococcus saccharolyticus
  Staphylococcus saprophyticus
  Staphylococcus warneri
  Staphylococcus xylosus
  Stenella araguata
  St. Louis encephalitis virus
  Streptobacillus moniliformis
  Streptococcus
  Streptococcus acidominimus
  Streptococcus aecium
  Streptococcus agalactiae
  Streptococcus anginosus
  Streptococcus avium
  Streptococcus bovis

pathogen *(continued)*
  Streptococcus constellatus
  Streptococcus durans
  Streptococcus equi
  Streptococcus equinus
  Streptococcus equisimilis
  Streptococcus faecalis
  Streptococcus faecium
  Streptococcus intermedius
  Streptococcus M antigen
  Streptococcus milleri
  Streptococcus mitis
  Streptococcus morbillorum
  Streptococcus mutans
  Streptococcus pneumoniae
  Streptococcus pyogenes
  Streptococcus salivarius
  Streptococcus sanguis
  Streptococcus uberis
  Streptococcus viridans
  Streptococcus zooepidemicus
  Streptomyces
  Streptomyces paraguayensis
  Streptomyces somaliensis
  Strong bacillus
  Strongyloides stercoralis
  Suipoxvirus (swinepox virus)
  swine influenza virus
  swinepox virus
  Tacaribe virus
  Taenia saginata
  Taenia solium
  Tahyna virus
  Tamiami virus
  tanapox virus
  Tatumella
  Tatumella ptyseos
  Teschen virus
  tetanus bacillus
  Theiler virus
  Thermoactinomyces sacchari
  tick-borne virus

pathogen *(continued)*
    timothy bacillus
    togavirus
    Torulopsis candida
    Torulopsis glabrata
    Toscana virus
    Toxocara canis
    Toxoplasma gondii
    Treponema
    Treponema buccale
    Treponema carateum
    Treponema pallidum
    Treponema pertenue
    Treponema vincentii
    Trichinella spiralis
    Trichomonas
    Trichomonas tenax
    Trichomonas vaginalis
    Trichophyton
    Trichophyton ajelloi
    Trichophyton concentricum
    Trichophyton equinum
    Trichophyton fisheri
    Trichophyton flavescens
    Trichophyton floccosum
    Trichophyton georgiae
    Trichophyton gloriae
    Trichophyton gourvilii
    Trichophyton longifusum
    Trichophyton mariatii
    Trichophyton megninii
    Trichophyton mentagrophytes
    Trichophyton phaseoliforme
    Trichophyton rubrum
    Trichophyton schoenleinii
    Trichophyton simii
    Trichophyton soudanense
    Trichophyton terrestre
    Trichophyton tonsurans
    Trichophyton vanbreuseghemii
    Trichophyton verrucosum
    Trichophyton violaceum

pathogen *(continued)*
    Trichosporon beigelii
    trichosporosis
    Trichuris
    Trichuris trichiura
    Trypanosoma
    Trypanosoma cruzi
    Trypanosoma gambiense
    Trypanosoma rhodesiense
    tumor virus
    2060 virus
    typhoid bacillus
    U echovirus
    Uganda S arbovirus
    ultravirus
    Uppsala virus
    Ureaplasma urealyticum
    vaccinia virus
    varicella-zoster virus (VZV)
    Varicellavirus
    variola virus (now extinct)
    Veillonella
    Veillonella parvula
    Vesiculovirus
    Vibrio alginolyticus
    Vibrio cholerae
    Vibrio damsela
    Vibrio fetus
    Vibrio fluvialis
    Vibrio hollisae
    Vibrio jejuni
    Vibrio metschnikovii
    Vibrio mimicus
    viridans streptococci
    vole bacillus
    Wangiella dermatitidis
    Weeks bacillus
    Welch bacillus
    Wesselsbron virus
    West Nile virus
    Whitmore bacillus
    Wolinella

pathogen *(continued)*
  Wucheraria bancrofti
  Wyeomyia melanocephala
    mosquito virus
  Wyeomyia virus
  Xanthomonas
  Xylohypha bantiana
  yabapox virus
  Yale SK poliovirus
  Yatapoxvirus
  yellow fever virus
  Yersinia
  Yersinia enterocolitica (formerly
    Pasteurella enterocolitica)
  Yersinia frederiksenii
  Yersinia intermedia
  Yersinia kristensenii
  Yersinia pestis (formerly
    Pasteurella pestis)
  Yersinia pestis comitans
  Yersinia pseudotuberculosis
    (formerly *Pasteurella*
    pseudotuberculosis)
  Zika virus
  zygomycetous fungus
pathogenic microorganism
pathogenic organism
  bacterium
  fungus
  parasite
  virus
pathologic atrophy
pathologic diagnosis
pathologic fracture
pathological
pathologist
pathology
  anatomic
  clinical
  forensic
  general
pathology report

pathophysiologic
pattern
  abdominal wall venous
  adenoid
  airspace-filling
  airway
  alveolar
  ballerina-foot
  basketweave
  bowel gas
  branching
  butterfly
  cartwheel
  chromatin
  cribriform
  elongate
  fibrotic
  fold
  frondlike
  gas
  ground-glass
  haustral
  honeycomb
  hourglass
  interstitial
  juvenile
  lamellated
  layered
  lobular
  micronodular fibrotic
  miliary
  mosaic
  mucosal
  nutmeg
  progestational
  proliferative
  rugal
  sawtooth
  signet ring
  speckled
  starry-sky
  stellate

pattern *(continued)*
   undifferentiated
   vesicular
   wax
patterned alopecia
Patterson test for uremia
patulous
Paul-Bunnell-Davidsohn test
Paul-Bunnell test
Pautrier abscess
Pautrier microabscess
Pauwels femoral neck fracture classifi-
   cation
Pavy test for urine glucose
Pawlik triangle
Pawlik trigone
Pb (lead)
PBC-associated antibody
PBI (protein-bound iodine) test
P blood group
PBS (phosphate-buffered saline)
P cell
PCI (protein C inhibitor)
PCO_2 (partial pressure of carbon
   dioxide)
PCP (plasma cell pneumonitis)
PCP (*Pneumocystis carinii*) pneumonia
PCR (polymerase chain reaction)
PCT (porphyria cutanea tarda)
PDW (platelet distribution width)
peak and trough level
peak, monoclonal
pearl
   enamel
   epithelial
   horn
   Laënnec
pearl cyst
pearlescent
pearl formation
pearly umbilicated papule
pear-shaped defect in the iris

pea soup stool
peau d'orange
pectinate ligament of iridocorneal angle
pectinate ligament of iris
pectinate line
pectineal ligament
pectoral artery
pectoral girdle
pectoral gland
pectoral muscle
pectoralis major muscle
pectoris, angina
pectus carinatum (pigeon chest)
pectus excavatum (funnel chest)
pectus recurvatum (funnel chest)
pedal bone
pedes (pl. of pes)
pedicle
pediculosis
pediculosis capitis
pediculosis corporis
pediculosis pubis
Pediculus
Pediculus humanus
Pediculus humanus capitis
Pediculus humanus corporis
Pediculus humanus humanus (yes)
pedis, tinea (athlete's foot)
peduncular ansa
peduncular loop
pedunculated fibroid
pedunculated myxoma
pedunculated papule
PEG (polyethylene glycol)
peg-and-socket articulation
peg-and-socket joint
pegs, rete (rete ridges)
Pelger-Huët anomaly
Pelger-Huët cell
pelgeroid
Pelizaeus-Merzbacher disease
pellagra

pellagra-preventing factor
pelleted stool
pelvic abscess
pelvic aperture
pelvic bone
pelvic brim
pelvic canal
pelvic colon
pelvic diaphragm, twigs to
pelvic fascia
pelvic floor, fibromuscular
pelvic inflammatory disease (PID)
pelvic kidney
pelvic organ
pelvic outlet
pelvic peritoneal cavity
pelvic peritoneum
pelvic sacral foramina
pelvic sidewall
pelvic splanchnic nerve
pelvic viscera
pelvirectal abscess
pelvis (pl. pelves, pelvises)
  android
  anthropoid
  assimilation
  beaked
  bony
  brachypellic
  caoutchouc
  contracted
  cordate
  cordiform
  Deventer
  dolichopellic
  dwarf
  false
  female
  flat
  frozen
  funnel-shaped
  greater

pelvis *(continued)*
  gynecoid
  hardened
  heart-shaped
  inverted
  juvenile
  kyphoscoliotic
  kyphotic
  lesser
  longitudinal oval
  lordotic
  male
  masculine
  mesatipellic
  Nagele
  osteomalacic
  platypelloid
  Prague
  pseudo-osteomalacic
  rachitic
  renal
  reniform
  Rokitansky
  scoliotic
  spider
  spondylolisthetic
  transverse oval
  true
  ureteric
pelvis major
pelvis minor
pemphigoid
  benign mucosal
  bullous
  cicatricial
  ocular
pemphigoid of Brunsting-Perry,
  localized
pemphigus
  benign familial chronic
  paraneoplastic
pemphigus antibodies

pemphigus erythematosus
pemphigus foliaceus
pemphigus gangrenosus
pemphigus leprosus
pemphigus vegetans, Hallopeau type
pemphigus vulgaris
pencil-like
pendulous pouch
penetrating trauma
penetrating ulcer
penetrating wound
penetration
penicillate artery
penicillinase test
Penicillium chrysogenum
Penicillium citrinum
Penicillium commune
Penicillium expansum
Penicillium lilacinum
Penicillium marneffei
Penicillium spinulosum
penile atrophy
penile raphe
penis
    bulb of
    bulbospongiosus muscle of
    clubbed
    concealed
    corpora cavernosa
    corpus spongiosum
    crura of
    deep fascia of
    dorsal artery of
    dorsal nerve of
    dorsum of
    double
    glans
    ischiospongiosus muscle of
    root of
    suspensory ligament of
    webbed
penis artery

penis bone
penis lacuna
pennate muscle
pennatus
pentagastrin
pentoses test
Penzoldt-Fischer test
Penzoldt test for acetone
pepsin
pepsin test
pepsinogen (PG I) test
peptic cell
peptic gland
peptic ulcer
    acute
    chronic
peptic ulcer disease
peptide
    adrenocorticotropic
    regulatory
    vasoactive intestinal (VIP)
peptide test
Peptococcus
Peptococcus niger
peptone test
Peptostreptococcus
Peptostreptococcus anaerobius
Peptostreptococcus asaccharolyticus
Peptostreptococcus indolicus
Peptostreptococcus lanceolatus
Peptostreptococcus magnus
Peptostreptococcus micros
Peptostreptococcus parvulus
Peptostreptococcus prevotii
Peptostreptococcus productus
Percoll separation
percutaneous
percutaneous epididymal sperm
    aspiration
Perdrau method of staining
perforans (pl. perforantes)
perforate

perforated tympanic membrane
perforating abscess
perforating artery of foot
perforating artery of internal mammary
perforating artery of peroneal
perforating artery of profunda femoris
perforating artery of thigh
perforating branch
perforating wound
perforation, frank
perforation of bowel
perfume dermatitis
perfusion, acid
Peria test
perianal region
perianal skin
periangitis
periaortic lymph node
periaortitis
periapical abscess
periappendiceal abscess
periarteritis nodosa
periarteritis, syphilitic
periarticular abscess
periarticular soft tissues
periarticular tissues
periaxial neuritis
Peria test for tyrosine
peribronchial
peribronchial connective tissue
pericallosal artery
pericapillary cell
pericardiacophrenic artery
pericardial artery
pericardial cavity
pericardial cyst
pericardial effusion
pericardial effusion fluid
pericardial fluid
pericardial sac
pericardial sinus
pericardioperitoneal canal

pericarditis
  acute benign
  acute fibrinous
  adhesive
  bacterial
  carcinomatous
  chronic constrictive
  constrictive
  dry
  fibrinous
  hemorrhagic
  internal adhesive
  obliterating
  postmyocardial infarction
  postpericardiotomy
  posttraumatic
  purulent
  rheumatic
  staphylococcal
  tuberculous
  viral
pericarditis with effusion
pericardium
  bread-and-butter
  calcified
  fibrous
  nerves of
  parietal
  serous
  shaggy
  veins of
  visceral
pericecal lymph node
pericellular
pericentral fibrosis
pericentric inversion
pericentromeric region
perichondral bone
perichondrium
perichondroma
pericolonic fat
pericoronal abscess

pericranium
pericyte
pericytial
pericytoma
peridental ligament
periductal inflammation and fibrosis
periductal mastitis
periductal stroma
periencephalitis
periependymal myelitis
periesophagitis
perifolliculitis capitis abscedens et
    suffodiens (dissecting cellulitis
    of scalp)
perifolliculitis, superficial pustular
perihepatitis chronica hyperplastica
perihepatitis, gonococcal
perikaryon
perilobar pancreatitis
perilobular duct
perimenopausal female
perimetrium
perimuscular fibrosis
perimysium
perineal artery
perineal branch of posterior femoral
    cutaneous nerve
perineal branch of pudendal nerve
perineal fascia
perineal membrane
perineal muscle
perineal nerve
perineal space, superficial
perineal tendon, central
perineovaginal fistula
perinephric abscess
perineum
perineural epithelium
perineurium
periocular dermatitis
periodate-lysing-paraformaldehyde
    fixative

periodic acid-Schiff (PAS) stain
periodic acid-Schiff test
periodic fever
period line
periodonal abscess
periodontal degeneration
periodontal ligament
periodontal membrane
periodontitis
perioplic band
perioral dermatitis
periorbital edema
periorbital tissues
periosteal artery
periosteal bone
periosteal nerve
periosteal osteosarcoma
periosteal sarcoma
periosteoma
periosteum, alveolar
periosteum of rib
periostitis, proliferative
periotic bone
peripancreatic area
peripartum myocarditis
peripelvic adipose tissue
peripheral aneurysm
peripheral blood
peripheral blood smear
peripheral embolism
peripheral hepatic necrosis
peripheral lesion
peripheral necrosis
peripheral nerve
peripheral neuritis
peripheral neuropathy
peripheral palisading
peripheral protein
peripheral smear
peripheral zone
periphery
peripleuritic abscess

peripolar cell
periportal area
periportal cellular component
periportal cirrhosis
periportal component
periportal fibrosis
perirectal abscess
perirectal fat
perirenal fat
perisigmoid colon
perisinusoidal space
perisplenic soft tissue
peristalsis
peristaltic contraction
peristaltic rushes
peristaltic wave
perithelial cell
perithelioma
peritoneal abscess
peritoneal band
peritoneal cavity
    greater sac of
    lesser sac of
peritoneal effusion fluid
peritoneal fluid
peritoneal fold
peritoneal gutter
peritoneal ligament
peritoneal recess
peritoneal reflection
peritoneal sac
peritoneal scarring
peritoneal seeding
peritoneal space
peritoneum
    double-layered sheets of
    parietal
    pelvic
    visceral
peritonitis
peritonsillar abscess
peritubular contractile cell

periungual desquamation
periureteral abscess
periurethral cellulitis
periurethral phlegmon
perivascular canal
perivascular cuffing
perivascular goiter
perivascular lymphocytic infiltrate
perivascular mononuclear infiltrate
perivascular round-cell infiltrate
perivascular space
perivascularity
periventricular zone
perlèche
Perls Prussian blue stain
Perls test
permanent molar, first
permanent section
permanent teeth
permeable
permissive cell
Permount mounting medium
pernicious anemia
pernicious malaria
pernicious myocarditis
peroneal artery
peroneal atrophy
peroneal bone
peroneal nerve phenomenon
peroxidase-antiperoxidase (PAP)
    labeling method
peroxidase stain
peroxidase test
perpendicular plate of ethmoid bone
per se
persistent atrioventricular canal
persistent common atrioventricular
    canal
persistent hematuria
persistent truncus arteriosus
Perspex
Perthes-Legg-Calvé disease

pertussis (whooping cough)
pertussoid eosinophilic pneumonia
per volume units
pessary cell
pesticide, organophosphate
Pestivirus
petechia (pl. petechiae)
petechial angioma
petechial fever
petechial hemorrhage of viscera
Petit canal
Petit ligament
Pétrequin ligament
Petri dish
Petri test for proteins
petrobasilar articulation
petrobasilar joint
petroleum distillates poisoning
petro-occipital joint
petro-occipital suture
petrosal artery, superficial
petrosal bone
petrosal sinus
petrous bone
petrous ridge
Pette-Döring panencephalitis
Pettenkofer test for bile acids in urine
Petzetaki test for typhoid fever
Peyer gland
Peyer patches in ileum
Peyer plaque
Peyronie disease
PF (parafascicular) nucleus
Pfeiffer bacillus
Pfeiffer phenomenon
P-50 blood gas
p53 oncogene
p53 protein
p53 tumor suppressor gene
pg (picogram)
pH scale
pH, urine

PHA (phytohemagglutinin)
PHA antigen
PHA assay
Phaeoannellomyces
Phaeoannellomyces elegans
Phaeoannellomyces werneckii
Phaeococcomyces
phage, beta
phage typing of organisms
phagocyte
phagocytic cell immunocompetence
    profile
phagocytic cells
phagocytic index
phagocytic stellate cell
phagocytosis
phalangeal bone
phalangeal cell
phalangeal joint
phalanx (pl. phalanges)
phantom aneurysm
phantom limb
phantom pregnancy
PharmChek sweat patch drug detection
    system
pharyngeal aponeurosis
pharyngeal arch
pharyngeal artery
pharyngeal canal
pharyngeal gland
pharyngeal orifice of auditory tube
pharyngeal ostium of auditory tube
pharyngeal plague
pharyngeal plexus
pharyngeal pouch
pharyngeal tonsil
pharyngitis
    atrophic
    exudative
    follicular
    gangrenous
    hypertrophic

pharyngitis *(continued)*
   phlegmonous
   streptococcal
pharyngoconjunctival fever
pharyngoconjunctival fever virus
pharyngoesophageal sphincter
pharyngopalatine arch
pharynx
   laryngeal part of
   nasal part of
   oral part of
phase
   catagen
   follicular
   inadequate luteal
   luteal
   proliferative
   secretory
   telogen
phase-contrast
phase-defect, luteal
Phaseolus vulgaris
phase reactants
phenacetin
phenacetin test in urine
phenanthridium dye
phenol/chloroform method
phenol (carbolic acid) poisoning
phenolphthalein test
phenol red test
phenolsulfonphthalein (PSP) test for
   kidney function (also, phenol red)
phenoltetrachlorophthalein test for liver
   function
phenomenon (pl. phenomena)
   Anderson
   aqueous-influx
   blood-influx
   booster (on TB test)
   Bordet-Gengou
   Cushing
   Danysz

phenomenon *(continued)*
   dawn
   Debré
   Denys-Leclef
   d'Herelle
   embolic
   fall-and-rise
   first-set
   Gengou
   glass-rod
   halisteresis
   Hamburger
   Hektoen
   Houssay
   Koch
   Koebner
   LAK (lymphokine-activated killer)
      cell
   Lewis hydrophagocytosis
   Liacopoulos
   Liesegang
   Lucio
   Lust peroneal nerve
   Meirowsky
   Neisser-Wechsberg
   no-reflow
   peroneal nerve
   Pfeiffer
   reclotting
   Rumpel-Leede
   satellite
   Schramm
   second-set
   Somogyi
   Staub-Traugott
   Sulzberger-Chase
   Theobald Smith
   Twort-d'Herelle bacteriophagia
phenothiazine
phenotype
phenylalanine
phenylhydrazine test

phenylketonuria (PKU)
  atypical
  classic
  maternal
  transient
phenylthiocarbamoyl protein
pheochrome cell
pheochromocytoma
pheresis
phialides, flask-shaped
Phialophora bubakii
Phialophora dermatitidis
Phialophora parasitica
Phialophora pedrosoi
Phialophora repens
Phialophora richardsiae
Phialophora verrucosa
Philadelphia chromosome
Philip gland
Philippine dengue
Philippine hemorrhagic fever
Phillips 300 transmission electron
  microscope
philtrum
phimosis
phlebitic induration
phlebitis
phlebolith
phlebothrombosis
phlebotomus fever
phlebotomy
Phlebovirus
phlegmon
  Holz
  pancreatic
  periurethral
phlegmonous abscess
phlegmonous mastitis
phlogocyte
phlogocytosis
phloxine
phlyctenule ("flick-ten'-yule")

phoenix abscess
Phoma cruris-hominis
Phoma eupyrena
Phoma glomerata
Phoma herbarum
Phoma hibernica
Phoma oculo-hominis
phosphatase
  acid
  alkaline
  leukocyte acid
  placental alkaline (PLAP)
  prostatic acid (PAP)
  serum alkaline
phosphate
  ammonium magnesium
  amorphous
phosphate-buffered saline (PBS)
phosphate diabetes
phosphofructokinase (PFK) in
  erythrocytes
phosphomolybdic acid
phosphoric acid test
phosphorus (P)
phosphorus necrosis
phosphorus poisoning
phosphorylation
phosphotungstic acid
phosphotungstic acid hematoxylin
  (PTAH)
"phossy jaw" (osteomyelitis of maxilla
  and mandible)
photoallergic contact dermatitis
photoallergy
photo cell
photodermatitis
photopheresis therapy for T-cell
  lymphoma
photoreceptor cells
photosensitivity
phototoxic dermatitis
phrenic artery

phrenic nerve
phrenicocolic ligament
phrenicoesophageal ligament
phrenicolienal ligament
phrenicosplenic ligament
phrenoesophageal ligament
phrenoesophageal membrane
phrenogastric ligament
phrenosplenic ligament
phrygian cap deformity
phthiriasis
Phthirus pubis
phthisis (tuberculosis)
phycobiliprotein
phycoerythrin
Phycomycetes
phycomycetosis
phyllodes, cystosarcoma
phyllolith
phyma
phymatorrhysin
physaliphorous cell
physical diagnosis
physical examination
Physick pouch
physiologic atrophy
physiologic hypertrophy
physiologic jaundice
physiologic proteinuria
phytoagglutinin
phytohemagglutinin (PHA) antigen
phytophotodermatitis
pia mater
pian (yaws)
Pichinde virus
Pick body
Pick cell
Pick disease
Picker nodule
Pick inclusion body
Pick-Niemann disease
picogram (pg)

picoliter (pL)
picometer (pm)
picomole (pmol)
picornavirus
picric acid
picrocarmine stain
picroformol fixative
picro-Mallory trichrome stain
picronigrosin stain
PID (pelvic inflammatory disease)
piecemeal necrosis
piedra
Piedraia hortae
piercer tissue
Pierre Robin syndrome
pigeon-breeder's lung
pigeon-breeder's pneumonitis
pigment
   anthracotic
   bile
   blood
   blotchy clumping of
   endogenous
   exogenous
   fatty
   hematogenous
   hemosiderin-like
   hepatogenous
   lipid
   malarial
   melanotic
   respiratory
   retinal
   visual
   wear and tear
pigmental degeneration
pigmentary atrophy
pigmentary degeneration
pigmentation
pigment cell of skin
pigment cirrhosis
pigmented epidermis

pigmented hair epidermal nevus
pigmented hairy nevus
pigmented lesion (melanotic)
pigmented melanocytic proliferation
pigmented mole
pigmented nevus
pigmented purpuric lichenoid dermatitis
pigmented villonodular synovitis
pigmentosa, retinitis
pilar cyst
pilar sheath
pile, sentinel
piles (hemorrhoids)
pillar
pillar cells of Corti
pillar of fauces, anterior
pillowlike consistency
piloleiomyoma
pilomatricoma
pilonidal cyst
pilonidal fistula
pilonidal sinus
pilosebaceous follicle
pilosebaceous unit
pilus (pl. pili)
Pincus test
pine wood test for indole
pineal body
pineal cells
pineal cyst
pineal gland
pineal hormone
pinealocyte
pinealocytoma
pinealoma
pineal teratoma
pineal ventricle
pineapple test for butyric acid in
    stomach
pineocytoma
ping-pong bone
pink eye

pink stria
pink urine
pinna
pinocyte
pinocytic mouth
pinocytosis
pinta
pinta fever
pinworm
pinworm infestation
pinworm preparation
PIP (proximal interphalangeal) joint
pipe bone
piperidine cleavage
pipestem artery
pipestem cirrhosis
pipestem fibrosis
pipestem stool
pipet (pipette)
pipette
Piria test for tyrosine
Pirie bone
piriform
piriform sinus
Piry virus
pisiform articulation
pisiform bone
pisiform bone articulation
pisiform joint
pisocuneiform articulation
pisohamate ligament
pisometacarpal ligament
pisotriquetral joint
pisounciform ligament
pisouncinate ligament
pit
    anal
    articular
    auditory
    central
    colonic
    costal

pit *(continued)*
  cutaneous
  gastric
  postanal
pit of stomach
pitted subcapsular surface
pitted surface
Pittsburgh pneumonia
pituicytes
pituitary cyst
pituitary dwarfism
pituitary failure
pituitary gigantism
pituitary gland
pituitary gonadotropic hormone
pituitary hormone
pituitary, hyperplasia of
pituitary sinusoid
pityriasis alba
pityriasis alba atrophicas
pityriasis capitis
pityriasis circinata
pityriasis, lichenoid
pityriasis lichenoides et varioliformis
  acuta (PLEVA)
pityriasis linguae
pityriasis maculata
pityriasis nigra
pityriasis rosea
pityriasis rotunda
pityriasis rubra
pityriasis rubra pilaris
pityriasis sicca (dandruff)
pityriasis versicolor (tinea versicolor)
pityrodes, alopecia
Pityrosporum
Pityrosporum orbiculare
PIVKA-II levels
pivot articulation
pivot joint
pixielike facial features
PiZZ alpha antitrypsin

PKU (phenylketonuria)
pL (picoliter)
placenta
  abnormal adherence of
  accessory
  adherent
  annular
  battledore
  bilobate
  chorioallantoic
  chorioamniotic
  cirsoid
  deciduate
  Duncan
  fetal
  fundal
  horseshoe
  incarcerated
  kidney-shaped
  maternal
  nondeciduate
  panduriform
  retained
  Schultze
  third-trimester
  velamentous
  villous
placenta accreta
placenta increta
placenta percreta
placenta previa
  central
  complete
  incomplete
  lateral
  marginal
  partial
  total
placenta protein
placental alkaline phosphatase (PLAP)
placental disk
placental grade

placental lactogen hormone
placental membrane
placental polyp
placental transfusion
placental villi
placental zone
placode, dorsolateral
plague
   ambulatory
   black
   bubonic
   hemorrhagic
   lung
   meningeal
   pharyngeal
   pneumonic
   pulmonic
   septicemic
   white
plague bacillus
plague meningitis
plane
   auriculo-infraorbital
   axiolabiolingual
   axiomesiodistal
   bite
   coronal
   datum
   eye-ear
   facial
   first parallel pelvic
   fourth parallel pelvic
   Frankfort
   Frankfort horizontal
   frontal
   horizontal
   interspinous
   median
   sagittal
   subcostal (SCP)
   supracristal (SCP)
   transpyloric

plane *(continued)*
   transtubercular (TTP)
   transumbilical (TUP)
plane joint
plane of fifth intercostal space
plantar
plantar aponeurosis
plantar arch
plantar artery
plantar calcaneocuboid ligament
plantar calcaneonavicular ligament
plantar cuboideonavicular ligament
plantar cuneocuboid ligament
plantar cuneonavicular ligament
plantar ligament
plantar metatarsal ligament
plantaris aponeurosis
planus, lichen
PLAP (placental alkaline phosphatase)
plaque
   argyrophil
   arteriosclerotic
   atheromatous
   bacteriophage
   calcific
   cutaneous
   dental
   eczematous
   fibromyelinic
   fibrous
   flat
   gastrointestinal
   Hollenhorst
   Hutchinson
   iliac
   infiltrating
   Lichtheim
   neuritic
   Peyer
   pleural
   Randall
   Redlich-Fisher miliary

plaque *(continued)*
   rock-hard
   senile
   yellowish-gray
plaque of glial fibrils as repair material
plaquing
plasma
   antihemophilic
   barium sulfate-absorbed
   blood
   celite-absorbed
   citrated
   consisting of
      dissolved gases
      electrolytes
      nutrients
      proteins
      wastes
      water
   fresh normal
   normal human
   oxalate
   pooled
   salt
   seminal
   supernatant
   true
plasma assay
plasma bicarbonate
plasmablast
plasma buffer
plasma cell (plasmacyte)
plasma cell granuloma
plasma cell hepatitis
plasma cell leukemia
plasma cell mastitis
plasma cell myeloma
plasma cell pneumonia
plasma cell pneumonitis (PCP)
plasma clotting factor
plasmacyte
plasmacytic infiltrate

plasmacytic leukemia
plasmacytoma
plasmacytosis
plasma fraction
plasma hemoglobin
plasma labile factor
plasma lactic acid
plasma leaks from capillaries and
   venules
plasma lipid
plasma lipoprotein level
plasma membrane
plasmapheresis
plasma pool
plasma protein
plasma protein fibrinogen
plasma protein fraction
plasma proteins
plasma renin activity (PRA)
plasmarrhexis
plasma stain
plasma thromboplastin component
   (PTC)
plasma volume
plasmid
   conjugative
   F
   oligomeric
   R
plasminogen
plasminogen activator inhibition (PAI)
   assay
plasmocyte
Plasmodium
plasmodium embolism
Plasmodium falciparum
Plasmodium malariae
Plasmodium ovale
Plasmodium vivax
plastic clot
plastic induration
plasticine

plastic pleurisy
plastic plug
plastic section stain
plastic trocar plug
plate
  agar
  alar
  anal
  auditory
  axial
  basal
  base
  blood
  bone
  bony
  budding
  cardiogenic
  cell
  chorionic
  clinoid
  cloacal
  cortical
  cough
  cribriform
  cutis
  end
  epiphyseal
  epiphyseal cartilage
  equatorial
  ethmovomerine
  frontal
  growth
  hilar
  liver cell
  streak
  tarsal
platelet-activating factor
platelet adhesion test
platelet aggregation
platelet aggregation inhibitor
platelet antibody
platelet count (thrombocyte count)

platelet-derived growth factor
platelet distribution width (PDW)
platelet factor
platelet function
  abnormal
  impaired
platelet indices
platelet metamorphosis
platelet-poor blood (PPB)
platelet-poor plasma (PPP)
platelet protein
platelet-rich plasma (PRP)
platelet, Thrombosphere synthetic
platelike cell
platypelloid pelvis
Plaut bacillus
pleiotropic gene
pleocytosis of cerebrospinal fluid
pleomorphic cell
pleomorphic lymphoma
pleomorphism
Plesiomonas shigelloides (formerly
  Aeromonas shigelloides)
pleura (pl. pleurae)
  biopsy of
  cervical
  costodiaphragmatic recess of
  diaphragmatic
  mediastinal
  mesothelioma of
  parietal
  visceral
pleuracentesis
pleural calculus
pleural canal
pleural cavity
pleural cupola
pleural effusion fluid
pleural fibroma
pleural fluid
pleural plaque
pleural recess

pleural reflection
  costal
  mediastinodiaphragmatic
  sternal
  vertebral
pleural space
pleural tuberculosis
pleurisy
  acute
  adhesive
  blocked
  cholesterol
  chronic
  chyliform
  chylous
  circumscribed
  costal
  diaphragmatic
  diffuse
  double
  dry
  encysted
  exudative
  fibrinous
  hemorrhagic
  ichorous
  indurative
  interlobular
  latent
  mediastinal
  metapneumonic
  plastic
  primary
  proliferating
  pulmonary
  pulsating
  purulent
  sacculated
  secondary
  serofibrinous
  serous
  single

pleurisy *(continued)*
  suppurative
  typhoid
  visceral
pleuritic pneumonia
pleuritis
pleurodynia, epidemic
pleurogenic pneumonia
pleurolith
pleuropericardial canal
pleuroperitoneal canal
pleuropericardial effusion
pleuroperitoneal membrane
pleuropneumonia
pleuropneumonia-like organism
  (PPLO)
plexiform
plexus (pl. plexuses)
  abdominal aortic
  aortic
  Auerbach
  Auerbach mesenteric
  autonomic
  axillary
  basilar
  biliary
  brachial
  cardiac
  cavernous
  celiac
  cervical
  choroid
  ciliary ganglionic
  coccygeal
  colic
  colonic myenteric
  common carotid
  coronary
  cystic
  deep
  deferential
  enteric

plexus *(continued)*
  facial
  femoral
  gastric
  gastroesophageal variceal
  hemorrhoidal
  hepatic nerge
  hypogastric
  inferior mesenteric
  intermesenteric
  lymph
  Meissner
  nerve
  pampiniform
  pharyngeal
  presacral
  prostatic venous
  rectal
  sacral
  solar
  submucosal venous
  superficial
  superior hypogastric
  superior mesenteric
  uterovaginal
  vaginal
  vascular
  vertebral
  vesical
  vesical venous
pliable tissue
plica semilunaris (semilunar fold)
plicae circulares (circular folds)
plicae transversales (transverse folds)
PLP (parathyroid hormonelike protein)
plug
  epithelial
  keratin
  meconium
  mucus
  plastic
  skin

plug of mucous membrane
Plugge test for phenol
plugging, follicular
plump nuclei
plunging goiter
plural pregnancy
pluripotential cell
pm (picometer)
PML (progressive multifocal
  leukoencephalopathy)
PMN (polymorphonuclear leukocyte)
pmol (picomole)
pneumatic bone
pneumatic cell
pneumococcal meningitis
pneumococcal myocarditis
pneumococcal pneumonia
pneumococcus nephritis
Pneumococcus
pneumoconiosis
pneumocystiasis
pneumocystis pneumonia
Pneumocystis carinii pneumonia (PCP)
pneumocytosis
pneumonia (see also *pneumonitis*)
  abortive
  acute
  acute eosinophilic
  alcoholic
  allergic
  amebic
  anthrax
  apex
  apical
  aspiration
  atypical
  atypical bronchial
  atypical interstitial
  bacterial
  bilious
  bronchial
  bronchiolitis obliterans organizing

pneumonia *(continued)*
Buhl desquamative
capillary
caseous
catarrhal
central
cerebral
cheesy
chronic
chronic eosinophilic
classic interstitial
cold agglutinin
community-acquired
consolidative
contusion
Corrigan
Cryptococcus neoformans
deglutition
delayed resolution of
desquamative
desquamative interstitial (DIP)
double
Eaton agent
embolic
endogenous lipoid
eosinophilic
ephemeral
Escherichia coli (*E. coli*)
exogenous
fibrinous
fibrous
Friedländer
fungal
gangrenous
giant cell
granulomatous
gray hepatization stage of
Haemophilus influenzae
Hecht
hypersensitivity
hypostatic
incomplete resolution of

pneumonia *(continued)*
indurative
infantile
influenzal virus
inhalation
interstitial
interstitial plasma cell
intrauterine
irradiation
Klebsiella
Legionella
lipoid
lobar
lobular
lymphoid interstitial
massive
metastatic
migratory
Mycoplasma
mycoplasmal
necrotizing
nonbacterial
nosocomial
obstructive
oil-aspiration
parenchymatous
passive
pertussoid eosinophilic
Pittsburgh
plague
plasma cell
pleuritic
pleurogenetic
pleurogenic
pneumococcal
pneumocystis
Pneumocystis carinii (PCP)
postobstructive
postoperative
post-traumatic
primary atypical
Proteus

pneumonia *(continued)*
  protozoal
  Pseudomonas
  purulent
  red hepatization stage of
  rheumatic
  rickettsial
  secondary
  segmental
  septic
  staphylococcal
  streptococcal
  Streptococcus
  subacute allergic
  superficial
  suppurative
  terminal
  toxemic
  toxic
  traumatic
  tuberculous
  tularemic
  typhoid
  unresolved
  vagus
  varicella
  viral
  wandering
  white
  woolsorter's
pneumonic plague
pneumonitis (see also *pneumonia*)
  acid aspiration
  acute interstitial
  aspiration
  bacterial
  chemical
  cholesterol
  chronic
  congenital rubella
  cytomegalovirus
  early

pneumonitis *(continued)*
  granulomatous
  hypersensitivity
  interstitial
  interstitial plasma cell
  lipoid
  lymphocytic interstitial
  malarial
  manganese
  Mycoplasma (mycoplasmal)
  pigeon-breeder's
  plasma cell (PCP)
  pneumocystis
  radiation
  staphylococcal
  trimellitic anhydritic
  uremic
  ventilation
pneumonocyte
  granular
  membranous
pneumonolipoidosis
pneumonolysis
pneumonomelanosis
pneumonomoniliasis
pneumonomycosis
pneumonophthisis
pneumorenal syndrome
pneumosepticemia
pneumosilicosis
pneumothorax
Pneumovirus
PNH (paroxysmal nocturnal
  hemoglobinuria) cell
PNH cell
PO_2 (partial pressure of oxygen in
  arterial blood)
podocyte
Pohl test for globulins
poikilocyte
poikilocyte in peripheral blood
poikilocytosis

poikiloderma
point
  Addison
  alveolar
  apophysary
  apophyseal
  auricular
  Boas
  cardinal
  Chauffard
  cold-rigor
  congruent
  craniometric
  Desjardins
  dorsal
  end
  Hartmann
  Lanz
  Mackenzie
  McBurney
  midinguinal
  Munro
  Ramond
  Robson
  Sudeck
pointed condyloma
Poirier gland
Poirier space
Poiseville space
poisoning
  acidic salts
  alcohol
  arsenic
  bacterial food
  benzene
  carbon monoxide
  chemical
  chloroform
  copper
  cyanide
  dinitrophenol
  fluoride

poisoning *(continued)*
  food
  heavy metal
  hydrogen sulfide
  insecticide
  lead
  mercury
  mushroom
  naphthalene
  nitrogen oxides
  organophosphate
  petroleum distillates
  phenol
  phosphorus
  shellfish food
  snake venom
  thallium
  tobacco
  zinc
poison ivy dermatitis
poison oak dermatitis
poison sumac dermatitis
pokeweed mitogen
polar cell
polar cushion (Polkissen)
polarity, cell
polarization
polarized light
polarizing microscope
pole
  abapical
  cephalic
  frontal
  germinal
  inferior
  superior
  temporal
poles of organ
poles of vessels
poliomyelitis
poliomyelitis virus
poliovirus

Pollacci test for urine albumin
pollens, inhaled
polyacrylamide gel
polyalveolar lobe
polyarteritis nodosa (PAN)
polyarthritis, migratory
polyaxial joint
polychromatic cell
polychromatophil cell
polychromatophilic normoblast
polychrome methylene blue stain
polychrome stain
polycystic kidney
polycystic ovary
polycystic ovary syndrome
polycyte
polycythemia
polycythemia vera
polyethylene glycol (PEG)
polygonal cell
polygonal chromophobe cell
polyhedral cell
polymastia
polymer
polymerase chain reaction (PCR)
polymer fume fever
polymerization
polymorphic fungi
polymorphocellular
polymorphocyte
polymorphonuclear infiltrate of dermis
polymorphonuclear leukocyte (PMN)
polymyalgia rheumatica
polymyositis, primary idiopathic
polymyositis-dermatomyositis
polyneuritis, acute idiopathic
polynuclear
Polyomavirus, polyomavirus
polyp
    adenomatous
    benign
    bleeding

polyp *(continued)*
    bronchial
    cardiac
    cellular
    cervical
    choanal
    colon
    colonic
    cystic
    dental
    endometrial
    fibrinous
    fibroepithelial
    gastric
    gelatinous
    Hopmann
    hydatid
    hyperplastic
    inflammatory
    juvenile
    laryngeal
    lipomatous
    lymphoid
    metastatic
    mucous
    multiple
    myomatous
    nasal
    osseous
    pedunculated masses of
    placental
    polypoid adenocarcinoma
    pulp
    regenerative
    retention
    sessile
    sigmoid
    single
    uterine
    vascular
    villous
polyp stalk

polypeptide
  gastric inhibitory (GIP)
  glucose-dependent
    insulinotropic (GIP)
  islet amyloid (IAPP)
  pancreatic (PP)
  parathyroid-like
  vasoactive intestinal (VIP)
polypeptide antigen
polypeptide chain
polyphrenic gene
polyplastic cell
polypoid mass
polyposis
  familial
  familial adenomatous (FAP)
  familial intestinal
  gastric
  multiple intestinal
polypropylene line
polyptychic gland
"polys" (slang for polymorphonuclear
  leukocytes)
polysaccharide
polytene chromosome
polythelia
polyuria
polyvinylidene difluoride membrane
Pompe disease
Pongola virus
pons
Pontamine sky blue stain
Pontiac fever
pontine
pontine artery
pontine cistern
pool
  abdominal
  bile acid
  blood
  plasma
pooled plasma

pooling, vallecular
poorly differentiated adenocarcinoma
poorly differentiated carcinoma
popliteal artery
porencephaly
pores of Kohn
Porges-Meier flocculation test
  for syphilis
porokeratosis
poroma
porphobilinogen (PBG)
porphyria
  acute
  acute intermittent (AIP)
  congenital
  congenital erythropoietic (CEP)
  cutaneous hepatic
  erythrohepatic
  erythropoietic
  hepatic
  hepatoerythropoietic (HEP)
  symptomatic
  variegate (VP)
porphyria cutanea tarda (PCT)
porphyrin
porphyrinemia
porphyrins in blood and urine
porphyrinuria
Porphyromonas asaccharolytica
portacaval anastomosis
porta hepatis
portal canal
portal cirrhosis
portal hypertension
portal lobule
portal pyemia
portal space
portal-systemic anastomotic area
portal system of veins
portal triad
portal vascular bed
portal vein

portal venous system
portal zone
Porter test for excess of uric acid
portion, intramural
port-wine nevus
port-wine stain
positive
    false
    gram
    Nitrazine
    Rh
positive charge
positive control
positive stain
positive test for occult blood
positive whiff
Posner test for albumin
"post" (postmortem examination)
postanal pit
postcoital bleeding
postcoital test
postcricoid area
postcricoid web
posterior abdominal wall
posterior alveolar artery
posterior annular ligament of wrist
posterior auricular artery
posterior auricular nerve
posterior auricular vein
posterior border of lung
posterior cell
posterior cerebral artery
posterior chamber
posterior clinoid process
posterior communicating artery
posterior cricoarytenoid ligament
posterior cruciate ligament
posterior cusp
posterior dental artery
posterior ethmoidal air cell
posterior ethmoidal sinus
posterior femoral cutaneous nerve

posterior fontanelle
posterior fornix of vagina
posterior fossa meningioma
posterior humeral circumflex artery
posterior inferior cerebellar artery
posterior intercostal artery
posterior interosseous artery
posterior intraoccipital joint
posterior layer of rectus sheath
posterior ligament of head of fibula
posterior ligament of incus
posterior ligament of knee
posterior longitudinal ligament
posterior mediastinum
posterior meniscofemoral ligament
posterior muscle, serratus
posterior occipitoaxial ligament
posterior pancreaticoduodenal artery
posterior papillary muscle
posterior recess of ischiorectal fossa
posterior rectus sheath
posterior sacroiliac ligament
posterior sacrosciatic ligament
posterior scapular artery
posterior scrotal artery
posterior semicircular canal
posterior spinal artery
posterior sternoclavicular ligament
posterior superior alveolar artery
posterior surface of pancreas
posterior surface of prostate
posterior synechiae
posterior talofibular ligament
posterior talotibial ligament
posterior tibial artery
posterior tibiofibular ligament
posterior tibiotalar ligament
posterior triangle
posterior uveitis
posterior vagal trunk
posterior wall
posterolateral fontanelle

posterolateral sclerosis
postfebrile neuritis
postganglionic fiber, unmyelinated
post-heparin lipolytic activity test
posthepatitic cirrhosis
posthitis
postinfectious myelitis
postinflammatory hypopigmentation
postinflammatory leukoderma
postischemic acute renal failure
postmenopausal atrophy
postmenopausal bleeding
postmenopausal osteoporosis
postmenopausal syndrome
postmenopausal women
postmortem clot
postmortem delivery
postmortem examination ("post")
postmortem hypostasis
postmortem livedo
postmortem lividity
postmortem pustule
postmortem rigidity
postmortem suggillation
postmortem thrombus
postmortem tubercle
postmortem wart
postmyocardial infarction pericarditis
postnecrotic cirrhosis
postobstructive pneumonia
postocular optic neuritis
postoperative diagnosis
postoperative infection
postoperative pneumonia
postoperative pressure alopecia
postpartum alopecia
postpartum hemorrhage
postpartum hypertension
postpartum pituitary necrosis
postpericardiotomy pericarditis
postprandial blood-sugar level,
    two-hour

postprandial glucose
postprandial lipemia
postprandial test
postprimary tuberculosis
post-radiation change
postrenal azotemia
postrenal proteinuria
postsphenoid bone
post-term pregnancy
post-transfusion hepatitis
post-traumatic atrophy of bone
post-traumatic osteoporosis
post-traumatic pericarditis
post-traumatic pneumonia
postural proteinuria
postvaccinal myelitis
postvertebral muscle
"post" (postmortem exam)
potassium (K)
potassium bichromate
potassium dichromate
potassium ferricyanide
potassium hydroxide (KOH)
potassium hydroxide (KOH) solution
potassium iodide test
potassium-losing nephritis
potassium metabisulfite
potassium permanganate
potential space
Pott abscess
Pott aneurysm
Pott disease
pouch
    antral
    apophyseal
    blind
    branchial
    Broca pudendal
    celomic
    deep perineal
    Denis Browne
    Douglas rectouterine

pouch *(continued)*
  endodermal
  gastric
  Hartmann
  haustral
  Heidenhain
  hepatorenal
  hypophysial
  ileoanal
  ileocecal
  jejunal
  Kock
  Morison
  paracystic
  pararectal
  paravesical
  pendulous
  pharyngeal
  Physick
  Prussak
  Rathke
  rectal
  rectouterine
  rectovaginal
  rectovaginouterine
  rectovesical
  renal
  Seessel (note: 2 e's, 2 s's)
  superficial inguinal
  superficial perineal
  ultimobranchial
  uterovesical
  vesicoureterine
  water-filled
  Zenker
pouchlike
pouch of Douglas
pounds per square inch (psi, p.s.i.)
Poupart ligament, shelving edge of
pour plate
Powassan virus
powder burn

power
  high (microscope)
  low (microscope)
  scanning
poxvirus (also, pox virus)
PPB (platelet-poor blood)
PP cell
PPD skin test
PRA (plasma renin activity)
PRA (progesterone receptor assay)
Prague pelvis
preampullary portion of bile duct
pre-B cell
precancerous dermatitis
precancerous lesion
precipitates (KPs), keratic
precipitation
precipitation reaction
precipitation test
precipitin
precipitin test
Precision-G handheld blood glucose
  test
precision of laboratory test
Precision Q-I-D handheld blood
  glucose test
preclinical diabetes
precocious sexual development
precursor cell
predator damage
predilection
predisposing factor
predominant
prefollicle cell
preganglionic fiber
preganglionic sympathetic fibers
pregangrenous
pregnancy
  abdominal
  aborted ectopic
  ampullar
  bigeminal

pregnancy *(continued)*
  broad ligament
  cervical
  combined
  compound
  cornual
  ectopic
  extrauterine
  fallopian
  false
  heterotopic
  hydatid
  hysteric
  interstitial
  intraligamentary
  intraperitoneal
  membranous
  mesenteric
  molar
  multiple
  mural
  nervous
  ovarian
  ovarioabdominal
  oviductal
  parietal
  phantom
  plural
  post-term
  prolonged
  pseudointraligamentary
  sarcofetal
  sarcohysteric
  spurious
  stump
  toxemia of
  tubal
  tuboabdominal
  tuboligamentary
  tubo-ovarian
  tubouterine
  twin

pregnancy *(continued)*
  uteroabdominal
  uterotubal
pregnancy cell
pregnancy diabetes
pregnancy gland
pregnancy test
pregnanetriol test
pregnenolone test
pregranulosa cell
prehyalin
prehyoid gland
preileal appendix
preinterparietal bone
Preisz-Nocard bacillus
prekallikrein
preliminary diagnosis
premalignant neoplasm
premammary abscess
premature alopecia
premature birth
premaxillary bone
premeasured reagent
premenstrual edema
premolar tissue
prenatal diagnosis
prenatal genetic diagnosis
prenatal sex determination
preoccipital notch
preoperative diagnosis
prepancreatic artery
prepapillary bile duct
preparation
  cytospin
  impression
  KOH (potassium hydroxide)
  LE cell
  Nuclepore prep
  sickle cell
  tissue
prepatellar bursitis
preperitoneal fat

preperitoneal space
prepuce of clitoris
preputial gland
prepyloric antrum
prepyloric sphincter
prepyloric vein
prerenal azotemia
prerenal proteinuria
presacral plexus
presacral space
presegmental artery
presphenoid bone
pressure alopecia
pressure atrophy
pressure cooker technique
pressure epiphysis
pressure, intrathoracic
pressure necrosis
pressure-type groove
pressure-volume loop
prestyloid recess
presumptive diagnosis
pre-T cell
preternatural anus
pretibial edema
pretibial fever
prevertebral artery
prevertebral ganglia
Prevotella bivia
Prevotella disiens
Prevotella intermedia
Prevotella loeschii
Prevotella melaninogenica
Prevotella oralis
Prevotella oris
Preyer test
prickle cell
prickle-cell layer of epidermis
primary aldosteronism
primary amyloidosis
primary atypical pneumonia
primary biliary cirrhosis

primary cartilaginous joints
primary center of ossification
primary disease
primary embryonic cell
primary hematuria
primary hypertension
primary idiopathic polymyositis
primary irritant dermatitis
primary lesion
primary lymphoma of central nervous
    system
primary malignancy
primary metabolism
primary methemoglobinemia
primary multiple myositis
primary myeloid metaplasia
primary pleurisy
primary progressive cerebellar
    degeneration
primary pyoderma
primary ramus
primary tuberculosis
prime movers
primipara (para 1)
primitive aorta
primitive cell
primitive gland
primitive granulosa cell
primitive reticular cell
primitive wandering cell
primordial cell
primordial cyst
primordial follicle
primordial germ cell
primordium
principal artery of pterygoid canal
principal artery of thumb
principal bronchus
principal cell
principal diagnosis
prion protein
pro time (prothrombin time)

proaccelerin
proactivator, C_3
probe patent
Probe Tech II
procedure
    diagnosis
    HPV genotyping
    immunoblot
    Northern blot (NB)
    Southern blot (SB)
    Western blot (WB)
process
    accessory
    acromial
    alar
    alveolar
    apical
    articular
    ascending
    auditory
    basilar
    calcaneal
    caudate
    ciliary
    clinoid
    cochleariform
    condyloid
    conoid
    coracoid
    costal
    dendritic
    ensiform
    ethmoidal
    falciforn
    fibroplastic
    frontal
    frontonasal
    frontosphenoidal
    transverse
    uncinate
    vertebral spinous
    xiphoid

processing of tissue specimen
process of fat, digital
process of maxilla, alveolar
process of pancreas, uncinate
process of vertebra, articular
proconvertin (Factor VII)
proctitis
production antibody
productive nephritis
products of conception
proerythroblasts in marrow
profile
    antigenic
    biochemical
    chemistry
    executive
    lipid
    liver
    phagocytic cell immunocompetence
    test
    thyroid
    20-channel chemistry
    urethral pressure
profuse sweat
progenitalis, herpes
progenitor
progestational endometrium
progestational hormone
progestational pattern
progesterone
progesterone hormone
progesterone receptor assay (PRA)
proglottid
prognosis, grave
programmed cell death
progranulocyte
progressive choroidal atrophy
progressive degeneration
progressive emphysematous necrosis
progressive multifocal leuko-
    encephalopathy (PML)
progressive muscular atrophy

progressive muscular dystrophy
progressive neural muscular atrophy
progressive ossifying myositis
progressive spinal muscular atrophy
progressive staining
progressive subcortical atrophy
progressive systemic sclerosis
progressive unilateral facial atrophy
progressive visual impairment
proinsulin
projectile horn
projection, enamel
prokaryotic cell
prolactin
prolactin anterior pituitary hormone
prolactin cell
prolactin hormone (hPRL)
prolactin-inhibiting factor
prolactin-inhibiting hormone
prolactin–insulin stimulation test
prolactin-releasing factor
prolactin-releasing hormone
prolactin, serum
prolactoliberin hormone
proliferans, retinitis
proliferating astrocytes
proliferating by mitosis
proliferating pleurisy
proliferation
  bony
  cellular
  fibroplastic
  nodular
  papillary
  pigmented melanocytic
proliferation of amastigotes in dermal
  cells
proliferation of fibroblasts
proliferation of fibrous tissue
proliferative dermatitis
proliferative endometrium
proliferative glomerulitis

proliferative glomerulonephritis
proliferative inflammation
proliferative myositis
proliferative pattern
proliferative periostitis
proliferative stage
proliferative synovitis
prolonged bleeding from wounds
prolonged pregnancy
prolymphocyte
prominent nucleus
prominent scalene tubercle
promontory
promyelocyte
promyelocytic anemia
pronormoblast
pronounced dead
proparathyroid hormone
properdin test
proper ligament of ovary
properitoneal fat
properitoneal flank stripe (on x-ray)
propidium iodide
Propionibacterium acnes (formerly
  Corynebacterium acnes)
Propionibacterium avidum
Propionibacterium freudenreichii
Propionibacterium granulosum
Propionibacterium jensenii
propionic acid
propria
  lamina
  substantia
  tunica
prorubricyte
prosector
prospective recipient
prostaglandin test
prostate
  adenocarcinoma of
  apex of
  inferolateral surfaces of

prostate *(continued)*
    lateral lobe of
    lymph vessels of
    median lobe of
    posterior surface of
prostate chip
prostate gland
prostate specific antigen (PSA)
prostatic abscess
prostatic acid phosphatase (PAP)
prostatic adenocarcinoma
prostatic calculus (pl. calculi)
prostatic capsule
prostatic carcinoma
prostatic concretion
prostatic cyst
prostatic duct
prostatic fluid
prostatic hyperplasia
prostatic malignancy
prostatic shaving
prostatic sinus
prostatic urethra
prostatic venous plexus
prostatitis
    acute
    chronic
Protargol
protection test
protective layer of fat
protective protein
protein
    abnormal mitochondrial
    acute phase
    acyl carrier
    alcohol-soluble
    amyloid A (AA)
    androgen binding (ABP)
    antitumor
    antiviral (AVP)
    autologous
    bacterial

protein *(continued)*
    bacterial cellular
    Bence Jones
    binding
    bone morphogenetic
    carrier
    cationic
    CD14 membrane
    c-erb
    cerebrospinal fluid
    C4 binding
    c-myc
    coagulated
    complete
    compound
    conjugated
    constitutive
    cord
    C-reactive (CRP)
    CSF (cerebrospinal fluid)
    deficiency
    denatured
    derived
    desmoplakin
    DNA tumor virus
    encephalitogenic
    fibrillar
    fibrous
    floating
    foreign
    G
    glial fibrillary acidic (GFAP)
    globular
    GM activator
    guanyl-nucleotide-binding
    heat shock
    Hektoen, Kretschmer, and Welker
    heterologous
    HIV
    homologous
    immune
    incomplete

protein *(continued)*
   insoluble
   integral
   intrinsic
   iodized
   iron-sulfur
   leukocyte adhesion (LAP)
   M
   macrophage inflammatory
   maintenance
   MCP-1 (monocyte chemoattractant)
   metabolism, disorders of
   microtubule-associated (MAP)
   mutant
   myelin basic (MBP)
   myeloblastic
   myeloma
   myofilament
   native
   neurofilament triplet
   neutrophil activating (NAP)
   non-heme iron
   nonspecific
   odorant binding
   p53
   parathyroid hormonelike (PLP)
   partial
   peripheral
   phenylthiocarbamoyl
   placenta
   plasma
   platelet
   prion
   protective
   pS2
   purified placental
   R
   racemized
   receptor
   retinol-binding (RBP)
   S100
   serum

protein *(continued)*
   serum amyloid A (SAA)
   simple
   sphingolipid activator (SAP)
   staphylococcal A
   stimulatory (SP1)
   strong silver
   structure
   synthetic
   Tamm-Horsfall
   thyroxine-binding (TBP)
   total
   transport
   troponin T
   uncoupling
   unwinding
   urinary
   vitamin D-binding (DBP)
   water-soluble
   whole
   Z-
   zinc finger
protein A
proteinaceous
proteinase, cysteine
proteinase enzyme
proteinase K
protein C
protein C deficiency
protein C inhibitor (PCI)
protein concentration of spinal fluid,
   total
protein electrophoresis
proteinemia, Bence Jones
protein factor
protein hyaline
protein hydrolysate
protein in spinal fluid
protein in urine
proteinosis
   lipoid
   pulmonary alveolar

protein phosphatase
protein-rich fluid
protein S (*not* S protein)
protein shell of virus particle
protein test
proteinuria
  accidental
  adventitious
  athletic
  Bence Jones
  colliquative
  dietetic
  effort
  emulsion
  enterogenic
  essential
  false
  febrile
  functional
  gestational
  globular
  gouty
  hematogenous
  intermittent
  isolated
  light-chain
  lordotic
  mixed
  nephrogenous
  nonisolated
  orthostatic
  overflow
  palpatory
  paroxysmal
  physiologic
  postrenal
  postural
  prerenal
  pyogenic
  regulatory
  renal
  serous

proteinuria *(continued)*
  transient
  true
proteinuria praetuberculosa
proteolytic enzyme
proteose test
Proteus
Proteus hydrophilus
Proteus inconstans subgroup B
Proteus mirabilis
Proteus morganii
Proteus Ox-19 antibody
Proteus Ox-2 antibody
Proteus Ox-K antibody
Proteus penneri
Proteus pneumonia
Proteus rettgeri
Proteus vulgaris
Proteus zenkeri
prothrombin
prothrombin consumption test (PCT)
prothrombin-proconvertin test
prothrombin test
prothrombin time (pro time, PT)
  one-stage (Quick)
  two-stage modified
    (Ware and Seegers)
prothrombin time ratio
protocol, GTC/silica beads
Protocult test
proto-oncogene
protoplasm
protoporphyrin
protozoa
protozoal myocarditis
protozoal pneumonia
protruded disk
protruding
protuberant
proudflesh
Proust space
Providencia

Providencia alcalifaciens
Providencia rettgeri
Providencia stuartii
provisional anatomic diagnosis
Prower-Stuart factor
proximal clot
proximal interphalangeal joint
proximal muscles
proximal part of dorsal pancreatic duct
proximal phalanges
proximal radioulnar articulation
proximal radioulnar joint
proximal tibiofibular joint
proximally
prurigo ("itch")
  Besnier
  Hebra
  melanotic
  nodular
  summer p. of Hutchinson
prurigo actinic
prurigo aestivalis (also, estivalis)
prurigo agria
prurigo chronica multiformis
prurigo ferox
prurigo gestationis
prurigo infantilis
prurigo mitis
prurigo simplex
pruritic eruption
pruritic urticarial papules of pregnancy
pruritus
  aquagenic
  essential
  senile
  symptomatic
  uremic
pruritus aestivalis (summer itch)
pruritus ani
pruritus at site of skin invasion
  (ground itch)
pruritus balnea (bath itch)

pruritus hiemalis
pruritus scroti
pruritus vulvae
Prussak pouch
Prussak space
Prussian blue stain
pS2 protein
PSA (prostate specific antigen)
psammoma body
psammomatous meningioma
psammous
Pseudallescheria boydii
pseudoatrophoderma colli
pseudobacillus
pseudobacterium
pseudocartilage
Pseudochaetosphaeronema larense
pseudochancre redux
pseudocholinesterase (PCHE)
pseudocoarctation
pseudocowpox virus
pseudocyst
  adrenal
  pancreatic
  pulmonary
pseudodiverticulum
pseudoepitheliomatous hyperplasia
pseudofollicular salpingitis
pseudofolliculitis
pseudogout, calcium pyrophosphate
  crystals in
pseudo-Gaucher cell
pseudogranulomatous aggregations of
  cells
pseudohermaphroditism
pseudohypertrophic muscular atrophy
pseudohypertrophy
pseudohyphae
pseudohypoparathyroidism
pseudointraligamentary pregnancy
pseudokeloidal band
pseudolymphoma

pseudomelanosis
pseudomembrane
pseudomembranous enterocolitis
pseudomembranous gastritis
pseudomembranous inflammation
pseudometaplasia
Pseudomonas
Pseudomonas acidovorans (formerly
  Comamonas terrigena)
Pseudomonas aeruginosa
Pseudomonas alcaligenes
Pseudomonas cepacia
Pseudomonas diminuta
Pseudomonas fluorescens
Pseudomonas-like bacteria
Pseudomonas mallei
Pseudomonas maltophilia
Pseudomonas paucimobilis
Pseudomonas pickettii
Pseudomonas pneumonia
Pseudomonas pseudoalcaligenes
Pseudomonas pseudomallei
Pseudomonas putida
Pseudomonas putrefaciens
Pseudomonas stutzeri
Pseudomonas testosteroni
pseudomucinous
pseudomyxoma peritonei
pseudo-osteomalacic pelvis
pseudopalisade formation
pseudopalisading
pseudoparenchyma
pseudophakic
pseudoplatelet
pseudopod
pseudopolyp
pseudoproteinuria
pseudopyogenic granuloma
pseudorabies virus
pseudosac
pseudosarcoma
pseudostoma

pseudostone
pseudostratification
pseudostratified columnar epithelium
pseudostratified epithelium
pseudostratified nuclei
pseudotubercle
pseudotuberculosis
pseudotumor cerebri
pseudotumor, inflammatory
pseudounipolar cell
pseudovacuole
pseudoxanthoma cell
pseudoxanthoma elasticum
psi, p.s.i. (pounds per square inch)
psi factor
psittacosis
psoas abscess
psoas fascia
psoas gap
psoas major muscle
psoas margin
psoas muscle
psoas muscle abscess
psoas shadow
psorelcosis
psorenteritis
psoriasis
  circinate
  diffused
  discoid
  exfoliative
  generalized pustular p. of
    Zambusch
  guttate
  gyrate
  inverse
  nummular
  ostraceous
  palmar
  pustular
  seborrheic
psoriasis geographica

psoriasis inveterata
psoriasis orbicularis
psoriasis punctata
psoriasis rupioides
psoriasis spondylitica
psoriasis universalis
PSP (phenolsulfonphthalein) test for
   kidney function (also, phenol red)
pS2 protein
PT (prothrombin time, pro time)
PTAH (phosphotungstic acid-
   hematoxylin) stain
PTC (plasma thromboplastin
   component)
pterion
pterygoid artery
pterygoid bone
pterygoid canal
pterygoid plate
pterygoid plexus
pterygoid process
pterygomandibular ligament
pseudomandibular raphe
pterygomaxillary fissure
pterygopalatine canal
pterygopalatine fossa
pterygopalatine ganglion
pterygospinal ligament
PTT (partial thromboplastin time)
p24 antigen
ptyocrinous cell
pubes
pubic arch
pubic artery
pubic bone
pubic hair line
pubic itching
pubic ligament
pubic louse
pubic ramus
pubic symphysis
pubic tubercle

pubis (slang for os pubis)
   mons
   pecten
   Phthirus
   ramus of
   symphysis
pubocapsular ligament
pubocervical ligament
pubococcygeal line
pubococcygeal muscle
pubofemoral ligament
pubo-obturator area
puboprostatic ligament
puborectalis loop
puborectalis muscle
pubovaginalis muscle
pubovesical ligament
puckered
Puchtler-Sweat stain
pudendal artery
pudendal canal
pudendal cleft
pudendal nerve
pudendal vein
pudendal vessel
puerperal fever
puerperal mastitis
puerperal osteomalacia
pulled tendon
pulmoaortic canal
pulmonale, cor
pulmonary alveolar proteinosis
pulmonary alveolus
pulmonary artery
pulmonary artery aneurysm
pulmonary cirrhosis
pulmonary congestion
pulmonary consolidation
pulmonary edema
pulmonary embolism
pulmonary emphysema
pulmonary endothelial cell

pulmonary epithelial cell
pulmonary excretion of carbon dioxide
pulmonary fibrosis
pulmonary function
pulmonary gas exchange
pulmonary gases
pulmonary hypertension
pulmonary infarct(ion)
pulmonary ligament
pulmonary macrophage
pulmonary nerve
pulmonary orifice
pulmonary osteoarthropathy
pulmonary parenchyma
pulmonary pleurisy
pulmonary retention of carbon dioxide
pulmonary segment
pulmonary stenosis
pulmonary tissue–blood barrier
pulmonary trunk, bifurcation of
pulmonary tuberculosis
pulmonary valve
pulmonary valvular leaflet
pulmonary venous–systemic air
    embolism
pulmonary vein
pulmonic plague
pulmonic valve
pulmonis, apex
pulp
    coronal
    dead
    dental
    dentinal
    devitalized
    digital
    enamel
    red
    splenic
    white
pulp abscess
pulp canal

pulp cavity
pulp chamber
pulpar cell
pulpitis, hyperplastic
pulposus, nucleus
pulp polyp
pulsating metastases
pulsating pleurisy
pulse (pl. pulses)
pulseless disease
pulsion diverticulum
pultaceous
pumped-dye laser
punch biopsy
punch, cylindrical
punctate hemorrhage
punctate infiltrate
punctate keratotic lesion
puncture
    arterial
    cisternal
    fingerstick
    lumbar (LP)
puncture diabetes
puncture ulcer
puncture wound
pupil (pupillae), dilator
pupillary zone
Purdy test for albumin
purified placental protein
Purkinje cell
Purkinje corpuscle
Purkinje fiber
purplish discoloration of skin
purplish rash
purpura
    acute vascular
    allergic
    anaphylactoid
    factitious
    fibrinolytic
    Henoch-Schönlein (Shoenlein)

purpura *(continued)*
  hyperglobulinemic
  idiopathic thrombocytopenic (ITP)
  immune thrombocytopenic
  iodic
  nonthrombocytopenic
  psychogenic
  Schönlein-Henoch (Shoenlein)
  thrombocytopenic (TP)
  thrombotic thrombocytopenic (TTP)
  Waldenström
purpura angioneurotica
purpura annularis telangiectodes
purpura fulminans
purpura hemorrhagica
purpura nervosa
purpura pulicans
purpura pulicosa
purpura rheumatica
purpura senilis
purpura simplex
purpura urticans
purpuric bleeding
purpuric cutaneous eruption
purpurinuria
purulence
purulent discharge
purulent exudate
purulent inflammation
purulent lesion
purulent material
purulent meningitis
purulent otitis media
purulent pancreatitis
purulent pericarditis
purulent pleurisy
purulent pneumonia
purulent salpingitis
purulent sinusitis
purulent subarachnoid exudate
purulent synovitis
purulosanguineous pus

pus
  anchovy sauce
  blue
  blue-green
  burrowing
  cheesy
  collagen
  creamy
  curdy
  discrete yellow masses in
  green
  ichorous
  laudable
  sanious
pus cell
pus corpuscle
pus-forming bacteria
pus in pleural cavity
pustular eruption
pustular exanthem and enanthem
pustular psoriasis
pustule
  acneiform
  multiloculated
  postmortem
  spongiform
  unilocular
pustules in lash follicles
putamen
Putnam-Dana syndrome
putrefaction of gases
putrefactive changes in dead body
putrefy
putrescence
putrescent
putrid
putty kidney
Puumala virus
Puusepp reflex
pyelocaliceal
pyelocaliectasis
pyelocalyceal

pyelocystitis
pyelolymphatic
pyelonephritic kidney
pyelonephritis
   acute
   ascending
   chronic
   descending
   hematogenous
   xanthogranulomatous
pyeloureterectasis
pyelovenous
pyemesis
pyemia
   cryptogenic
   portal
pyemic abscess
pyesis
pyknosis
pyknotic nucleus
pylephlebitis
pyloric antrum
pyloric antrum cardiacum
pyloric artery
pyloric canal
pyloric channel
pyloric gland
pyloric mucosa
pyloric orifice
pyloric outlet
pyloric ring
pyloric sphincter
pyloric stenosis
pyloroduodenal junction
pylorostenosis
pylorus (pl. pylori)
pyocele
pyocephalus, circumscribed
pyochezia
pyocin
pyococcus
pyocolpocele

pyocolpos
pyocyanic
pyocyanogenic
pyocyst
pyocystis
pyocyte
pyoderma
   chancriform
   primary
   secondary
pyoderma gangrenosum
pyoderma vegetans
pyodermatitis
pyodermatosis
pyogen
pyogenesis
pyogenic bacteria
pyogenic fever
pyogenic granuloma
pyogenic infection of sweat glands
pyogenic meningitis
pyogenic organism
pyogenic proteinuria
pyogenous
pyohemothorax
pyoid
pyometra
pyometritis
pyomyositis
pyonephritis
pyonephrolithiasis
pyonephrosis
pyo-ovarium
pyopericarditis
pyopericardium
pyoperitoneum
pyoperitonitis
pyophysometra
pyopneumocholecystitis
pyopneumohepatitis
pyopneumoperitoneum
pyopneumoperitonitis

pyopneumothorax, subphrenic
pyopoiesis
pyopoietic
pyopyelectasis
pyorrhea
pyorrhea alveolaris
pyosalpingitis
pyosalpingo-oophoritis
pyosalpinx
pyosemia
pyosepticemia
pyosis, Manson
pyostomatitis vegetans
pyramid
pyramidal bone
pyramidal cell
pyramidal decussation

pyramidal eminence
pyramidal tract
Pyramidon test for occult blood
   in urine
pyridoxilated stroma-free hemoglobin
   (SFHb)
pyriform (piriform) sinus
pyrogen, endogenous
pyrogenicity
pyrogenic proteins
pyroglobulin
pyrosis
pyrrol blue stain
pyrrol cell
pyruvic acid
pyuria

Q, q

Q band
Q-banding stain
Q-b band
Q fever
Qiaex bead
QNS (quantity not sufficient)
Q-Prep staining system
quadrant
   left lower (LLQ)
   left upper (LUQ)
   left upper outer
   right lower (RLQ)
   right upper (RUQ)
   right upper outer
quadrate ligament
quadrate lobe of liver
quadrate muscle
quadriceps artery of femur
quadrigeminal cistern
quadrilateral bone
qualitative
qualitative analysis
quantitative

quantitative analysis
quantity not sufficient (QNS)
quantum
Quaranfil virus
quartan fever
quartan malaria
quenching of fluorescence intensity
Quervain disease
Queyrat, erythroplasia of
Quick prothrombin test
Quick test
QuickVue Chlamydia test
quiescent cell
quinacrine fluorescent method
   of staining
Quincke edema
Quincke meningitis
quinine
quinine carbacrylic resin test
   for gastric anacidity
Quinlan test for bile
quinsy
quotidian malaria

R, r

Raabe test for albumin
rabbit stool
rabies
rabies-like viruses
rabies virus
Rabuteau test for hydrochloric acid
   in urine
RA (ragocyte) cell
racemized protein
racemose aneurysm
racemose gland
rachitic pelvis
rachitis
rad (radiation absorbed dose)
radial artery
radial bone
radial carpal artery
radial cells of Mueller
radial collateral ligament
radial groove
radial immunodiffusion (RID)
radial neck groove
radial sclerosing lesion
radial sigmoid notch
radial styloid
radiant energy
radiate ligament

radiate sternocostal ligament
radiation
   diagnostic
   ionizing
   ultraviolet
radiation absorbed dose (rad)
radiation cell change
radiation colitis
radiation cystitis
radiation dermatitis
radiation gastritis
radiation necrosis
radiation neuritis
radiation pneumonitis
radiation therapy
radical
   free
   biliary
   intrahepatic
   tertiary
radicular abscess
radicular artery
radicular neuritis
radicular odontoma
radiculitis
radioactive chromium
radioactive cobalt

radioactive iodide uptake test
radioactive iodinated serum albumin
(RISA) test
radioactive isotope
radioactively tagged
radioallergosorbent test (RAST)
radiocarpal articulation
radiocarpal joint
radiocarpal ligament
radiocarpal portal
radioceptor assay
radiodermatitis
radiohumeral articulation
radiohumeral joint
radioimmunoassay (RIA)
   direct
   indirect
radioimmunosorbent test (RIST)
radioisotopically tagged antihuman
   antibody
radiolunotriquetral ligament
radioneuritis
radioscaphocapitate ligament
radioscapholunate ligament
radioulnar articulation
radioulnar joint, articular disk of distal
radioulnar ligament, anterior
radium
radius, annular ligament of
ragocyte
raised flap
Raji cell
Raji cell assay
rales, basilar
Ralfe test for acetone in urine
Rambourg chromic acid-
   phosphotungstic acid stain
Rambourg periodic acid-chromic
   methenamine-silver stain
rami (pl. of ramus)
Ramon flocculation test
Ramón y Cajal stain

Ramond point
Ramsay Hunt syndrome
Ramularia
ramus (pl. rami)
   dorsal
   dorsal primary
   inferior pubic
   ischiopubic
   pubic
   ventral
   ventral primary
ramus bone
ramus communicans
   gray
   white
ramus of ischium, ascending
ramus of os pubis, ascending
RANA (rheumatoid-associated nuclear
   antigen)
Randall plaque
Randolph test for peptones in urine
random blood glucose
random blood sugar
range
   normal
   reference
   therapeutic
ranine artery
Ranke complex
Rankine scale
Ranson pyridine silver stain
Rantzman test
Ranvier node
raphe
   abdominal
   amniotic
   anococcygeal
   anogenital
   longitudinal
   median
   palpebral
   penile

raphe *(continued)*
   pterygomandibular
   scrotal
   tendinous
raphe anococcygea
raphe corpus callosi
raphe palati
raphe penis
raphe pharyngis
rapid absorption of dietary glucose
rapid flow cytometry assay
rapid mucin stain
rapid plasma reagin (RPR) test
rapid serum amylase test
Rapoport differential ureteral
   catheterization test
Rappaport lymphoma classification
Rasmussen aneurysm
ras oncogenes
rash
   butterfly
   lilac
   maculopapular
   malar
   purplish
RAST (radioallergosorbent test)
rate
   erythrocyte sedimentation (ESR)
   glomerular filtration (GFR)
   mitotic
   sed (sedimentation)
   sedimentation
   Westergren sedimentation
rat-bite fever
Rathke pouch
ratio
   A/G (albumin/globulin)
   BUN/creatinine
   cytoplasmic
   cytoplasmic/nuclear
   erythroid/myeloid
   international normalized (INR)

ratio *(continued)*
   inversion of
   inversion of A/G
   lecithin/sphingomyelin (L/S)
   leukocyte/erythrocyte
   M/E (myeloid/erythroid)
   nuclear/cytoplasmic
   prothrombin time
   reversal
   reversal of A/G
   T4/T8
   T_4/TBG (thyroxine/thyroxine-
      binding globulin)
rat-mite dermatitis
RAV (Rous-associated virus)
ray, medullary
Raynaud phenomenon
R band
R-banding stain
R-b band
RBC (red blood cell)
RBC/hpf (red blood cells per
   high-power field)
RB1 tumor suppressor gene
RBP (retinol-binding protein)
RCA (right coronary artery)
RDW (red cell distribution width)
reabsorbed
reabsorption of aqueous humor
reactant
   acute phase
   phase
reaction
   acetowhite
   acid base
   allergic
   antigen-antibody
   Arias-Stella
   Bence Jones
   biochemical
   chromaffin
   colorless

reaction *(continued)*
   diffuse fibrotic
   fibrotic
   focal fibrotic
   foreign body
   Forssman
   glial
   hemolytic
   hypersensitivity
   inflammatory
   insulin
   leukemoid
   nitroprusside
   nodular fibrotic
   polymerase chain (PCR)
   precipitation
   sunburn-like
   transfusion
   urine
   white-graft
reactive airways disease (RAD)
reactive cell
reactive hyperplasia
reactive mesothelial cell
reagent
   ninhydrin
   premeasured
reagin
Rebuck skin window test
recanalization
recanalized area
recanalized occlusion
receptor
   acetylcholine
   adrenergic
   alpha-adrenergic
   aortic
   B cell antigen
   beta-adrenergic
   cholinergic
   epidermal growth factor (EGFR)
   estrogen

receptor *(continued)*
   low-density lipoprotein (LDL)
   progesterone
   T cell antigen (TCR)
receptor protein
recess
   attic
   cecal
   cerebellopontine
   cochlear
   costodiaphragmatic
   costomediastinal
   duodenojejunal
   epitympanic
   hepatorenal
   ileocecal
   inferior duodenal
   intersigmoid
   paraduodenal
   peritoneal
   pleural
   prestyloid
   retrocecal
   retroduodenal
   splenorenal
   subphrenic
   superior duodenal
recessive gene
recess of ischiorectal fossa
recess of pleura, costodiaphragmatic
recipient
   prospective
   transfusion
   universal
recipient cells
recipient serum
reciprocal reception, articulation by
reciprocal transfusion
reciprocal translocation
Recklinghausen, canal of
Recklinghausen disease of bone
reclotting phenomenon

recombinant antihemophilic factor
recombinant DNA
recombinant hemoglobin (rHb1.1)
recombinant human erythropoietin
  (rhEPO)
recombinant tissue plasminogen
  activator (rtPA, rt-PA)
recruitable collaterals
rectal ampulla
rectal artery
rectal fold
  inferior transverse
  superior transverse
rectal mucosa
rectal muscle cuff
rectal nerve
rectal plexus
rectal polyp
rectal pouch
rectal prolapse
rectal shelf
rectal stricture
rectal stump
rectal valve
rectal vault
rectal vein
rectosigmoid carcinoma
rectosigmoid junction
rectouterine fold
rectouterine pouch
rectovaginal fistula
rectovaginal pouch
rectovaginal septum
rectovaginouterine pouch
rectovesical fistula
rectovesical pouch
rectovesical septum
rectum, ampulla of
rectus abdominis muscle
rectus sheath
recurrent abortion
recurrent aphthous stomatitis

recurrent bleeding
recurrent canal
recurrent embolism
recurrent interosseous artery
recurrent intravascular thrombosis
recurrent laryngeal nerve
recurrent radial artery
recurrent ulnar artery
red algae
red atrophy
red blood cell (pl. cells) (RBC, rbc)
  fragility of
  hemolyzed
  nucleated
  packed
  urinary
red blood cell cholinesterase level
red blood cell count
red blood cell fragility
red blood cell indices
red blood cell mass
red blood cell precursor
red blood cells per high-power field
  (RBC/hpf)
"red cell" (slang for red blood cell)
red cell adherence test
"red count" (slang for red blood cell
  count)
red cell clot
red cell distribution width (RDW)
red cell indices
red cell survival, ^{51}Cr
red cell volume
red degeneration of uterine leiomyoma
red hepatization stage of pneumonia
red induration
Redlich-Fisher miliary plaque
red marrow
redness of bone
redness of skin
redox equilibrium
red phenolsulfonphthalein test

red pulp
red pulp of spleen
red test
reduced hemoglobin
reducing substance in stool
reducing sugar
reduction deformity
reduction division
reduplication, chromosomal
  abnormality of
reduplication of a kidney
reduplication of a ureter
redwater fever
Reed cells
Reed-Sternberg cell
Reese-Ellsworth classification of
  retinoblastoma
Rees test for albumin
re-excreted
reference laboratory
reference range
reflected
reflected inguinal ligament
reflected light
reflecting edge of ligament
reflection
  costopleural
  hepatoduodenal-peritoneal
  hepatoduodenoperitoneal
  mediastinodiaphragmatic pleural
  peritoneal
  sternal pleural
  vertebral pleural
reflex
  abdominal
  abdominocardiac
  accommodation
  acquired
  acromial
  adductor
  anal
  arc

reflex *(continued)*
  auricular
  cardiac
  costal arch
  crossed
  deltoid
  depressor
  digital
  dorsum of foot
  dorsum pedis
  elbow
  epigastric
  erector spinal
  esophagosalivary
  external oblique
  eye-closure
  facial
  faucial
  femoral
  finger-thumb
  flexor
  forced grasping
  fundus
  gag
  gastrocolic
  gastroileac
  involuntary
  Moro startle
  nasolabial
  nasomental
  neck
  neck righting
  nociceptive
  nostril
  obliquus
  oculoauricular
  oculocardiac
  oculocephalogyric
  oculopharyngeal
  oculopupillary
  oculosensory
  oculovagal

reflex *(continued)*
    open loop
    Oppenheim
    opticofacial winking
    orbicularis
    orbicularis oculi
    orbicularis pupillary
    orienting
    palatal
    palatine
    palmar
    palm-chin
    palmomental
    paradoxical pupillary
    patellar
    patelloadductor
    pathologic
    pectoral
    penile
    perianal
    periosteal
    peristaltic
    peritoneointestinal
    pharyngeal
    phasic
    Philippson
    pilomotor
    Pilitz
    placing
    plantar
    platysmal
    postural
    pressor
    Preyer
    proprioceptive
    psychic
    psychocardiac
    psychogalvanic
    pulmonocoronary
    pupillary
    Puusepp
    quadriceps

reflex *(continued)*
    quadrupedal extensor
    radial
    rectal
    red
    regional
    Remak
    renointestinal
    renorenal
    retrobulbar pupillary
    reversed pupillary
    Riddoch mass
    righting
    Roger
    rooting
    Rossolimo
    Ruggeri
    Saenger
    scapular
    scapulohumeral
    Schäffer (Schaeffer)
    scratch
    scrotal
    segmental
    senile
    sexual
    shot-silk
    simple
    skin
    skin pupillary
    Snellen
    sole
    somatointestinal
    spinal
    stapedial
    startle
    static
    statotonic
    stepping
    Stookey
    stretch
    Strümpell (Struempell)

reflex *(continued)*
   sucking
   superficial
   supinator longus
   supraorbital
   suprapatellar
   suprapubic
   supraumbilical
   swallowing
   tapetal light
   tarsophalangeal
   tendon
   testicular compression
   threat
   Throckmorton
   tibioadductor
   toe
   tonic neck
   trained
   triceps
   triceps surae
   trigeminus
   ulnar
   unconditioned
   urinary
   vagus
   vascular
   vasopressor
   vertebra prominens
   vesical
   vesicointestinal
   vestibular
   vestibulo-occular
   virile
   visceral
   viscerocardiac
   visceromotor
   viscerosensory
   viscerotrophic
   voluntary
   von Mering
   water-silk

reflex *(continued)*
   Weiss
   Westphal pupillary
   withdrawal
   zygomatic
reflex inguinal ligament
refract
refracted light
refractile
refractile medium
refraction, angle of
refractive index
Regan isoenzyme
Regaud fixative
regeneration
regeneration of damaged tissues
regenerative polyp
region
   abdominal
   anal
   ankle
   axillary
   buccal
   calcaneal
   deltoid
   epigastric
   femoral
   frontal
   gluteal
   hypochondriac
   hypogastric
   inguinal
   lumbar
   paraumbilical
   perianal
   scapular
   suprapubic
   umbilical
   urogenital
regional enteritis
regional ileitis
regional lymph nodes

registry, tumor
regressive staining
regular connective tissue
regulator gene
regulatory peptide
regulatory proteinuria
regurgitant fraction
regurgitation
Rehberg test
Reichert canal
Reichl test for proteins
Reil ansa
Reil band
Reinke crystals
Reinke space
Reinsch test for heavy metals
Reiter complement fixation test
   for syphilis
Reiter syndrome
rejection
   acute cellular renal
   acute renal
   cellular
   chronic
   first-set
   hyperacute
   second-set
   transplant
   vasculitic
relapsing febrile nodular nonsuppurative panniculitis
relapsing fever
relapsing malaria
relative lymphocytosis
relative molecular mass
relaxation factor
relaxin
release of fluid into intercellular tissues
releasing factor (RF)
releasing hormone (RH)
remittent fever
remittent malaria

remnant, gastric
remnant of ductus arteriosus
remnant of processus vaginalis
remodeling process
renal abscess
renal agenesis
renal amino acid diabetes
renal amyloidosis
renal artery
renal artery dilatation
renal atrophy
renal calix (pl. calices)
renal calyces
renal calyx
renal capsule
   fatty
   fibrous
renal cell carcinoma
renal cholesterol embolism
renal column
renal cortex
renal cyst
renal degeneration
renal diabetes
renal disease
renal dwarfism
renal edema
renal excretion of hydrogen ion
renal failure
renal fascia
renal fat
renal function test
renal glycosuria
renal hematuria
renal hilum
renal hilus
renal hypertension
renal impression on liver
renal infarction
renal insufficiency
renal labyrinth
renal medulla

renal nerve
renal obstruction
renal osteitis fibrosa
renal osteodystrophy
renal papilla
renal parenchyma
renal pelvis
renal plasma flow (RPF) test
renal pouch
renal proteinuria
renal pyramids
renal rickets
renal shutdown
renal sinus
renal sodium
renal tuberculosis
renal tubular acidosis
renal tubular degeneration
renal tubular epithelial cast (RTE cast)
renal tubular necrosis
renal tubular osteomalacia
renal tubule
renal vein
renal vessel
Rendu-Osler-Weber disease
reniform pelvis
renin (*not* rennin)
renin hormone
rennin test (not renin)
renovascular hypertension
Renshaw cells
REO (respiratory enteric orphan) virus
reovirus
repair
    cellular
    fracture
    process
    wound
repair in inflammation
repair of fracture
repair or bridging of defects with
    fibrous scar tissue

reparative
replacement bone
replacement fibrosis
replicate
replication
report
    cytologic
    gross
    laboratory
    macroscopic
    pathology
repressor gene
reproducibility
reptilase test for blood clotting time
requisition
resection
    limit of
    line of
    margin of
    transurethral
reserve cell
reservoir, chromatin
residential cell
residual abscess
residual capacity
residual flaccid paralysis
residual stool
resilient
resin
resistance
resistance factor
resistance-inducing factor
resistance-transfer factor
resorbed
resorcinol–hydrochloric acid test for
    fructose
resorption, bone
resorption of calcium
respirator brain
respiratory acidosis
respiratory alkalosis
respiratory apparatus

respiratory area of nose
respiratory arrest
respiratory bronchiole
respiratory capacity
respiratory depression
respiratory distress
respiratory disturbance of acid-base
    balance
respiratory droplets
respiratory epithelium
respiratory failure
respiratory lobule
respiratory metabolism
respiratory nodule
respiratory obstruction
respiratory paralysis
respiratory pigment
respiratory syncytial disease
respiratory syncytial virus (RSV)
respiratory system
respiratory virus
response, desmoplastic
Response GM handheld device
    to test granulocyte count
rest (mass of cells)
resting cell
resting wandering cell
restructured cell
results of fracture
resurrection bone
resuscitation, artifacts of
retained dead fetus
retained placenta
retained products of conception
retained root
rete (pl. retia)
rete mirabile
rete pegs of epidermis
rete ridges
rete testis
retention cyst
retention defect

retention meal
retention of carbon dioxide, pulmonary
retention polyp
reticular cell
reticular colliquation
reticular connective tissue
reticular dermis
reticular fiber
reticular layer
reticulated bone
reticulated tissue
reticulin stain
reticulocyte
reticulocyte count
reticulocytosis
reticuloendothelial cell
reticuloendothelial organ
reticuloendotheliosis
reticulohistiocytic granuloma
reticulohistiocytosis
reticulonodular pattern
reticulosis
reticulum
    agranular
    Chiari
    cistern of endoplasmic
    Ebner
    endoplasmic
    granular endoplasmic
    sarcoplasmic
    stellate
    trabecular endoplasmic
    vesicle of endoplasmic
reticulum cell
reticulum cell sarcoma
retina
    amacrine cells of
    capillary microaneurysms of
    central artery of
    coarctate
    deeply pigmented lesions in
    detached

retina *(continued)*
  leopard
  necrotic lesions in
  pigmentary degeneration of
  shot-silk
  tessellated
  tigroid
  watered-silk
retinaculum, caudal
retinal artery
retinal cone
retinal degeneration
retinal detachment
retinal dysplasia
retinal ganglion cells, degeneration of
retinal pigment
retinal rod
retinal tumor
retinitis pigmentosa
retinitis proliferans
retinoblastoma
retinoblastoma hereditary human
  cancer
retinol-binding protein
retraction clot
retraction, stromal
retroauricular nodes
retrobulbar abscess
retrobulbar optic neuritis
retrocecal abscess
retrocecal appendix
retrocecal recess
retrocolic appendix
retrocostal artery
retroduodenal artery
retroduodenal recess
retroesophageal subclavian artery
retroflexed uterus
retroverted uterus
retrograde degeneration
retrograde metamorphosis
retroileal appendix

retrolental fibroplasia
retromammary mastitis
retromolar gland
retropancreatic tunnel
retroperitoneal cavity
retroperitoneal fibrosis
retroperitoneal organ
retroperitoneal region
retroperitoneal space
retroperitoneum
retropharyngeal abscess
retropubic space
retrorectal lymph node
retrotonsillar abscess
retrovascular goiter
retrovirus
Retzius
  ligament of
  line of
  space of
  system of
  vein of
Retzius space
Reuss test for atropine
Reverdin needle
reversal of A/G ratio
reversal of ratio
reverse triiodothyronine (rT_3) test
Rex-Cantli-Serege line
Reye syndrome
Reynolds test for acetone
Reynold lead citrate
rhabdoid
rhabdomyolysis
rhabdomyoma
rhabdomyosarcoma
rhabdovirus
rhagiocrine cell
Rh (Rhesus)
Rh antibody
Rh antigen
Rh blocking

Rh blood system
Rh blood type
rheumatic atrophy
rheumatic endocarditis
rheumatic fever
rheumatic granuloma
rheumatic myocarditis
rheumatic pericarditis
rheumatic pneumonia
rheumatoid (rheumatology) panel
rheumatoid arthritis
rheumatoid arthritis test
rheumatoid-associated nuclear antigen
  (RANA)
rheumatoid factor (RF)
rheumatoid myositis
rheumatoid nodule
rheumatoid spondylitis
rheumatology panel
Rh factor
Rhinocladiella aquaspersa
rhinoscleroma bacillus
Rhinosporidium seeberi
Rhinovirus, rhinovirus
Rhizoctonia
Rhizoctonia solani
Rhizomucor pusillus
Rhizopus
Rhizopus arrhizus
Rhizopus microsporus
Rhizopus nigricans
Rhizopus rhizopodiformis
Rhizopus stolonifer
Rh negative
Rh negative blood type
rhodopsin
Rhodotorula
Rhodotorula rubra
rhomboid
rhomboid ligament
Rh positive
Rh positive blood type

Rh test
rhubarb test in urine
rhus dermatitis
RIA (radioimmunoassay)
rib
  angle of
  bicipital
  bifid
  cervical
  facet for head of
  false
  first
  floating
  fused
  head of
  inferior margin of superior
  lumbar
  neck of
  notching of
  periosteum of
  shaft of
  superior
  superior margin of inferior
  true
  tubercle of
  typical
  vertebrocostal
  vertebrosternal
ribbon stool
riboflavin test
ribonucleoprotein particle
ribosome
ribovirus
rib shears, Gluck
rib tubercle
rice-water stool
Richter syndrome
rickets, renal
ricketts
Rickettsia
Rickettsia akari
Rickettsia australis

Rickettsia conorii
Rickettsia mooseri
Rickettsia prowazekii
Rickettsia rickettsii
Rickettsia sibirica
Rickettsia tsutsugamushi
Rickettsia typhi
rickettsiae
rickettsial infection
rickettsial myocarditis
rickettsial pneumonia
rickettsialpox
RID (radioimmunodiffusion)
rider's bone
rider's tendon
ridge
   alveolar
   apical ectodermal
   basal
   bicipital
   buccocervical
   buccogingival
   bulbar
   cutaneous
   dental
   epidermal
   epipericardial
   ganglion
   genital
   sagittal
   supraorbital
riding embolism
Riedel lobe
Riedel struma
Rieder cell
Rieder cell leukemia
Riegler test for albumin
Rift Valley fever virus
right atrium
right auricle
right border of heart
right colic artery

right colic (or colonic) flexure
right colon
right coronary artery (RCA)
right crus (pl. crura)
right dominant coronary artery
right gastric artery
right gastroepiploic artery
right gutter
right heart
right hemisphere
right lobe of liver
right lower quadrant (RLQ)
right shift on WBC count
right-sided pneumonia
right triangular ligament
right upper outer quadrant
right upper quadrant (RUQ)
right ventricle of heart
rigid canal
rigidity
   muscle
   nuchal
   postmortem
rigor mortis
rim degeneration
Rimini test
rim of fascia
Rindfleisch cell
ring
   abdominal
   amnion
   anorectal
   benzene
   Cabot
   choroidal
   ciliary
   common tendinous
   conjunctival
   crural
   distal esophageal
   external
   femoral

ring *(continued)*
  fibrinocartilaginous
  fibrous
  Fleischer-Kayser
  ilioinguinal
  iliopsoas
  inguinal
  internal abdominal
  internal inguinal
  intrahaustral contraction
  Kayser-Fleischer
  Ochsner
  pyloric
  Schatzki
  sphincter contraction
  superficial inguinal
  Waldeyer
ring abscess
ringbone, false
ring chromosome
Ringer's solution
ring ligament
ring of esophagus, B
ring precipitin test
ring-shaped cluster
ring test for antibiotic activity
ring test for protein
ring-wall lesion
ringworm (tinea corporis)
ringworm of groin
ringworm of scalp
ringworm of skin
Riolan, arc of
Riolan bone
RISA (radioactive iodinated serum
  albumin) test
risk factor
RIST (radioimmunosorbent test)
Ritter disease
Rivinus canal
Rivinus gland
riziform

RLQ (right lower quadrant)
RNA (ribonucleic acid)
RNA tumor virus
RNA virus (ribovirus)
Rnase
RNAzolB method of RNA extraction
Ro (SS-A) autoantibody
Robert ligament
robertsonian translocation
Roberts test for albumin
Robinson index
Robinson-Kepler test for adrenocortical
  insufficiency
Robson point
Rochalimaea
Rochalimaea henselae
Rochalimaea quintana
Rocio virus
rock-hard plaque
rocking microtome
Rocky Mountain spotted fever
rod
  Auer
  basal
  Corti
  germinal
  gram-negative
  gram-positive
  retinal
rod cell of retina
rod neutrophil
rod nuclear cell
rod-shaped granule
rodent ulcer
Rohon-Beard cell
Rokitansky-Aschoff sinus
Rokitansky pelvis
Rolando cell
Rolando zone
roll of erythrocytes
rolled margin
Romaña sign

Romanovsky blood stain
Ronchese test for ammonia in urine
roof of abdomen
root
    anatomical
    cochlear
    cranial
    dental
    facial
    lingual
    motor
    nerve
    palatine
    retained
    sensory
    spinal
    ventral
root abscess
root canal of tooth
root cell
rooting reflex
root of lung
root of mesentery
root of penis
ropy bile
rose bengal radioactive (^{131}I) test
rose bengal test for liver function
Rose-Bradford kidney
Rosenbach-Gmelin test for bile
    pigment
Rosenmüller fossa
Rosenmüller gland
Rosenthal canal
Rosenthal degeneration
Rosenthal fibers in astrocytomas
Rosenthal test for blood in urine
roseola
roseola infantum
rose spot
rosette formation
rosette-forming cell
rosette, Homer-Wright

rosette test
Rose-Waaler agglutination test
    for rheumatoid factor
Rosin test for indigo red
Ross-Jones test
Ross River fever
Ross River virus
rostrum (pl. rostra)
Rotalex
rotary joint
rotary microtome
rotator cuff tear
rotavirus
rotavirus antigen
rotavirus DNA virus
rotavirus in stool specimen
Rotex cutting biopsy needle
Rothera nitroprusside test for ketone
    bodies
Rothera test for acetone
Roth spot
Rouget bulb
Rouget cell
roughened epithelium
roughening
rough texture
rouleau (pl. rouleaux)
rouleaux formation
round cell
round cell sarcoma
round ligament, artery of
round ligament of elbow joint
round ligament of femur
round ligament of liver
round ligament of uterus
rounded keratin inclusions
roundworm, human intestinal
Roughton-Scholander apparatus
Rous-associated virus (RAV)
Rous sarcoma
Rous sarcoma virus (RSV)
Roussin test

Rous test for hemosiderin
Rous virus
route, collateral
Roux-en-Y jejunal limb
Roux stain
Rowntree and Geraghty test
R plasmid
R protein
RPR (rapid plasma reagin) test
   for syphilis
RSV (respiratory syncytial virus)
RSV (Rous sarcoma virus)
RTE (renal tubular epithelium)
RTE cast
rubbery consistency
rubbery gray mass
rubbery nodule
rubbery texture
rubella
rubella HI (hemagglutination
   inhibition) test
rubella titer
rubella virus
rubeola
rubescent
rubifacient
Rubivirus
Rubner test for carbon monoxide
   in blood
Rubner test for lactose or glucose
   in urine
rubor
rubriblast (red blood cell precursor)
rubricyte
rudimentary bone
ruga (pl. rugae)

rugal pattern
rugate
Ruge solution
Ruhemann test for uric acid in urine
rule of nines
rumble (bowel sounds)
Rumpel-Leede phenomenon
Rumpel-Leede test
Rumpel-Leede tourniquet
Runeberg disease
runner's knee
runny stool
ruptured aneurysm
ruptured appendix
ruptured disk
ruptured fallopian tube
ruptured follicle
ruptured hernia
ruptured intraperitoneal viscus
ruptured membranes
ruptured perineum
ruptured spleen
rupture of congenital aneurysm
rupture, spo ntaneous
RUQ (right upper quadrant)
rushes (bowel sounds), peristaltic
Russell body
Russian autumn encephalitis virus
Russian spring-summer encephalitis
   virus
rust-colored papule
Rust disease
rusty sputum
Ruttan and Hardisty test for blood
Rye histopathologic classification
   of Hodgkin disease

S, s

SA (sinoatrial) node
SA virus (simian virus SV5)
SAA (serum amyloid A) protein
Saathoff test for fat in stools
saber shin
Sabin-Feldman dye test
Sabouraud agar
Sabouraud culture medium
sabra dermatitis
sac
    abdominal
    air
    allantoic
    alveolar
    amniotic
    anal
    aneurysmal
    aortic
    chorionic
    conjunctival
    cupular blind
    dental
    embryonic
    endolymphatic
    fluid-filled
    gestational
    greater peritoneal

sac *(continued)*
    hernial
    lacrimal
    lesser peritoneal
    pericardial
    peritoneal
    thecal
    wide-mouth
saccharimeter test
Saccharomyces cerevisiae
sacciform kidney
saccular aneurysm
saccular gland
sacculated pleurisy
sacculation
sacculocochlear canal
sacculoutricular canal
Sachs bacillus
Sachsse test for glucose in urine
Sachs-Tay disease (also, Tay-Sachs)
Sacks-Libman endocarditis
sacral artery
sacral bone
sacral canal
sacral foramina
sacral meningocele
sacral nerve

sacral parasympathetic outflow
sacral plexus
sacral promontory
sacral vertebra
sacred bone
sacroabdominoperineal
sacrococcygeal joint
sacrococcygeal junction
sacrococcygeal symphysis articulation
sacrococcygeal symphysis joint
sacrodural ligament
sacrogenital fold
sacroiliac articulation
sacroiliac joint
sacroiliac ligament
sacrospinous ligament
sacrotuberous ligament
sacrovertebral angle
sacrum
    alae of
    assimilation
    cornua of
    promontory of
    scimitar
    tilted
sacrum and coccyx articulation
sacrum and coccyx joint
saddle articulation
saddle embolus
saddle joint
safranin
sagittal fontanelle
sagittal limb
sagittal plane
sagittal ridge
sagittal section
sagittal suture
sago-grain stool
Sahli-Nencki test for lipolytic activity
    of pancreas
Sainte-Marie method of alcoholic
    fixation and paraffin embedding

saint (see *St.*)
Saint triad
Sakaguchi test for arginine
Saksenaea vasiformis
Sala cell
salicylate
salicylic acid
salicylic acid test
saline solution
Salinem infection
Salisbury common cold virus
saliva
salivary gland
salivary gland atrophy
salivary gland hormone
salivary gland stone
salivary gland tumor
salivary gland virus
salivary stone
Salkowski and Schipper test for bile
    pigments
Salkowski-Ludwig test for uric acid
Salkowski test
salmon-patch hemorrhage
salmonella food poisoning
salmonella osteomyelitis
Salmonella
Salmonella arizonae
Salmonella choleraesuis
Salmonella enteritidis
Salmonella typhi
salmonellosis
salpingitis
    chronic interstitial
    follicular
    gonococcal
    hemorrhagic
    interstitial
    pseudofollicular
    purulent
    tuberculous
salpingo-oophorectomy

salt (pl. salts)
   bile
   bone
   inorganic
   mercuric
salt-losing defect
salt-losing nephritis
salt plasma
sampling, endometrial
S&A (sugar and acetone)
sandal strap dermatitis
sand, brain
sandfly fever–Naples virus
sandfly fever–Sicilian virus
sandfly fever virus
sandpaper gallbladder
Sandrock test for thrombosis
Sandström gland
sand test for bile and hemoglobin
   in urine
sanguineous fluid
sanguineous infiltration
sanguinopurulent
sanguinoserous
sanguinoseropurulent
sanious pus
San Joaquin Valley fever
Saõ Paulo fever
Santorini canal
Santorini, duct of
Santorini labyrinth
Santorini ligament
SAP (sphingolipid activator protein)
saphenous artery
saphenous opening
saphenous vein
saponification
Sappey ligament
Sarastro-2000 confocal scanning
   microscope
sarcofetal pregnancy
sarcogenic cell

sarcohysteric pregnancy
sarcoid, Boeck
sarcoidosis, hepatic
sarcolemma
sarcoplasmic reticulum
sarcoma
   Abernethy
   alveolar soft part
   ameloblastic
   angiolithic
   botryoid
   endometrial stromal
   Ewing
   fascicular
   giant cell
   giant cell monstrocellular
   granulocytic
   immunoblastic
   Jensen
   juxtacortical osteogenic
   Kaposi
   leukocytic
   lymphatic
   medullary
   mixed cell
   multiple idiopathic hemorrhagic
   myelogenic
   myeloid
   neurogenic
   osteogenic
   periosteal
   reticulum cell
   round cell
   Rous
   spindle cell
   synovial
   telangiectatic osteogenic
sarcomere
sarcophagic syndrome
sarcoplasm
sarcoplasmic matrix
sarcoplasmic reticulum

Sarcoptes scabiei
satellite abscess
satellite cell of skeletal muscle
satellite, chromosome
satellite lesion
satellite metastasis
satellite phenomenon
satellite structure
satellite virus
satellitism
satellitosis
saturated solution
saturation index (SI) of bile
saturation recovery technique
saturnine nephritis
saucerize
saucer-like crusts of favus
Saundby test for blood in stool
sausage finger
sawtooth configuration
saw-toothed acanthosis
saw-toothed gland
scabbard trachea
scab of exudate
scabies
scalded skin syndrome
scale (pl. scales)
    absolute
    absolute temperature
    Baumé
    Bloch
    Celsius
    centigrade
    coma
    extensive shedding of
    Fahrenheit
    French
    gray
    hardness
    interval
    Karnofsky
    Kelvin

scale *(continued)*
    pH
    Rankine
    Sörensen
    temperature
    Zubrod
scale formation
scalelike cell
scalene tubercle, prominent
scalenus anterior
scalenus anterior muscle
scalenus medius
scalenus minimus
scaling
    dry
    greasy
    moist
scalloped
scalp hair
scalp infection
scalp, occipital
scaly dermatosis
scaly erythematous dermatitis
scaly erythematous patches of face
scaly erythematous patches of scalp
scanning power
scant cellularity
scant discharge
scanty cytoplasm
scaphoid abdomen
scaphoid bone
scaphoid facet
scaphoid fossa
scaphoid waist
scapholunate joint
scapholunate ligament
scaphotrapezoid trapezial (STT) joint
scapula (pl. scapulae)
scapula bone
scapular artery
scapular circumflex artery
scapular region

scapuloclavicular articulation
scapuloclavicular joint
scapulohumeral
scar
  astroglial
  excised
  flank
  keloid
  postnecrotic
  surgical
  traumatic
scar formation
scarification test
scarified duodenum
scarlatina
scarlatinal nephritis
scarlet fever
scarlet red
Scarpa
  canal of
  fascia of
  ligament of
Scarpa fascia
Scarpa triangle
scarring
  hypertrophic
  keloid
  peritoneal
  postnecrotic
scarring alopecia
scarring of cornea
scarring of uterine tube
scar tissue
scar tissue reaction
SCAT (sheep cell agglutination test)
scavenger cell
Scedosporium apiospermum
S cell
SCFA (short chain fatty acid)
Schäffer-Fulton stain (Schaeffer)
Schäffer test for nitrites in urine
Schalfijew test

Schällibaum solution
Schamberg dermatitis
Scharlach R
Schatzki ring
Schaudinn fixative
Schaumann body
Scherer test
Scheuermann disease
Schick test
Schiff reagent
Schiff solution
Schilder disease
Schiller test for cervical cancer
Schilling band cell
Schilling monocytic leukemia
Schilling test
schindylesis (wedge-and-groove joint)
  articulation
schindylesis articulation
schindylesis joint
schistocyte (keratocyte)
Schistosoma
Schistosoma haematobium
Schistosoma japonicum
Schistosoma mansoni
schistosome dermatitis
schistosomiasis, cutaneous
Schivoletto test for hydrochloric acid
  in urine
Schlatter-Osgood disease
Schlemm canal
Schlemm ligaments
Schlesinger test for urobilin
Schlichter test
Schmitz bacillus
Schmorl bacillus
Schmorl ferric-ferricyanide reduction
  stain
Schmorl node
Schmorl nodule
Schmorl picrothionin stain
Schönbein test for blood

Schönberg-Albers disease
 (also, Schoenberg)
Schönlein-Henoch purpura (Schoenlein)
Schramm phenomenon
Schroeder test for urea
Schüffner dots (Schueffner)
Schüller (Schueller)
Schüller-Christian-Hand disease
Schüller gland
Schulte test for proteins
Schultze cell
Schultze placenta
Schultze test
Schultz stain
Schumm test
Schwalbe space
Schwann cell
Schwann, sheath
schwannoma, vestibular
sciatic artery
sciatic foramen (pl. foramina)
 greater
 lesser
sciatic nerve, companion artery of
sciatic neuritis
sciatic notch
 greater
 lesser
scirrhous carcinoma of breast
scirrhous lesion
scirrhous tumor
SCLC (small cell lung carcinoma)
sclera (pl. sclerae)
scleral canal
sclerenchyma cell
sclerocorneal junction
sclerodactyly
scleroderma antibody
scleromyxedema
sclerosing hemangioma
sclerosing hepatic carcinoma (SHC)
sclerosing inflammation

sclerosing myeloma
sclerosing nonsuppurative osteomyelitis
sclerosing osteitis
sclerosis
 amyotrophic lateral
 combined
 focal glomerular
 gastric
 Mönckeberg
 multiple
 posterolateral
 progressive systemic
 tuberous
 valvular
sclerosis of brain
sclerosis of pubic bones
sclerotic bone
sclerotic degeneration
sclerotic kidney
sclerotic vein
scoliotic pelvis
Scopulariopsis brevicaulis
score, Gleason
Scotch tape technique
Scott solution
scraping
 conjunctival
 fungal
 skin
 surgical
 vesical
scratch test
screen
 fluorescent
 Glucola
 Monospot
 strep
 TORCH
 toxicology
screening test
screening, toxicology
screw joint

scroll bones
scrotal artery
scrotal raphe
scrotal swelling
scrotal vein
scrotum, lymphatics of
scrub typhus
scurvy
scutulum (pl. scutula)
scutum
scybalous stools
SDS (sodium dodecyl sulfate)
Se (selenium)
seabather's eruption
sea-blue histiocyte
seal-fin deformity
seatworm
sebaceous cyst
sebaceous gland
sebaceous nevus
seborrhea
seborrhea corporis
seborrheic dermatitis
seborrheic eczema
seborrheic keratosis
sebum
sec (second)
second (sec)
secondary aldosteronism
secondary amyloidosis
secondary anemia
secondary biliary cirrhosis
secondary cartilaginous joint
secondary center of ossification
secondary degeneration
secondary diabetes
secondary disease
secondary hypertension
secondary infection
secondary metabolism
secondary methemoglobinemia
secondary myeloid metaplasia

secondary pleurisy
secondary pneumonia
second-look laparotomy
second-set phenomenon
secretin test
secretion
   cytocrine
   gastric acid
   nasal
   nasopharyngeal
   serous
   thin
   vaginal
   watery
secretor
secretor factor
secretory cell
secretory endometrium
secretory epithelium
secretory granule
secretory phase
secretory stage
section
   abdominal
   celloidin
   cesarean
   coronal
   cross-
   cryostat
   deep
   fresh frozen
   frontal
   frozen
   longitudinal
   paraffin
   perineal
   permanent
   Pitres
   plastic
   representative
   Saemisch
   sagittal

section *(continued)*
  semithin
  serial
  serosal
  serous fluid
  serpiginous
  step
  transverse
  ultrathin
sectioning a block of tissue
sectioning of tissue specimen
secundipara (para 2)
"sed rate" (slang for erythrocyte
  sedimentation rate)
sediment
  amorphous
  urinary
sedimentation rate ("sed rate")
seeding, peritoneal
Seessel pouch (2 e's, 2 s's)
"seg" (slang for segmented neutrophil)
segment
  apical
  apicoposterior
  bronchopulmonary
  cardiac
  liver
  pulmonary
  vaterian
segmental artery
segmental bronchi
segmental colonic resection
segmental demyelination
segmental necrotizing glomerulonephritis
segmental neuritis
segmental neuropathy (demyelination)
segmental pneumonia
segmental resection
segmental zone
segmented cell
segmented neutrophil ("seg")

"segmenter" (slang for segmented
  neutrophil)
segregation analysis
SeHCAT (selenium-labeled
  homocholic acid conjugated
  with taurine) test
Seidel test for inositol
seizure
Seldinger needle
selective stain
selenium (Se)
self-limited inflammatory response
Selivanoff test
sella turcica
Seller stain
semen
semen analysis (sperm count)
semicircular canal
semiformed stool
semilunar bone
semilunar fold
semilunar ganglion artery
semilunar lobule
semilunar-shaped fold
semilunar valve, aortic
seminal cell
seminal colliculus
seminal fluid
seminal gland
seminal plasma
seminal vesicle
seminiferous tubule
seminoma
semiquantitative test
semisolid material
semisolid sebaceous debris
semisolid stool
semisynthetic
semithin section
Semliki Forest virus
Semunya virus
Sendai virus

Senear-Usher disease
senile arteriosclerosis
senile atrophy
senile cataract
senile degeneration
senile hemangioma
senile keratosis
senile lentigo
senile myocarditis
senile myocardium
senile nephrosclerosis
senile osteomalacia
senile osteoporosis
senile plaque
senile pruritus
senile vaginitis
senilis
    arcus
    circus
senna test in urine sensitivity
sensitivity index
sensitivity of laboratory test
sensitized cell
sensory cell
sensory fiber
sensory ganglion
sensory root
sentinel cell
sentinel fold
sentinel gland
sentinel loop
sentinel lymph node
sentinel pile
Seoul virus
separator tube
Sephadex
sepsis
    catheter
    gram-negative
    incarcerated
    intestinal
    intra-abdominal (IAS)

sepsis *(continued)*
    oral
    puerperal
sepsis syndrome
septa (pl. of septum)
septal artery of nose
septal bone
septal cartilage
septal cell
septal cirrhosis, diffuse
septal cusp
septal defect
septal mucosa
septal panniculitis
septal papillary muscle
septal tissue
septal wall
septate uterus
septic abortion
septic arthritis
septic embolism
septic embolus
septicemia
    meningococcal
    viral
septicemic abscess
septicemic plague
septic fever
septic infarct
septic myocarditis
septic necrosis
septic pneumonia
septic pulmonary embolism
septic shock
septic splenitis
septic wound
septomarginal band
septomarginal trabecular
septicopyemia
    cryptogenic
    metastatic
    spontaneous

septum (pl. septa)
  alveolar
  anal intermuscular
  aortic
  aortopulmonary
  bulbar
  cartilaginous
  crural
  distal bulbar
  femoral
  fibroelastic
  gingival
  interatrial
  interventricular
  nasal
  rectovaginal
  rectovesical
septum pellucidum (translucent)
septum secundum
sequela (pl. sequelae)
sequence analysis
Sequential Multiple Analyzer (SMA)
Sequential Multiple Analyzer plus
  Computer (SMAC)
sequestered disk
sequestrum
Sereny test to determine invasiveness
  of bacteria
serial cardiac isoenzymes
serial CK enzyme study (also, CPK)
serial dilutions
serial hemoglobin
serially sectioned
serial sections
seroculture
serocystic
serofibrinous inflammation
serofibrinous pleurisy
serologic cross-reactivity
serologic markers for hepatitis
serologic test(ing)
serologic test for syphilis (STS)

serologic titer
"serology" (slang for serologic test for
  syphilis or lues)
seromucous cell
seromucous gland
seromuscular layer
seronegative
seroplastic inflammation
seropositive
serosa (serous membrane)
serosal cyst
serosal puckering
serosal section
serosal surface
serosanguineous discharge
serosanguineous fluid
serosanguinopurulent
serotonin test
serotype
serous adenocarcinoma
serous atrophy
serous cell
serous cystadenocarcinoma
serous cystadenoma
serous cystoma
serous effusion
serous exudate
serous fluid
serous gland of tongue
serous infiltration
serous inflammation
serous ligament
serous membrane (serosa)
serous meningitis
serous otitis
serous pericardium
serous pleurisy
serous proteinuria
serous secretion
serous synovitis
serovar
serpentine aneurysm

serpentine appendix
serpiginous ulceration
serrate bone
Serratia
Serratia liquefaciens
Serratia marcescens
Serratia rubidaea
serratus anterior muscle
serratus posterior inferior muscle
serratus posterior superior muscle
Serres gland
Sertoli cell
serum
   acidified
   acute
   aged normal
   antivenomous
   convalescent
   donor
   Löffler
serum albumin
serum alkaline phosphatase
serum amylase
serum amylase level
serum bactericidal activity test
serum bilirubin
serum chloride
serum cholesterol
serum electrolytes
serum gamma-glutamyl transpeptidase
   (SGGT)
serum glutamic-oxaloacetic
   transaminase (SGOT) (now AST)
serum glutamic-pyruvate transaminase
   (SGPT) (now ALT)
serum hemoglobin
serum hepatitis
serum hepatitis (SH) antigen
serum leucine aminopeptidase (SLAP)
serum lipase
serum marker
serum neuritis

serum neutralization test
serum osmolality
serum prolactin
serum protein
serum protein electrophoresis
serum recipient
serum sickness
sesamoid bone
sessile hydatid
sessile papule
sessile polyp
seton wound
set point
sex cell
sex chromatin analysis
sex chromatin mass
sex factor
sex hormone
sex-linked recessive trait
sexual development, precocious
sexual gland
sexually transmitted disease (STD)
Seyderhelm solution
Sézary cell
SFHb (pyridoxilated stroma-free
   hemoglobin)
Sgambati reaction test
SGGT (serum gamma-glutamyl
   transpeptidase)
SGOT (serum glutamic-oxaloacetic
   transaminase) (now AST)
SGPT (serum glutamic-pyruvate
   transaminase) (now ALT)
shadow cell
shaft
shaft of rib
shaggy aorta
shaggy pericardium
shake test
shallow funnel
shallow mucosal ulcers
shank bone (tibia)

shape
  boat
  oval
  sickle
  spherical
shaped spindle
sharp, intermittent pain
Sharpey fiber
shave biopsy
SHb (sulfhemoglobin)
SHC (sclerosing hepatic carcinoma)
sheath
  carotid
  caudal
  common synovial flexor
  crural
  dentinal
  dural
  extensor carpi ulnaris
  fascial
  femoral
  fenestrated
  fibrous
  myelin
  nerve
  pilar
  rectus
  Schwann
  tendon
sheathing canal
sheath ligament
sheath of artery
Sheehan syndrome
sheep cell agglutination test (SCAT)
sheep red blood cells (sRBC)
sheet, areolar
sheetlike connection
sheetlike tendon
shelf
  buccal
  dental
  mesocolic

shelf *(continued)*
  palatine
  rectal
shellfish, contaminated
shell vial
shelving edge of Poupart ligament
S, hemoglobin (*not* S hemoglobin)
shield, embryonic
shift to the left on WBC count
shift to the right on WBC count
shifting dullness
Shiga bacillus
Shiga-Kruse bacillus
Shigella
Shigella boydii
Shigella dysenteriae
Shigella flexneri
Shigella sonnei
shin bone
shingles (herpes zoster)
shirt-stud abscess
shock
  anaphylactic
  electrical
  hemorrhagic
  hypovolemic
  septic
shock absorption
shock kidney
shock syndrome, toxic
Shorr trichrome
short bone
short chain fatty acid (SCFA)
short ciliary artery
short gastric artery
short palpebral fissures
short root
short stature
shortening lifespan
shortening of muscle
shot-silk retina
shotty lymph node

shoulder articulation
shoulder bone
shoulder joint
shoulder-girdle neuritis
shoulder muscles
"shower" of emboli
shrinkage and cavitation of basal
    ganglia
shrinkage of cells
shriveled or pitted surface
shrunken eye
shuleri articulation
shuleri joint
shunt, AV (arteriovenous)
SI (saturation index) of bile
Sia test for macroglobulinemia
sialic acid, lipid-associated (LASA)
sialolithiasis
sialorrhea
sialosyl-Tn
"sibilous" (see *scybalous stool*)
Sibson groove
Sicard-Cantelouble test
sicca, keratoconjunctivitis
sickle cell
sickle cell anemia
sickle cell disease
sickle cell hemoglobin
sickle cell preparation
sickle cell test
sickle cell trait
Sickledex test for hemoglobin S
Sicklequik rapid screening test
sickle shape
sickle-shaped erythrocytes
sickling
sickling test
sickness
    African sleeping
    serum
sideroblast
sideroblastic anemia

siderocyte
siderophage
siderophilin
sidewall, pelvic
SIDS (sudden infant death syndrome)
Siebold and Bradbury test for salicylic
    acid in urine
sieve bone
SIF, SRIF (somatotropin releasing-
    inhibiting factor)
sigma factor
sigmoid artery
sigmoid colon
sigmoid curve
sigmoid flexure
sigmoid fold
sigmoid kidney
sigmoid mesocolon
sigmoid notch of radius
sigmoidovesical fistula
sigmoid sinus
Sigmund gland
sign
    fronding
    Nikolsky
    Romana
    Winterbottom
signet-ring cell
signet-ring cell carcinoma
signet ring pattern
SIH (somatotropin release-inhibiting
    hormone)
silane-coated slide
Silastic band
silent gallstone
silhouette, cardiovascular
siliceous earth
silicosis
silicotic granuloma
silk suture
silo filler disease
silver (Ag)

silver cell
silver-fork deformity
silver nitrate
silver protein stain
silver stool
silver test for glucose in urine
Silverman needle
Simbu virus
simian immunodeficiency virus (SIV)
simian virus 40 (SV40)
simian virus SV5
Simmonds disease
Simonart band
Simonart ligament
Simplate
simple articulation
simple atrophy
simple columnar epithelium
simple cuboidal epithelium
simple epithelium
simple gland
simple goiter
simple inflammation
simple joint
simple obesity
simple protein
simple squamous epithelium
simplex, herpes
Simplexvirus
Sims test
Sindbis virus
singer's nodule
Singh-Vaughn-Williams arrhythmia
    classification
single-breath diffusing capacity of lung
    ($DLCO_{SB}$)
single human leukocyte antigen
single phase
single pleurisy
single ventricle
sinilis arch
sinoatrial node

sinus
    anal
    aortic
    Aschoff-Rokitansky
    barber's pilonidal
    basilar
    carotid
    cervical
    circular
    coccygeal
    coronary
    costomediastinal
    cranial
    dermal
    dural
    ethmoidal
    frontal
    Guérin
    lymph node
    marginal
    medullary
    oblique pericardial
    paranasal
    pilonidal
    piriform
    prostatic
    pyriform (piriform)
    renal
    Rokitansky-Aschoff
    sphenoidal
    thin-walled venous
    thrombosis of a venous
    transverse pericardial
    valve of coronary
    venous
sinus histiocytosis
sinus hyperplasia
sinus of epididymis
sinusitis
sinusoid
    hepatic
    pituitary

sinusoidal capillary
sinusoidal lymphocyte
SISI (small increment sensitivity index)
Sister Joseph nodule
sitosterolemia
situ, in
situs inversus viscerum
situs perversus
situs solitus
situs transversus
SIV (simian immunodeficiency virus)
Siwe-Letterer disease
6-phosphatase-glucose
6-phosphate dehydrogenase-glucose
65-2A6 monoclonal antibody
Sjögren antibody
Sjögren syndrome
skein cell
skeletal abnormalities
skeletal defects
skeletal deformity
skeletal muscle
skeletal muscle fiber
skeletal muscle, striated
skeletomuscular system
skeleton
 appendicular
 articulated
 axial
 cardiac
 fibrous
 gill arch
 visceral
Skene glands
skin
 abnormal whiteness of
 absence of pigment from
 biopsy of
 color and consistency of
 deciduous

skin *(continued)*
 elastic
 keratinized
 microabscess of
 perianal
 premature wrinkling of
 purplish discoloration of
 redness of
 ringworm of
 stretchability of
 thin
 yellow discoloration of
skin crease
skin laceration
skin lesion
Skinny needle
skin pigment, reduced
skin puncture test for Behçet syndrome
skin slip
skin tag
skin test
skin window test
skull bone
skullcap
skull-type joint
slant, agar
SLAP (serum leucine aminopeptidase)
"slapped cheek" erythema
SLE (systemic lupus erythematosus)
slender body habitus
slender elongated cell
slide
 gelatin-chrome
 organosilane-coated glass
 preparation of
 silane-coated
 Superfrost/Plus Fisherbrand glass
 urine dip
slide clumping factor test
slide coagulase test
slide test
sliding microtome

slime fungus
sling muscle fibers
sling, volar ulnar
slipped intervertebral disk
slipped tendon
slit-scan measurement
slough
sloughing
slow virus
sludge
  bile
  biliary
  blood
  gallbladder
sludged blood
slurry of stool
SMA (smooth muscle antibody)
SMA (Sequential Multiple Analyzer)
SMAC ("smack") (Sequential Multiple
  Anayzer plus Computer) analyzer
SMA-6 chemistry panel*
  BUN
  chloride
  creatinine
  glucose
  potassium
  sodium
SMA-12 chemistry panel*
  bilirubin
  BUN
  calcium
  chloride
  cholesterol
  creatinine
  glucose
  phosphorus
  potassium
  sodium
  total protein
  uric acid

*The tests included may vary from lab to
 lab. The tests listed here are an example.

SMA-20 chemistry panel*
  albumin
  alkaline phosphatase
  ALT
  AST
  bilirubin
  BUN
  calcium
  chloride
  cholesterol
  creatinine
  direct bilirubin
  glucose
  iron
  LDH
  phosphorus
  potassium
  sodium
  total protein
  triglycerides
  uric acid
small B-cell lymphoma
small bowel
small canal of chorda tympani
small cardiac vein
small cell carcinoma
small cell lung carcinoma (SCLC)
small cell osteosarcoma
small cleaved cell
small cleaved cell lymphoma
small eye muscle
small granule cell
small gut
small increment sensitivity index (SISI)
small intestine
small intestine gland
small lymphocytic lymphoma
small noncleaved cell lymphoma
smallpox (variola)
smallpox-like disease
small round cell carcinoma
small round cell infiltrate

Sm antigen
SMAP (systemic mean arterial
    pressure)
smear (see also *stain, test*)
    AFB (acid-fast bacillus)
    air-dried
    alimentary tract
    bacteriologic
    blood
    bronchoscopic
    buccal
    buffy coat
    cervical
    cul-de-sac
    cytologic
    endocervical
    endometrial
    eosinophil
    fast
    feces
    FGT (female genital tract) cytologic
    fungal
    lateral vaginal wall
    lower respiratory tract
    malaria
    nasal
    oral
    pancervical
    PAP (Papanicolaou)
    peripheral
    peripheral blood
    pus
    sputum
    stool
    Tzanck
    urine
    vaginal
    VCE (vagina, ectocervix,
        endocervix)
    wet
smear immersed in fixative
smear sprayed with fixative

smear test
smegma bacillus
Smith test for bile pigments
smoker's lung
smoker's palate
smooth muscle
smooth-muscle antibody (SMA)
smooth-muscle hypertrophy
smooth texture
smudge cell
snake venom poisoning
snakelike
snap-frozen
SNOMED (Standard Nomenclature of
    Medicine)
Snook reticulum stain
snuff box, anatomical
soaplike material
socket
socket joint
SOD (superoxide dismutase)
sodium
sodium bicarbonate
sodium bisulfite
sodium chromate ^{51}Cr sterile solution
sodium dodecyl sulfate (SDS)
sodium hydroxide
sodium test
sodium thiosulfate
sodoku (spirillary rat-bite fever)
Soemmering crystalline
Soemmering ligament
softening of bone
soft palate
soft papilloma
soft spot, capitate
soft stool
soft tissue
solar cheilitis
solar degenerative change
solar dermatitis
solar elastosis

solar irradiation
solar keratosis
solar lentigo
solar plexus
Soldaini test for glucose in urine
Solera test for thiocyanates
solid matrix
solid ovarian teratoma
solid-phase extraction tube
solid teratoma
solid tissue specimen
solitary bone cyst
solitary cells of Meynert
solitary glands of large intestine
solitary glands of small intestine
solitary lesion
solitary lymph node
solitary myeloma
solitary nodule
solubility screening test for sickle cell
   hemoglobin
solution (see also *fixative*, *stain*)
   acid alcohol
   alcoholic
   anticoagulant heparin
   aqueous
   astringent
   Bouin
   buffered
   Burow
   DAKO target retrieval
   Depex mounting
   Drabkin
   Flemming
   formalin
   formol-Zenker
   Gilson
   Gowers
   half-normal
   Hamdi
   Ham F-10
   Hayem

solution *(continued)*
   heparin lock flush
   Hollande
   iodine topical
   lactated Ringer
   Lugol
   mordant
   normal
   Orth
   pyridoxilated stroma-free
      hemoglobin
   Ringer
   Ruge
   saline
   saturated
   Schällibaum
   Seyderhelm
   sodium chromate ^{51}Cr sterile
   stroma-free hemoglobin
   TAC (tetracaine, epinephrine,
      and cocaine)
   Toison
   Zamboni
   Zenker fixative
somatic artery
somatic cell
somatic death
somatic nerve
somatic tissue
somatomedin-C polypeptide hormone
somatostatin cell
somatotropic hormone (STH)
somatotropin release-inhibiting
   hormone (SIH)
somatotropin-releasing factor (SRF)
somatotropin-releasing hormone (SRH)
somatotropin releasing–inhibiting factor
   (SRIF, SIF)
Somogyi effect
Somogyi phenomenon
Sondermann canal
S100 protein

sonicator
Sonne-Duval bacillus
Sonnenschein test
sorbent
Sörensen scale
sore, Oriental
sorehead (filarial dermatosis)
Soret band
sorter, fluorescence-activated cell
  (FACS)
SOS gene
sounds, bowel
South American blastomycosis
Southern blot (SB) analysis
Southern blot test
Southern blotting
soy bean test for urease
sp. (species)
space
  alveolar dead
  anatomical dead
  antecubital
  apical
  axillary
  Baros
  Berger
  Bogros
  Böttcher
  Bowman
  Burns
  capsular
  cartilage
  Chassaignac
  Cloquet
  Colles
  corneal
  Cotunnius
  dead
  Disse
  epidural
  episcleral
  epitympanic

space *(continued)*
  filtration
  Fontana
  gingival
  Henke
  His
  intercellular
  intercostal
  Kiernan
  Kretschmann
  Kuhnt
  Lesgaft
  Magendie
  Malacarne
  Meckel
  Mohrenheim
  Nuel
  Parona
  perineal
  perisinusoidal
  peritoneal
  plane of fifth intercostal
  Poiseuille
  potential
  preperitoneal
  presacral
  Proust
  Prussak
  Reinke
  retroperitoneal
  retropubic
  Retzius
  Schwalbe
  subperitoneal
  suprahepatic
  supralevator
  Tarin
  Tenon
  tissue
  Traube semilunar
  Trautmann triangular
  vesicovaginal

space *(continued)*
   Virchow-Robin
   Waldeyer
   Westberg
   zonular
space of Mall, periportal
space of Poirier
space of Retzius
spade finger
spaghetti-like tangles of basophilic
   connective tissue fibers
spastic
spasticity
spasticity and rigidity, muscular
spatula, Ayre
specialized cell
species (sp.)
specific gravity, decreased in:
   diabetes insipidus
   ingestion or infusion of fluid
   renal failure
specific gravity, increased in:
   acute glomerulonephritis
   congestive heart failure
   dehydration
   diabetes mellitus with glycosuria
   toxemia
specific gravity test
specific gravity, urinary
specific inflammation
specificity of laboratory tests
specimen
   autopsy
   biopsy
   blood
   catheterized
   clean-catch urine
   clean-voided urine
   dimensions of
   fingerstick
   first-voided urine
   gross description

specimen *(continued)*
   histologic
   identification
   laboratory
   midstream urine
   processing of tissue
   sectioning of tissue
   solid tissue
   stool
   surgical
   tissue
   24-hour urine
speck finger
speckled appearance
speckled fluorescence
speckled pattern
speckling with fine dots
spectrophotometric test
spectrophotometry
S peptide
sperm
   donor
   frozen
   motile
   washed
sperm penetration assay
sperm allergy
sperm antibody
sperm motility study
sperm washing
spermatic abscess
spermatic artery
spermatic cord
spermatid
spermatogenesis
spermatogenic cell
spermatogenic granulomatous orchitis
spermatozoa
sperm cell
S-phase fraction
sphenoethmoidal recess
sphenoid biopsy

sphenoid bone
sphenoid cell
sphenoid fontanelle
sphenoid mucosa
sphenoidal ridge
sphenoidal roof of nasal cavity
sphenoidal sinus
sphenoidal turbinated bone
sphenomandibular ligament
spheno-occipital joint
sphenopalatine artery
sphenopalatine canal
sphenopalatine foramen
sphenopalatine ganglia
sphenopalatine vein
sphenopharyngeal canal
sphenoturbinal bone
spherical shape
spherocytosis, hereditary
spheroid or spheroidal (ball-and-socket)
spheroid articulation
spheroid joint
spheroplast
Spiegler test
Spielmeyer swelling
sphincter
    antral
    basal
    bicanalicular
    Boyden
    canalicular
    choledochal
    colic
    cricopharyngeal
    duodenal
    duodenojejunal
    external anal
    extrinsic
    first duodenal
    hypertensive lower esophageal
    Hyrtl
    inferior esophageal

sphincter *(continued)*
    lower esophageal (LES)
    Lutkens
    Nélaton
    O'Beirne
    pancreatic duct
    pancreaticobiliary
    pharyngoesophageal
    prepyloric
    pyloric
    upper esophageal (UES)
sphincter contraction ring
sphincter of anal canal, involuntary
sphincter of bile duct
sphincter of hepatopancreatic ampulla
sphincter of Oddi
sphincter urethral muscle
sphincteric mechanism
sphingolipid activator protein (SAP)
sphingomyelin
sphingomyelin accumulation in liver
    and spleen
sphingomyelinase deficiency
sphingomyelin in marrow histiocytes,
    accumulation of
spiculated
spicule
spider angioma (pl. angiomata)
spider cell
spider hemangioma
spider nevus (pl. nevi)
spider-web clot
Spiegler test for albumin
spillage of tumor cells
spina bifida cystica
spina bifida occulta
spinach stool
spinal artery of Adamkiewicz
spinal canal
spinal cord
spinal cord tissue
spinal defect

spinal degeneration
spinal fluid
   bloody
   cloudy
   frankly purulent
   glucose level of
   milky
   protein in
   total protein concentration of
spinal ganglion
spinal marrow
spinal meninges
spinal meningitis
spinal meningocele
spinal muscular atrophy
spinal nerve
spinal neuron
spinal part of accessory nerve
spinal roots
   C1-7 (cervical)
   Co. 1 (coccygeal)
   L1-5 (lumbar)
   S1-5 (sacral)
   T1-12 (thoracic)
spinal stenosis
spinal tap
spindle
   aortic
   cleavage
spindle cell
spindle cell nevus
spindle cell sarcoma
spindle colonic groove
spindle-shaped cell
spindle-shaped fibroblasts replacing
   osteoblasts
spindle-shaped incision
spindle-shaped structure
spine
   alar
   anterior superior iliac
   anteroposterior iliac

spine *(continued)*
   cervical (C)
   dorsal (D)
   iliac
   ischial
   lumbar (L)
   lumbosacral (LS)
   posterior column of
   posterior-inferior
   sacral (S)
   thoracic (T)
   thoracolumbar
spine cell
spinelike projection
spinnbarkeit
spinoglenoid ligament
spinothalamic tract
spinous processes, vertebral
spiral artery
spiral band of Gosset
spiral canal of cochlea
spiral canal of modiolus
spiral fashion
spiral fold
spiral fracture
spiral joint
spiral ligament of cochlea
spirals, Curschmann
spiral-shaped bacteria
spiral wound
spirillary rat-bite fever
Spirillum
Spirillum minus
spirochetal myocarditis
spirochete
spironolactone test
Spiro test
Spitz nerve
splanchnic artery
splanchnic nerve
splanchnomegaly
splatter

spleen
  accessory
  deep purple
  floating
  function
  inflammation
  long axis of
  red pulp of
  soft
  white pulp of
spleen tip
splenic abscess
splenic artery
splenic atrophy
splenic capsule
splenic cell
splenic congestion
splenic engorgement
splenic flexure
splenic hilum
splenic hyperplasia
splenic hypertrophy
splenic notch
splenic parenchyma
splenic pulp
  red
  white
splenic-renal angle
splenic tissue
splenic vein
splenic vessel
splenitis, acute septic
splenium
splenocolic ligament
splenogastric omentum
splenoid gland
splenomegaly
splenoportal hypertension
splenorenal anastomosis
splenorenal angle
splenorenal ligament
splenorenal recess

splint bone
split brain
split-brain syndrome
split gene
split-renal function test
splitting bone
spoke bone
Spondweni virus
spondylitis
  ankylosing
  rheumatoid
  tuberculous
spondylolisthesis
spondylolisthetic pelvis
sponge kidney
spongiform degeneration of gray
  matter
spongiform encephalopathy
spongiform leukodystrophy
spongiform pustule
spongioblast
spongiosis
spongiosum penis, corpus
spongy bone
spongy degeneration of central nervous
  system
spongy degeneration of white matter
spongy urethra
spontaneous abortion
spontaneous bacterial myositis
spontaneous rupture
spore stain
Sporothrix schenckii
sporotrichosis
Sporotrichum schenckii
spot
  blue
  café au lait
  capitate soft
  coffee-colored
  cotton-wool
  germinal

spot *(continued)*
  Koplik
  red
  rose
  soft
  violet
  white
spot test for infectious mononucleosis
spout, ileal
Sprengel deformity
spring ligament
S protein (*not* protein S)
sprue
spur, calcaneal
spur cell (acanthocyte)
spur-cell anemia
spurious meningocele
spurious pregnancy
Spurr medium
Sputasol
sputum (pl. sputa)
  albumoid
  blood-tinged
  bloody
  gelatinous
  globular
  grayish
  green
  icteric
  moss-agate
  mottled
  nummular
  opalescent
  prune-juice
  reddish brown
  rusty
  yellow
sputum aeroginosum
sputum cruentum
sputum in rounded disks
SQ (subcutaneous)
squama alveolaris

squamate
squamocellular
squamocolumnar junction
squamocolumnar mucosal junction
squamo-occipital bone
squamous alveolar cell
squamous bone
squamous cell
squamous cell carcinoma
squamous cell carcinoma of cervix
squamous cell carcinoma of digestive
  tract
squamous cell carcinoma of lung
squamous cell carcinoma of penis
squamous cell carcinoma of skin
squamous cell carcinoma of uterine
  cervix
squamous cell carcinoma of vagina
squamous cell carcinoma of vocal cord
squamous epithelial cell
squamous epithelium
squamous intraepithelial lesion
squamous metaplasia of bronchus
squamous metaplasia of cervix
squamous-type bone
squeeze, tussive
sRBC (sheep red blood calls)
sRBC and phenylethyl alcohol
SS-A antibody
SS-B antibody
SSPE (subacute sclerosing
  panencephalitis)
stab (neutrophil)
stab cell
stable factor (Factor VII)
stab wound
staff cell
stage
  end-
  menstrual
  proliferative
  secretory

staghorn calculus
staging
  cancer
  Dukes
  FIGO
  malignancy
  malignant melanoma
  metastasis
  neoplasm
  tumor
staging of tumor, TNM
  T (primary tumor)
  N (regional nodes)
  M (metastasis)
stagnation mastitis
stagnation of urine
Stahr gland
stain (see also *method*, *solution*)
  acetic acid
  acid
  acid alcohol
  acid-fast
  acid-fast bacilli (AFB)
  acid fuchsin
  acid phosphatase
  Alcian blue
  alizarin
  alpha-naphthol esterase
  alum-carmine
  Alzheimer
  ammoniacal silver
  ammonium silver carbonate
  amyloid
  aniline blue
  argentaffin
  auramine-rhodamine
  auramine-rhodamine fluorescent
  auramine rhodamine fluorochrome
  azocarmine
  azure
  basic
  basic fuchsin

stain *(continued)*
  Best
  Best carmine
  Betke-Kleihauer
  Biebrich scarlet
  Bielschowsky
  blue aniline
  Bodian
  Bowie
  Brown-Brenn Gram
  Brown-Hopp tissue Gram
  Bullard hematoxylin
  Cajal gold sublimate
  Cajal trichrome
  carbolfuchsin
  carmine
  Celani method
  Congo red
  contrast
  counter
  cresyl blue
  cresyl blue brilliant
  cresyl fast violet
  crystal violet
  Dane and Herman keratin
  Darrow red
  Davenport
  Del Rio Hortega method
  Delafield
  Delafield hematoxylin
  Dieterle
  Dieterle silver
  differential
  DOPA (dihydroxyphenylalanine)
  double
  Ehrlich acid hematoxylin
  Ehrlich neutral
  Ehrlich triacid
  elastic (elastin)
  elastica-van Gieson
  elastic fibers
  electron

stain *(continued)*
    eosin
    eosin azure
    eosin-phloxine
    fast blue
    fast green
    fast red
    ferric ammonium sulfate
    ferric chloride
    Feulgen
    Feulgen method
    Fite-Faraco
    F method
    Fontana-Masson
    Fontana methenamine-silver
    Foot reticulum
    Fouchet reagent
    fuchsin
    Gallego method
    gentian orange
    gentian violet
    Giemsa
    Giemsa-Wright
    Gill hematoxylin
    Gimenez
    GMS (Gomori methenamine-silver)
    gold
    gold chloride
    Golgi method
    Gomori aldehyde fuchsin
    Gomori methenamine-silver (GMS)
    Gomori-Takamatsu
    Gram
    Gridley
    Grocott-Gomori methenamine-
        silver nitrate
    Grocott methenamine-silver
    H&E (hematoxylin and eosin)
    Hale iron
    Hanks
    Hansel
    Harris hematoxylin

stain *(continued)*
    heavy-metal
    Heidenhain iron hematoxylin
    Heinz body
    hemalum
    hematoxylin
    hematoxylin and eosin (H&E)
    hematoxylin-malachite green–
        basic fuchsin
    hematoxylin-phloxine B
    Hirsch-Peiffer
    Hiss capsule
    Holmes silver nitrate
    Holzer method
    Hortega neuroglia
    Hucker-Conn
    hydrochloric acid
    immunofluorescent
    immunoperoxidase
    India ink
    India ink capsule
    indigo carmine
    intravital
    iodine
    iron
    iron hematoxylin
    Isamine blue
    Janus green B
    Jenner method
    Jones kidney
    Kasten fluorescent Feulgen
    Kernechtrot
    Kinyoun
    Kinyoun acid-fast
    Kinyoun carbolfuchsin
    Kleihauer-Betke
    Kluver-Barrera
    Kossa (von Kossa)
    Kronecker
    Langeron iodine
    Laquer
    lead hydroxide

stain *(continued)*
   Leder
   Leifson flagella
   Leishman
   Lendrum phloxine-tartrazine
   Lepehne-Pickworth
   Levaditi
   Levine alkaline Congo red method
   Lillie
   Lillie allochrome connective tissue
   Lillie azure-eosin
   Lillie ferrous iron
   Lillie sulfuric acid Nile blue
   lipoid
   Lison-Dunn
   lithium carbonate
   lithium-carmine
   Löffler (Loeffler)
   Löffler caustic
   Lorrain Smith
   Lugol
   Luna-Ishak
   Luna modification of Bodian
   Luxol fast blue
   Macchiavello
   MacNeal tetrachrome blood
   malachite green
   Malbin-Sternheimer
   Maldonado-San Jose
   Mallory aniline blue
   Mallory-Azan
   Mallory collagen
   Mallory hemofuchsin
   Mallory iodine
   Mallory iron
   Mallory phloxine
   Mallory phosphotungstic acid–
     hematoxylin
   Mallory trichrome
   Mallory triple
   Mancini iodine technique
   Mann methyl blue–eosin

stain *(continued)*
   Marchi method
   Masson argentaffin
   Masson–Fontana ammoniacal silver
   Masson trichrome
   Maximow
   May-Grünwald
   May-Grünwald-Giemsa
   Mayer
   Mayer mucicarmine
   meconium
   metachromatic
   methyl green–pyronin
   methyl violet
   methylene blue
   Michaelis
   Milligan trichrome
   Mowry colloidal iron
   MSB trichrome
   mucicarmine
   mucin
   multiple
   myeloperoxidase
   Nakanishi
   naphthol-ASD chloroacetate
     esterase
   naphthol green B
   naphthol yellow S
   Nauta
   negative
   Neisser
   neutral
   neutral red
   Nicolle
   Nile blue fat
   ninhydrin-Schiff
   Nissl
   Nobel
   nuclear
   nuclear fast red
   oil red O
   orange G

stain *(continued)*
orcein
Orth
osmic acid
osmium tetroxide
oxalic acid
Padykula-Herman
Paget-Eccleston
panoptic
PAP (Papanicolaou)
Pappenheim
paracarmine
Paragon
PAS (periodic acid-Schiff)
Perdrau method
periodic acid-Schiff (PAS)
Perls Prussian blue
peroxidase
phloxine
phosphomolybdic acid
phosphotungstic acid
phosphotungstic acid-hematoxylin
    (PTAH)
picrocarmine
picro-Mallory trichrome
picronigrosin
plasma
plasmatic
plastic section
polychrome
polychrome methylene blue
Pontamine sky blue
port-wine
positive
potassium metabisulfite
potassium permanganate
protoplasmic
Protargol
Prussian blue
PTAH (phosphotungstic acid-
    hematoxylin)
Puchtler-Sweat

stain *(continued)*
pyrrol blue
Q-banding
quinacrine fluorescent method
Rambourg chromic acid–
    phosphotungstic acid
Rambourg periodic acid–
    chromic methenamine–silver
Ramón y Cajal stain
Ranson pyridine silver
rapid mucin
R–banding
reticulin
reverse Giemsa method
Romanowsky
Romanowsky blood
Roux
safranin
scarlet red
Schaeffer–Fulton
Scharlach R
Schiff solution
Schmorl ferric–ferricyanide
    reduction
Schmorl picrothionin
Schultz
Scott solution
selective
Seller
Shorr trichrome
silver
silver nitrate
silver protein
Snook reticulum
sodium bicarbonate
sodium bisulfite
sodium hydroxide
sodium thiosulfate
spore
Sternheimer–Malbin
Stirling modification of Gram
Sudan

stain *(continued)*
  Sudan black
  Sudan black B fat
  Sudan III
  supravital
  Taenzer
  Takayama
  telomeric R–banding
  tetrachrome
  thioflavine T
  thionin
  Tilden
  Tizzoni
  T method
  T-staining method
  Toison
  toluidine blue
  trichrome
  Truant auramine-rhodamine
  trypsin G-banding
  tumor
  Turnbull blue
  Unna
  Unna-Pappenheim
  Unna-Taenzer
  uranium nitrate
  uranyl acetate
  urate crystals
  van Ermengen
  van Gieson
  Verhoeff
  Verhoeff elastic
  vital
  von Kossa
  von Kossa calcium
  Warthin-Starry
  Wayson
  Weigert
  Weigert-Gram
  Weigert iron hematoxylin
  Weigert-Pal method
  Weil

stain *(continued)*
  Weil myelin sheath
  Wilder reticulum
  Williams
  Wirtz-Conklin spore
  Wright
  Ziehl-Neelsen
  Ziehl-Neelsen acid-fast
stainable iron
staining (see also *stain*)
  acid-fast
  bipolar
  differential
  double
  fluorescent
  intravital
  multiple
  negative
  polar
  postvital
  preagonal
  progressive
  regressive
  relief
  simple
  substantive
  supravital
  telomeric
  terminal
  T method
  triple
  vital
staining antibody
staining of tissue sections
stalk
  allantoic
  body
  polyp
standard, calibration
standard cell
Standard Nomenclature of Medicine
  (SNOMED)

standard serologic test for syphilis (STS)
standing plasma test
Stanley bacillus
Stanley cervical ligament
stapedial artery
stapes bone
staph sepsis
staphyline gland
staphylococcal myocarditis
staphylococcal pericarditis
staphylococcal pneumonia
staphylococcal pneumonitis
staphylococcal protein A
staphylococcal scalded skin syndrome
staphylococcus
Staphylococcus albus
Staphylococcus aureus
Staphylococcus auricularis
Staphylococcus capitis
Staphylococcus cohnii
Staphylococcus epidermidis
Staphylococcus haemolyticus
Staphylococcus hominis
Staphylococcus pyogenes
Staphylococcus saccharolyticus
Staphylococcus saprophyticus
Staphylococcus warneri
Staphylococcus xylosus
staphyloma
star cell
starch granules
starch-iodine test
starch test
Stargardt macular degeneration
starry-sky pattern
star-shaped cell
starvation acidosis
starvation diabetes
stasis
  circulatory
  venous

stasis dermatitis
stasis gallbladder
stasis cirrhosis
stat (statim)
stat test
stature, abnormally increased
status asthmaticus
status post
Staub-Traugott phenomenon
STD (sexually transmitted disease)
steady state diffusing capacity of lung ($DLCO_{SS}$)
steamy appearance
steatorrhea
Stein-Leventhal syndrome
stellar nevus
stellate abscess
stellate cell
stellate cells of cerebral cortex
stellate cells of liver
stellate configuration
stellate ganglia
stellate granuloma
stellate ligament
stellate pattern
stellate reticulum
stem cell
stem cell assay
stem cell marrow harvesting
Stenella araguata
stenosis
  aortic valve
  arterial
  bowel
  bronchial
  cardiac valvular
  cervical
  esophageal
  mitral
  pulmonary
  pyloric
  spinal

Stensen canal
Stensen duct
step section
stephanofiliariasis
stercoraceous abscess
stercoral abscess
stereospecific enzyme
stereotactic biopsy
sterile lancet
sterile abscess
sterile hyphae
sterile meningitis
sterility
sternal angle
sternal articulation
sternal joint
sternal pleural reflection
Sternberg cell
Sternberg giant cell
Sternberg-Reed cell
sternebra (pl. sternebrae)
Sterneedle tuberculin test
Sternheimer-Malbin stain
sternoclavicular articulation
sternoclavicular joint, articular disk of
sternoclavicular ligament
sternocleidomastoid artery
sternocleidomastoid muscle
sternocostal articulation
sternocostal hiatus
sternocostal joint
sternocostal junction
sternomanubrial junction
steroid diabetes
steroid fever
steroidogenic diabetes
Stirling modification of Gram stain
St. Louis encephalitis
St. Louis encephalitis virus
Stock test
Stokvis test
Stoll test

stoma
stomach
   aberrant umbilical
   antrum of
   bilocular
   canal of
   cardia of
   cardiac
   cascade
   convex border of
   coronary artery of
   cup-and-spill
   distal blind
   dumping
   greater curvature of
   hourglass
   leather bottle
   lesser curvature of
   miniature
   Pavlov
   pit of
   scaphoid
   sclerotic
   thoracic
   trifid
   upside-down
   waterfall
   water-trap
stomach bed
stomach calculus
stomach fundus
stomatitis
   allergic
   aphthous
   bismuth
   catarrhal
   gonococcal
   gonorrheal
   herpetic
   infectious
   lead
   membranous

stomatitis *(continued)*
   mercurial
   mycotic
   nonspecific
   recurrent aphthous
   syphilitic
   trophical
   ulcerative
   uremic
   vesicular
   Vincent
stomatitis exanthematica
stomatitis medicamentosa
stomatitis nicotina
stomatitis scarlatina
stomatitis scorbutica
stomatitis venenata
stomatocyte
stone (also, calculus, gallstone)
   barrel-shaped
   bile duct
   biliary tract
   bilirubinate
   black faceted
   bladder
   blue
   bosselated
   calcium bilirubinate
   chalk
   common bile duct (CBD)
   cholesterol
   cystine
   gallbladder
   intrahepatic
   intraluminal
   kidney
   lung
   metabolic
   noncalcified
   renal
   residual
   salivary

stone *(continued)*
   skin
   staghorn
   struvite
   tear
   ureteric
   urinary
   vein
   womb
stonelike mass
stone mole
stool
   acholic
   bilious
   black tarry
   bloody
   brown
   bulky
   caddy (dark, sandy mud)
   caliber of
   clay-colored
   color and caliber
   consistency of
   currant jelly
   dark
   dark-green
   diarrhea
   fatty
   flattened
   floating
   foamy
   formed
   foul-smelling
   frank blood in
   frequency of
   green
   guaiac-negative
   guaiac-positive
   hard
   heme-negative
   heme-positive
   impacted

stool *(continued)*
  lienteric
  light gray
  liquid
  loose
  mahogany-colored
  malodorous
  maroon-colored
  melenic
  mucoid
  mucous
  mushy
  nonbloody
  occult blood in
  oily
  pale
  pea soup
  pelleted
  pencil-like
  pipe-stem
  rabbit
  reducing substance in
  residual
  ribbon
  rice-water
  runny
  sago-grain
  scybalous
  semiformed
  semisolid
  silver
  slurry of
  soft
  spinach
  tarry black
  undigested food in
  unformed
  watery
  white fatty
stool color
stool consistency
stool culture

stool for occult blood
stool for ova and parasites (O&P)
stooling
stool osmotic gap
stool smear
stool specimen
stool urobilinogen
storage disease
store (pl. stores)
  hepatic glycogen
  glycogen
  iron
  liver iron
storiform
straddling embolism
straight-chain fatty acid
straight sinus
straight tubule
strand, complementary
strangulated bowel
strangulation of hernia
strap cell
straplike connection
straplike muscle
strap muscle
Strassburg test for bile acids in
  albumin-free urine
stratification
stratified clot
stratified columnar epithelium
stratified cuboidal epithelium
stratified epithelium
stratified squamous epithelium
stratified squamous mucosa
stratified squamous submucosa
stratified transitional epithelium
stratographic analysis
straw itch
strawberry gallbladder
strawberry hemangioma
strawberry nevus
strawberry tongue

straw-colored fluid
straw-colored urine
streak
streaking, atheromatous
streak plate
Streeter band
strep (slang for streptococcus)
strep screen
strep throat
streptavidin-biotin peroxidase complex
streptavidin-horseradish peroxidase
streptobacillary rat-bite fever
Streptobacillus moniliformis
streptococcal antigen
streptococcal disease of newborn
streptococcal enzyme hyaluronidase
streptococcal pharyngitis
streptococcal pneumonia
streptococcus
    alpha-hemolytic
    anhemolytic
    beta-hemolytic
    gamma-hemolytic
    hemolytic
    group A beta-hemolytic (GABHS)
    nonhemolytic
Streptococcus acidominimus
Streptococcus aecium
Streptococcus agalactiae
Streptococcus anginosus
Streptococcus avium
Streptococcus bovis
Streptococcus constellatus
Streptococcus durans
Streptococcus equi
Streptococcus equinus
Streptococcus equisimilis
Streptococcus faecalis
Streptococcus faecium
Streptococcus intermedius
Streptococcus M antigen
Streptococcus milleri

Streptococcus mitis
Streptococcus morbillorum
Streptococcus mutans
Streptococcus pneumoniae
Streptococcus pyogenes
Streptococcus salivarius
Streptococcus sanguis
Streptococcus uberis
Streptococcus viridans
Streptococcus zooepidemicus
Streptomyces
Streptomyces paraguayensis
Streptomyces somaliensis
Streptozyme serologic test
stretchability of skin
stria (pl. striae)
    acoustic
    auditory
    brown
    dermal
    pink
striate artery
striated cardiac muscle
striated muscle
striated skeletal muscle
striation, basal
striations
striatonigral degeneration
string cell carcinoma
stringency
stringent factor
stringy mucous exudate
strip
stripe, properitoneal flank
striped muscle
stripped
stripper, vein
stroke
stroma
    abnormally scanty
    connective-tissue
    desmoplastic

stroma *(continued)*
    endometrial
    fibrofatty
    fibrous
    fibrovascular
    nonmalignant
    ovarian
    periductal
    synovial
stroma-free hemoglobin solution
stromal ganglion
stromal hemorrhage
stromal invasion
stromal necrosis
stromal retraction
strong silver protein
strong trichrome staining method
Strongyloides stercoralis
strongyloidiasis
Strong bacillus
structural lesion
structure
    biliary
    cord
    denture-supporting
    elongated
    glandular
    hollow
    organoid
    satellite
    subcutaneous
structure of cell
structure protein
struma ovarii
struma, Riedel
strumous abscess
Strümpell (Struempell)
Strümpell-Leichtenstern encephalitis
Strümpell-Marie disease
Struthers
    arcade of
    ligament of

Struve test for blood in urine
struvite
STS (serologic test for syphilis)
STT (scaphotrapezoid trapezial) joint
Stuart factor
Stuart medium
Stuart-Prower factor
study
    serial CK enzyme
    sperm motility
stump
    appendiceal
    cervical
    duodenal
    gastric
    limb
    rectal
stump pregnancy
stunned myocardium
stunting of growth
stupor
stye
styloglossus muscle
stylohyoid ligament
styloid, radial
stylomandibular ligament
stylomastoid foramen
stylomaxillary ligament
Stypven time test
subacromial bursitis
subacute allergic pneumonia
subacute atrophy of liver
subacute bacterial endocarditis
subacute combined degeneration of
    spinal cord
subacute granulomatous thyroiditis
subacute hepatitis
subacute hepatic necrosis
subacute inflammation
subacute myelitis
subacute myoendocarditis
subacute necrotic myelitis

subacute nephritis
subacute nodular migratory panniculitis
subacute sclerosing panencephalitis (SSPE)
subacute thyroiditis
subadventitial fibrosis
subaponeurotic abscess
subarachnoid cistern
subarachnoid exudate
subarachnoid hemorrhage
subarachnoid space
subareolar abscess
subauricular gland
subcapsular
subcarinal node
subcecal appendix
subchronic atrophy of liver
subclavian artery
subclavian loop
subclavian vein
subclinical diabetes
subclinical infection
subcostal artery
subcostal muscle
subcostal nerve
subcostal plane (SCP)
subcu (subcutaneous)
subculture
subcutaneous (SQ, subcu)
subcutaneous annulus
subcutaneous connective tissue
subcutaneous emphysema
subcutaneous fascia
subcutaneous fat
subcutaneous fat necrosis
subcutaneous inflammation
subcutaneous layer
subcutaneous nodule
subcutaneous pannus
subcutaneous structure
subcutaneous tissue
subcutaneous wound

subcutis
subdeltoid bursitis
subdiaphragmatic abscess
subdural abscess
subdural clot
subdural effusion
subdural hematoma, encapsulated
subdural hemorrhage
subdural space
subendocardial
subepicardial myocarditis
subepidermal abscess
subepithelial
subfascial abscess
subgaleal abscess
subhepatic abscess
subhepatic area
subhepatic cecum
subintimal fibrosis
subjacent
sublingual artery
sublingual gland
sublingual salivary gland
subluxation of lens
submammary mastitis
submandibular duct
submandibular ganglion
submandibular gland
submandibular lymph node
submandibular node
submandibulary salivary gland
submassive hepatic necrosis
submassive pulmonary embolism
submaxillary artery
submaxillary gland
submaxillary glandular artery
submental artery
submental lymph node
submucosa
submucosal venous plexus
submucous leiomyoma
submuscular

subpectoral abscess
subperiosteal abscess
subperitoneal fatty areolar tissue
subperitoneal space
subphrenic abscess
subphrenic pyopneumothorax
subphrenic recess
subpubic angle
subsartorial canal
subscapular abscess
subscapular angle
subscapular artery
subserosa
subserosal fibrosis
subserosal hemorrhage
subserosal layer
substance
    amorphous ground
    anterior pituitary-like
    basophil
    beta
    cement
    central gray
    chromophil
    cortical
    exophthalmos-producing
    ground
    lipoid
    medullary
    Nissl
substantia nigra (black substance)
substantia propria (proper substance)
substernal goiter
substitution bone
substrate
subtalar articulation
subtalar joint
subungual
subungual abscess
subungual melanoma
subunit
subvesical duct

subxiphoid
succulent
succumb
sucking wound
Sucquet-Hoyer canal
sucrose hemolysis test
sucrose lysis test
sucrose test
suction artifact
suction pipette
Sudan black
Sudan black B fat stain
sudanophilic leukodystrophy
Sudan III (oil red O)
sudden cardiac death
sudden infant death syndrome (SIDS)
Sudeck atrophy
Sudeck point
sudoriferous gland
sudoriparous abscess
SUDS (Single Use Diagnostic System)
suffocative goiter
sugar
    blood
    brain
    differential
    fasting blood
    random blood
    reducing
    threshold
    two-hour postprandial
    urine
sugar and acetone (S&A)
sugar-icing liver
suggillation, postmortem
Suipoxvirus (swinepox virus)
sulcal artery
sulcus (pl. sulci)
sulfate, keratan
sulfhemoglobin
sulfhemoglobinemia
sulfosalicylic acid turbidity test

sulfur granules
sulfuric acid
sulfur test for protein
Sullivan test for cysteine
Sulzberger-Chase phenomenon
summer prurigo
sunburn-like reaction
sunlight radiation
superciliary arch
superficial abscess
superficial brachial artery
superficial cardiac dullness
superficial cell
superficial cervical artery
superficial dorsal sacrococcygeal
    ligament
superficial epigastric artery
superficial external pudendal artery
superficial fascia
superficial iliac circumflex artery
superficial inguinal lymph node
superficial inguinal pouch
superficial inguinal ring
superficial layer, fatty
superficial lymph vessel
superficial necrosis
superficial palmar arch artery
superficial plexus
superficial perineal artery
superficial perineal pouch
superficial petrosal artery
superficial pneumonia
superficial posterior sacrococcygeal
    ligament
superficial pustular perifolliculitis
superficial spreading melanoma
superficial temporary artery
superficial transverse metacarpal
    ligament
superficial transverse metatarsal
    ligament
superficial transverse perineal muscle

superficial volar arch artery
superficial volar artery
Superfrost/Plus Fisherbrand glass slide
superimposed
superior alveolar artery
superior articular artery of knee
superior articular process
superior border of heart
superior bronchus
superior cerebellar artery
superior cistern
superior colliculi
superior costotransverse ligament
superior deep cervical lymph node
superior demifacet
superior duodenal fold
superior duodenal recess
superior epigastric artery
superior gluteal artery
superior gluteal vessel
superior hemorrhoidal artery
superior hypogastric plexus
superior intercostal artery
superior labial artery
superior laryngeal artery
superior ligament of epididymis
superior ligament of incus
superior ligament of malleus
superior lobe
superior lobe bronchus
superior longitudinal muscle of tongue
superior margin of inferior rib
superior meatus
superior mediastinum
superior mesenteric artery
superior mesenteric ganglion
superior mesenteric plexus
superior mesenteric vein
superior nasal concha
superior orbital fissure
superior pancreaticoduodenal artery
superior pelvic aperture

superior phrenic artery
superior pole
superior profunda artery
superior pubic ligament
superior pulmonary vein
superior radioulnar joint
superior rectal artery
superior rectal vein
superior rib, inferior margin of
superior sagittal sinus
superior thoracic aperture
superior thoracic artery
superior thyroid artery
superior tibial articulation
superior tibiofibular joint
superior transverse rectal fold
superior transverse scapular ligament
superior turbinated bone
superior tympanic artery
superior ulnar collateral artery
superior vena cava
superior vesical artery
supermedial surface
supernatant
supernatant plasma
supernumerary bone
supernumerary kidney
supernumerary nipple
superoxide dismutase (SOD)
supply
    motor
    nerve
supporting cell
suppressor cell
suppressor gene tumor
suppressor T cell
suppuration, frank
suppurativa, hidradenitis
suppurative infection
suppurative mastitis
suppurative nephritis
suppurative pleurisy

suppurative pneumonia
supraceliac aorta
supraciliary canal
supraclavicular lymph node
supraclavicular nerve
supraclinoid aneurysm
supracolic compartment
supracristal plane (SCP)
supraduodenal artery
suprahepatic abscess
suprahepatic caval cuff
suprahepatic space
suprahepatic vena cava
suprahyoid aponeurosis
suprahyoid artery
suprainterparietal bone
supralevator space
supranuclear lesion
supraoccipital bone
supraoptic anastomosis
supraoptic canal
supraorbital artery
supraorbital canal
supraorbital ridge
suprapharyngeal bone
suprapleural membrane
suprapubic region
suprarenal artery
suprarenal gland
suprarenal impression
suprascapular artery
suprascapular ligament
suprasellar meningioma
supraspinous ligament
suprasternal bone
supratrochlear artery
supravaterian duodenum
supravital stain
supravital staining of blood specimen
supreme nasal concha
supreme turbinated bone
sural artery

surface
  acromial articular
  anterolateral
  anteromedial
  articular
  articulating
  arytenoidal articular
  auricular
  axial
  basal
  buccal
  calcaneal articular
  carpal articular
  cerebral
  colic
  costal
  cuboidal articular
  denture basal
  denture foundation
  denture impression
  denture occlusal
  denture polished
  diaphragmatic
  distal
  facial
  fibular
  fibular articular
  gastric
  glenoid
  mucous
  occlusal
  posterior
  supermedial
surface biopsy
surface epithelium
surface mucous cells of stomach
surface of heart
  diaphragmatic
  sternocostal
surface of liver bed
surfactant
surfactant protein A concentration

surfer's knee
surfer's knot
surfer's nodule
surgery, Mohs
surgical margin
surgical neck
surgical scar
surgical scraping
surgical specimen
surgical wound
surveillance, medical
susceptibility test
suspensory ligament
suspensory muscle of duodenum
sustentacular cell of ear
sustentacular cell of testis
Sutter blood group
Sutton nevus
sutural bones
sutural ligament
suture (fibrous joint)
  coronal
  cranial (joint)
  dentate
  ethmoidolacrimal
  ethmoidomaxillary
  false
  frontal
  frontoethmoidal
  frontolacrimal
  frontomaxillary
  frontonasal
  frontozygomatic
  lambdoid
  metopic
  sagittal
suture joint
suture line
Suzanne gland
SVR (systemic vascular resistance)
swab, throat
swaged needle

swallowing center
swallowing mechanism
swan-neck deformity
sweat
  bloody
  blue
  drenching
  fetid
  green
  night
  phosphorescent
  profuse
sweat chloride
sweat electrolytes
sweat gland
sweat test
sweep, duodenal
Sweet disease
swelling (see also *edema*)
  ankle
  arytenoid
  brain
  Calabar
  capsular
  cloudy
  fugitive
  genital
  glassy
  hunger
  Kamerun
  labial
  labioscrotal
  Neufeld capsular
  scrotal
  Soemmering crystalline
  Spielmeyer
  tropical
swimmer's dermatitis
swimmer's ear
swimmer's itch
swimming pool granuloma
swine influenza virus

swinepox virus
swirls and tangles
swordfish test
sycosis nuchae
sylvian aqueduct
Sylvius, aqueduct of
Symmers fibrosis
symmetric
symmetrical distribution
symmetry
sympathetic abscess
sympathetic fibers, preganglionic
sympathetic formative cell
sympathetic ganglion
sympathetic hormone
sympathetic nerve
sympathetic ophthalmia
sympathetic system
sympathetic trunk
sympathicotropic cell
sympathochromaffin cell
symphysis cartilaginous joint
symphysis pubis
symptomatic porphyria
symptomatic pruritus
synapse
  axoaxonic
  axodendritic
  electrotonic
synarthrodial joint
synarthrosis articulation
synarthrosis joint
synchondrosis articulation
synchondrosis, cranial
synchondrosis joint
synchronous multicentric osteosarcoma
syncope
syncytial knot
syncytial meningioma
syncytium
  circular
  horseshoe-shaped

syncytium formation
syndesmosis
syndesmosis joint
syndrome
   acquired immune deficiency (AIDS)
   adrenogenital
   antiphospholipid
   aortic arch
   aplastic anemia
   autoerythrocyte sensitization
   Banti
   Barré-Guillain
   Behçet
   Bloom
   carcinoid
   Chédiak-Steinbrinck-Higashi
   Churg-Strauss
   Conn
   CREST
   Crigler-Najjar
   CRST
   crush
   Curtis–Fitz-Hugh
   Cushing
   dengue shock
   double-crush
   Down
   Dresbach
   Dubin-Johnson
   dumping
   dysplastic nevus
   Ehlers-Danlos
   Ellison-Zollinger
   empty sella
   Fanconi
   fetal alcohol
   Fitz-Hugh–Curtis
   fragile X
   Friderichsen-Waterhouse
   Goodpasture
   Gougerot-Blum
   Griscelli

syndrome *(continued)*
   Guillain-Barré
   Hantavirus pulmonary (HPS)
   hemolytic-uremic
   Henoch-Schönlein (Schoenlein)
   Hurler
   hyper-IgE
   inherited malformation
   Job
   Johnson-Dubin
   Klinefelter
   Leventhal-Stein
   Lichtheim
   Li-Fraumeni (LFS)
   locked-in
   Lutembacher
   malabsorption
   Mallory-Weiss
   Marfan
   Meigs
   Mikulicz
   mucocutaneous lymph node
   Najjar-Crigler
   nephrotic
   nutritional deficiency
   Omenn
   paraneoplastic
   Pierre Robin
   pneumorenal
   polycystic ovary
   postmenopausal
   Putnam-Dana
   Reiter
   Reye
   sarcophagic
   scalded skin
   sepsis
   Sheehan
   Sjögren
   staphylococcal scalded skin
   Stein-Leventhal
   testicular feminization

syndrome *(continued)*
   toxic shock
   Treacher Collins
   Turner
   Waterhouse-Friderichsen
   Weiss-Mallory
   Wiskott-Aldrich
   Zollinger-Ellison
syndrome of fever, urticaria, and joint
   inflammation due to allergy
synechia (pl. synechiae)
synergic
synergist
synostosis
synovia
synovial articulations of cranium
synovial cell
synovial fluid
synovial fluid differential count
   clasmatocytes
   lymphocytes
   monocytes
   polymorphonuclear cell
   synovial cell
   unclassified
synovial fluid lactic acid
synovial frost
synovial gland
synovial joint
synovial ligament
synovial-like
synovial lining
synovial membrane
synovial osteochondromatosis
synovial sarcoma
synovitis
   local
   localized nodular
   pigmented villonodular
   purulent
   serous
   villonodular

synovium, hyperplastic
synthase
synthesis of ammonia
synthetic azo dye
synthetic protein
syphilis
   congenital
   serologic test for (STS)
   tertiary
   VDRL test for
syphilitic abscess
syphilitic aneurysm
syphilitic aortitis
syphilitic arteritis
syphilitic chancre
syphilitic cirrhosis
syphilitic fever
syphilitic leukoderma
syphilitic meningitis
syphilitic myelitis
syphilitic myocarditis
syphilitic necrosis
syphilitic nephritis
syphilitic neuritis
syphilitic osteochondritis
syphilitic periarteritis
syphilitic stomatitis
syringobulbia
syringomyelia
system
   alimentary
   articular
   automatic nervous
   bulbosacral
   cardiovascular
   caudal neurosecretory
   cell-free
   central nervous
   cerebrospinal
   chromaffin
   circulatory
   colloid

system *(continued)*
  conducting
  craniosacral
  cytochrome
  dermal
  dermoid
  digestive
  endocrine
  esthesiodic
  excretory
  exterofective
  extrapyramidal motor
  female reproductive
  gamma motor
  genital
  genitourinary
  glandular
  haversian
  hemolymphatic
  intrahepatic duct
  lymphatic
  male reproductive
  nervous

system *(continued)*
  parasympathetic
  portal
  portal venous
  respiratory
  sympathetic
  venous
systematized nevus
Système International (SI) units
systemic and topical hypothermia
systemic effects
systemic fungal infection
systemic lesion
systemic lupus erythematosus (SLE)
systemic mean arterial pressure
  (SMAP)
systemic mycosis
systemic necrotizing vasculitis
systemic vascular resistance (SVR)
systemic vein
systemic zygomycosis
system of Retzius
Szabo test

T, t

T (temperature)
T (tesla)
T_3 (triiodothyronine)
T_4 (thyroxine, tetraiodothyronine)
TA (therapeutic abortion)
TAC (tetracaine, epinephrine, and cocaine) solution
Tacaribe virus
tachypnea
tactile cell
taenia (also, tenia)
Taenia saginata
Taenia solium
taeniae of Valsalva
Taenzer stain
tag
  skin
  toe
  wrist
tagged antibody, fluorescently
tagged, radioactively
Tahyna virus
tail bone
tail of epididymis
tail of pancreas
Takayama stain
Takayasu disease

tall columnar epithelium
talocalcaneal articulation
talocalcaneal ligament
talocalcaneonavicular articulation
talocalcaneonavicular joint
talocrural articulation
talocrural joint
talonavicular articulation
talonavicular joint
talonavicular ligament
talotibial ligament, anterior
talus bone
Tamiami virus
Tamm-Horsfall mucoprotein
Tamm-Horsfall protein
tamponade, cardiac
tanapox virus
T and B lymphocyte subset assay
T&C (type and crossmatch)
tangentially
tangential wound
tangles, neurofibrillary
tanned red cell (TRC)
tanning
Tanret test for albumin
tapeworm
tapeworm infestation

tapeworm segments and ova in stool
Taq Dye
target cell
target gland
target lesion
Tarin space
tarry black stools
tarsal artery
tarsal bone
tarsal canal
tarsal cyst
tarsal gland
tarsal ligament
tarsal plate
tarsal tunnel
tarsoconjunctival glands
tarsometatarsal articulation
tarsometatarsal joint
tarsometatarsal ligaments
tartaric acid
tart cell
tartrate resistant leukocyte acid
    phosphatase
taste bud
taste cell
TAT (thrombin-antithrombin III
    complex)
tattoo
Tatumella
Tatumella ptyseos
taurine test
Taylor test
Tay-Sachs disease
TB (tuberculin; tuberculosis)
TBG (thyroxine-binding globulin)
TBII (TSH-binding inhibitory
    immunoglobulins)
TBP (thyroxine-binding protein)
TBPA (thyroxine-binding prealbumin)
Tc (technetium)
T (thymus-dependent) cell
T (thymus-derived) cell

T cell activation marker
    CD25
    CD26
    CD69
T cell growth factor
T cell lymphoma
    convoluted
    cutaneous
    small lymphocytic
TCMI (T cell-mediated immunity)
TCPI Rapid Test for HIV
TCR (T cell antigen receptor)
T cytotoxic cell
TDA (TSH-displacing antibody)
T-dependent antigen
TdT (terminal deoxynucleotidyl
    transferase)
TDTH cells
teacher nodule
tear (laceration)
    full-thickness
    Mallory-Weiss
    partial-thickness
teardrop cell
teardrop-shaped erythrocyte
tear in articular cartilage
tearing of a muscle
technetium (Tc)
technetium 99m (^{99m}Tc)
technique (see also *method*, *staining*)
    PAP (peroxidase-antiperoxidase)
        technique for detecting antigen
        or antibody in tissue sections
    pressure cooker
    Scotch tape
teeth
    Hutchinson
    incisor
    milk
    primary
    secondary
    wisdom

teeth of Huschke, auditory
T effector cell
Teichmann test for blood
teichoic acid antibody
T-8 suppressor cell
tela (weblike tissue)
tela subcutanea (subcutaneous fascia)
telangiectasia
   generalized essential
   hemorrhagic
   hereditary
   hereditary hemorrhagic
   spider
   unilateral nevoid
telangiectasis
telangiectatic angioma
telangiectatic osteogenic sarcoma
telangiectatic osteosarcoma
Tellyesniczky solution
telogen phase
telomeric R-banding stain
temperate virus
temperature, basal body (BBT)
temperature scale
temporal arteritis
temporal artery
temporal bone
temporal canal
temporal fascia
temporal fossa
temporal muscle
temporal pole
temporomandibular articulation
temporomandibular joint
temporomandibular ligament
tenacious
tenderness, cervical motion (CMT)
tendineae, chordae
tendinitis
tendinous arch of pelvic fascia
tendinous band
tendinous fibers, interlacing

tendinous intersection
tendinous raphe
tendo Achillis
tendo calcaneus (calcaneal tendon)
tendon
   Achilles
   biceps
   bowed
   brachioradialis
   calcanean
   central (of diaphragm)
   central perineal
   common
   conjoined
   conjoint
   contracted
   coronary
   cricoesophageal
   Gerlach annual
   hamstring
   heel (tendo calcaneus)
   intermediate (of diaphragm)
   patellar
   pulled
   rider's
   sheetlike
   slipped
   Todaro
   trefoil
   Zinn (common tendinous ring)
tendon cell
tendon of Achilles
tendon of diaphragm, center
tendon of Hector (heel tendon)
tendon sheath
tendon sheath of ganglion
Tenon capsule
Tenon space
tenosynovitis of digital tendon sheath
tension, carbon dioxide
tension pneumothorax
tensor fasciae latae

tensor tympani muscle canal
tensor veli palatini (tensor palati)
tentative diagnosis
tentorial incisure
tentorial meningioma
tentorium cerebelli
teratocarcinoma of ovary
teratocarcinoma of testis
teratogen
teratogenic
teratology
teratoma
    cystic
    ovary
    pineal
    solid
    solid ovarian
    testis
teres, ligamentum
terminal artery
terminal bile duct
terminal bronchiole
terminal deletion
terminal deoxynucleotidyl transferase
    (TdT)
terminal hematuria
terminal ileum
terminal infection
terminal pneumonia
terminal sulcus
terminal ventricle of spinal cord
termination factor
territorial matrix
Terson gland
tertian malaria
tertiary radicle
tertiary syphilis
Teschen virus
tesselated retina
test (see also *smear* and *stain*)
    acetaldehyde
    acetoacetate

test *(continued)*
    acetone
    acetowhite
    acid clearance (ACT)
    acid elution (for fetal hemoglobin)
    acidification of stool
    acidified serum (for paroxysmal
        nocturnal hemoglobinuria)
    acid-lability
    acid perfusion
    acid phosphatase (for semen)
    acid reflux
    acid serum
    acoustic immittance
    ACTH stimulation
    activated coagulation time (ACT)
    activated partial thromboplastin
        time (APTT)
    Addis
    adrenocorticotropic hormone
        (ACTH)
    adrenocorticotropic hormone stimu-
        lation test
    agglutination
    alanine
    AlaSTAT latex allergy
    Albarran
    albumin
    aldolase
    aldosterone
    alkali denaturation
    alkaline phosphatase
    Allen
    Allen-Doisy
    Almén (for blood)
    AL patch
    alpha-fetoprotein
    ALT (alanine aminotransferase)
        (formerly SGPT)
    Ames assay
    amino acid nitrogen (AAN)
    aminolevulinate dehydratase

test *(continued)*
   aminolevulinic acid (ALA)
   aminopyrine breath
   ammonia nitrogen
   ammonium chloride loading
   amylase
   Anderson and Goldberger
   Anderson-Collip
   androstenedione
   angiotensin I
   angiotensin II
   anion gap
   anoxemia
   antibiotic sensitivity
   antichymotrypsin
   anticytoplasmic antibody (ACPA)
   anti-deoxyribonuclease B titer
      (anti-DNAse titer)
   antidiuretic hormone (ADH)
   antidiuretic hormone-water
      deprivation stimulation test
   anti-DNA antibodies
      Farr
      Ginsberg-Keiser
      indirect fluorescence
   anti-double-stranded DNA
   antiglobulin (AGT)
   antiglobulin consumption
   antihuman globulin
   antihyaluronidase titer (AH titer)
   anti-LA/SS-B
   anti-Ro/SS-A
   anti-Sm
   anti-streptolysin-O titer (ASO titer)
   antithrombin III (AT-III)
      amidolytic (chromogenic)
      radioimmunodiffusion (RID)
   antitrypsin
   Apt
   argentaffin reaction
   arsenic
   arylsulfatase

test *(continued)*
   Ascoli precipitin (for anthrax)
   ascorbate-cyanide
   ascorbic acid
   aspirin tolerance
   AST (aspartate aminotransferase)
      (formerly SGOT)
   ASTRA profile
   atropine
   augmented histamine (of gastric
      function)
   autoerythrocyte sensitivity
   autohemolysis
   Autolet blood glucose
   automated reagin (ART)
   Autopath QC
   Bachman
   Bachman-Pettit
   bacteriolytic
   Bárány caloric
   basal secretory flow rate (BSFR)
   base excess
   baseline
   basophil degranulation
   battery of
   BEI (butanol-extractable iodine)
   bench
   Benedict (for glucose)
   bentiromide
   bentonite flocculation
   benzidine
   Bernstein acid perfusion
   Bernstein esophageal acid infusion
   Berson
   betazole stimulation
   Bettendorff (for arsenic)
   Bial
   bicarbonate
   bile acid breath
   bile acid tolerance
   bile acids, total
   bile esculin

test *(continued)*
  bile solubility
  bilirubin
    conjugated
    direct
    indirect
    total
  Binz (for quinine in urine)
  biuret (for serum proteins)
  bleeding time (BT)
    Duke
    Ivy
    Mielke
    Simplate
  blood (see Table, pp. 576-590)
  blood sugar
  blood volume
  bone marrow, differential count
  borderline
  Bozicevich
  breath analysis
  breath-holding
  breath hydrogen
  bromosulfophthalein (BSP)
  bromphenol
  brucellosis agglutinins
  buffy coat smear
  CA15-3 RIA
  CA 19-9 (carbohydrate antigen)
  calcitonin (hCT)
  calcitonin–calcium infusion
    stimulation
  calcium
    ionized
    total
  Calmette
  caloric
  CAMP (Christie, Atkins, and
    Munch-Petersen) factor
  cancer antigen 125 (CA125)
  C&S (culture and sensitivity)
  capillary fragility

test *(continued)*
  capillary resistance
  carbohydrate utilization
  carbon dioxide
    partial pressure (PCO_2)
    total (TCO_2)
  carbon monoxide
  carbon 13-labeled ketoisocaproate
    breath
  carboxyhemoglobin
  carcinoembryonic antigen (CEA)
  cardiac enzymes
  cardiac isoenzymes
  Cardiac T Rapid Assay
  carotene
  carotene absorption
  carotid sinus
  Carr-Price
  Casoni intradermal (for hydatid
    disease)
  Casoni skin
  catalase
  catecholamines
    fractionated
    free
    plasma
    total
    urinary
  CEA (carcinoembryonic antigen)
  cephalin-cholesterol flocculation
  cerebrospinal fluid pressure
  cerebrospinal fluid volume
  ceruloplasmin
  CF (complement fixation)
  C-glycocholic acid breath
  "chem" (chemical profile)
  chemical
  Chemstrip bG
  chenodeoxycholic acid, total
  chenodeoxycholylglycine,
    conjugated
  Chick-Martin

test *(continued)*
  Chlamydiazyme
  chloride
  cholecystokinin
  cholesterol, total
  cholic acid, total
  cholinesterase II
  chorionic gonadotropin
  chromatin
  chromium red blood cell
  chromogenic enzyme substrate
  citrate
  citrulline
  C lactose
  Clinitest stool
  clomiphene
  CLOtest
  clot lysis
  clot retraction
  clotting time
    Lee-White
    plasma
  coagulase
  coagulation factor assay
  coagulation time
  coccidioidin
  cold pressor
  cold water calorics
  colloidal gold
  Coloscreen Self
  competitive binding assay
  complement fixation (CF)
  concentration (for renal function)
  conglutinating complement
    absorption (CCAT)
  Congo red (for amyloidosis)
  conjunctival
  contact patch
  contraction stress (CST)
  copper
  copper-binding protein
  coproporphyrin

test *(continued)*
  Corner-Allen
  corticobinding globulin (CBG)
  corticosterone
  cortisol
  cortisol, free
  CO_2-withdrawal seizure
  C-peptide
  creatinine
  C-reactive protein
  creatine kinase (CK)
    total
    isoenzymes
  creatinine
  creatinine clearance
  CSF glutamine
  Cult-Dip Plus bacteriological
    culture
  culture and sensitivity (C&S)
  cutaneous
  cutaneous tuberculin
  cyanide
  cyanide-nitroprusside
  cyclic AMP
  cysteine (also, cystine)
  cytotropic antibody
  DA pregnancy
  Davidsohn differential absorption
  Day
  d-dimer
  deferoxamine mesylate infusion
  Dehio
  dehydrocholate
  dehydroepiandrosterone (DHEA)
  dehydroepiandrosterone sulfate
    (DHEA-SO_4)
  deoxycholic acid, total
  11-deoxycortisol (Compound S)
  11-deoxycorticosterone (DOC)
  deoxyribonuclease (DNase)
  deoxyuridine suppression
  dexamethasone single dose
    overnight suppression

test *(continued)*
    dexamethasone suppression
    dextrose
    DFA-TP (direct fluorescent
        antibody-*Treponema pallidum*)
    diabetes
    diacetyl
    diagnostic
    Dick intracutaneous
    differential
    differential count
    differential renal function
    differential ureteral catheterization
    dihydrotestosterone (DHT)
    1,25-dihydroxycholecalciferol assay
        $(1,25\text{-}OH\text{-}D_3)$
    dinitrophenylhydrazine
    diphtheria
    direct antiglobulin
    direct Coombs
    direct fluorescent antibody
    discontinuation
    disk-diffusion
    Donath-Landsteiner
    double glucagon
    Dragendorff (for bile)
    Ducrey intradermal
    Duke bleeding time
    D-xylose absorption
    D-xylose tolerance
    dye exclusion
    edrophonium
    ELISA titer
    Ellsworth-Howard
    eosinophil count
    E-rosette
    erythrocyte adherence
    erythrocyte count
    erythrocyte protoporphyrin (EP)
    erythrocyte sedimentation rate
        (ESR)
    erythropoietin

test *(continued)*
    esophageal acid infusion
    esophageal function
    estradiol
    estriol (E_3)
        free
        total
    estrogen receptor assay (ERA)
    estrogens, total
    estrone (E_1)
    euglobulin clot lysis
    ExacTech blood glucose meter
    executive profile
    Farber
    Farr
    fat, fecal
    fatty acid profile
    fatty acids
        nonesterified (free)
        total
    FDL (fluorescein dilaurate)
    fecal alpha$_1$-antitrypsin
    fecal leukocyte count
    fecal occult blood
    Felix-Weil
    fermentation
    fern
    ferric chloride
    ferritin
    ferrohemoglobin solubility
    alpha$_1$-fetoprotein
    fibrin degradation products
    fibrin lysis time
    fibrinogen
    fibrin stabilizing factor (FSF)
    FIGLU excretion
    Finn chamber patch
    Fishberg concentration
    Fishman-Doublet
    fluorescent antibody (FA)
    fluorescent antinuclear antibody
        (FANA)

test *(continued)*
  fluorescent treponemal antibody
    (FTA)
  fluorescent treponemal antibody
    absorption (FTA-ABS)
  fluoride
  folate
  folate absorption
  follicle-stimulating hormone
    (FSH)
  follicle-stimulating hormone-
    releasing (FSH-RH)
  Foshay (for tularemia)
  Fouchet (for bilirubin in urine)
  fragility
  Francis
  free thyroxine index (FT_4I)
  free triiodothyronine (T_3)
  Frei intracutaneous diagnostic
  fructose challenge
  fructose loading
  fructose tolerance
  FTA-ABS (fluorescent treponemal
    antibody-absorption)
  function
  Gaddum and Schild
  galactose tolerance
  gastric acid
  gastric content
  gastric emptying
  gastric function
  gastric secretion rate
  gastric secretory
  gastrin
  gastrin-secretin stimulation
  gastrin stimulation
  Gastroccult
  GBIA (Guthrie bacterial inhibition
    assay)
  gel diffusion
  gel (double) diffusion precipitin
    in one or two dimensions

test *(continued)*
  gel diffusion reaction
  Geraghty
  Gerhardt (for acetoacetic acid)
  Gerhardt (for urobilin in urine)
  germ tube
  Gerrard
  GGTP liver function
  Gies biuret
  Gilchrist skin
  globulin
  glomerular selectivity
    (IgG/albumin clearance)
  glucagon stimulation
  glucose
  glucose oxidase paper strip
  glucose-6-phosphate dehydrogenase
    (G-6-PD)
  glucose tolerance (GTT)
  glucose tolerance with cortisone
  glucose, two-hour postprandial
  glutamine
  glutamyltransferase (GGT)
  glutathione reductase in
    erythrocytes
  glycerol, free
  glycerophosphate
  glycine
  glycogen storage
  glycolic acid
  glycosylated hemoglobin
  glycyltryptophan
  glyoxylic acid
  Gmelin
  Gofman
  gold
  gonadotropins
  Gordon
  Gothlin capillary fragility
  Graham-Cole cholecystography
  Gram stain of stool
  Gravindex pregnancy

test *(continued)*

Gregerson and Boas
Grigg
Gross
growth hormone–arginine
stimulation
growth hormone–glucagon
stimulation
growth hormone, human (hGH,
somatotropin)
growth hormone–L-dopa
stimulation
G-6-PD (glucose-6-phosphate
dehydrogenase)
guaiac (for occult blood)
Gunning
Gunning-Lieben
Günzberg (Guenzberg)
Guthrie bacterial inhibition assay
(GBIA)
Gutzeit
Ham acidified serum
hamatein
Hamel
Hammarsten
hamster egg penetration assay
hapten inhibition
haptoglobin (Hp)
Harding and Ruttan
Harris and Ray
Harrison spot
Hart
HATTS (hemagglutination
treponemal test for syphilis)
Hay
H_2 breath
HDL cholesterol (HDLC)
Heaf
heat coagulation
heat instability
heavy metal screening

test *(continued)*

Heinz body
Helicobacter pylori urease
Helisal rapid blood
Heller
hemadsorption
hemadsorption virus
hemagglutination
hemagglutination inhibition
(HI, HAI)
Hematest
hematocrit (HCT, Hct)
hemin (for blood)
Hemoccult II
hemoglobin (Hb)
hemoglobin A
hemoglobin A_{IC}
hemoglobin A_2 (HbA$_2$)
hemoglobin electrophoresis
hemoglobin F
hemoglobin H (HbH)
HemoQuant fecal blood
hemosiderin
hepatic function
Herzberg
Hess capillary
heterophile agglutination
Hickey-Hare
Hildebrandt
Hines-Brown cold pressor
Hinton
Histalog
Histalog stimulation
histamine
histamine flare
histidine loading
histoplasmin-latex
HIVAGEN
HIV-antibody test on blood
HIV Blot 2•2
Hoffmann

test *(continued)*
  Hofmeister
  Hollander
  homocystine
  homovanillic acid (HVA)
  Hooker-Forbes
  Hopkins-Cole
  Hopkins thiophene
  Hoppe-Seyler
  Horsley
  Howard
  Howell prothrombin
  Huddleson agglutination
  Huhner
  Huppert
  Huppert-Cole
  Hurtley
  hydrochloric acid
  hydrogen breath
  hydrogen peroxide
  hydroxybutyric acid
  17-hydroxycorticosteroids
    (17-OHCS)
  5-hydroxyindole acetic acid
    (5-HIAA)
  hydroxylamine (for glucose)
  17-hydroxyprogesterone (17-OHP)
  hydroxyproline
  25-hydroxyvitamin D assay
    (25-OH-D)
  hyperventilation
  hypoxemia
  ice water calorics
  Ilosvay
  immobilization
  immune adhesion
  immunoglobulin A (IgA)
  immunoglobulin D (IgD)
  immunoglobulin G (IgG)
  immunoglobulin G/albumin ratio
  immunoglobulin G synthesis rate
  immunoglobulin M (IgM)

test *(continued)*
  immunologic pregnancy
  immunoperoxidase
  IMViC metabolic
  indigo carmine
  indigo red
  indirect antiglobulin
  indirect Coombs
  indirect fluorescent antibody
  indirect hemagglutination
  indole
  indophenol
  inhibition
  insulin (12 hours fasting)
  insulin antibodies
  insulin and glucose suppression
  insulin clearance test
  insulin hypoglycemia
  insulin with oral glucose tolerance
  insulin tolerance
  intracutaneous
  intracutaneous tuberculin
  intradermal
  intraductal secretin (IDST)
  intraesophageal acid
  intraesophageal pH
  intrinsic factor, vitamin B_{12}
  iodine
  iodoform
  iron
  iron-binding capacity, total (TIBC)
  iron saturation
  islet cell antibody screening (ICA)
  isocitrate dehydrogenase (ICD)
  isoleucine
  isopropanol precipitation
  Ito-Reenstierna
  [131]I uptake (thyroid function)
  Ivy bleeding time
  Jacquemin
  Jaffe
  Johnson

test *(continued)*

- Jolles
- Jones and Cantarow urea concentration
- Jones fluorescein instillation
- Jorissen
- Kantor and Gies
- Kaplan
- Kapsinow
- Katayama
- Kentmann
- Kerner
- 17-ketogenic steroids (17-KGS)
- 17-ketosteroid (17 KS) fractions
- ketone bodies
- kidney function
- Killian
- Kirby-Bauer
- Kjeldahl
- Kleihauer acid elution
- Kleihauer-Betke
- Kleihauer-Betke acid elution
- Klimow
- Knapp
- Knott
- Kober
- Kobert
- KOH (potassium hydroxide)
- Kolmer
- Kondo
- Korotkoff
- Kossel
- Kowarsky
- Krokiewicz
- Kurzrok-Miller
- Kurzrok-Ratner
- Kveim intradermal
- lactic acid
- lactose
- lactose breath hydrogen
- Ladendorff
- lamellar body number density

test *(continued)*

- Lancefield precipitation
- Lang (for taurine)
- Lange (for acetone in urine)
- LAP (leucine aminopeptidase)
- latex agglutination
- latex fixation
- LDL cholesterol (LDLC)
- lead
- LE cell
- Lechini
- Lee
- Lee-White clotting time
- Legal
- leishmanin
- Leo
- lepromin
- Lesser
- leucine
- leukocyte adherence assay
- leukocyte bactericidal assay
- leukocyte esterase (LET)
- Levinson
- Lieben
- Lieben-Ralfe
- Liebermann
- Liebermann-Burchard
- Liebig
- limulus
- *Limulus* amebocyte lysate assay
- Lindemann
- line (for rickets)
- lipase
- lipoprotein electrophoresis
- litmus milk
- liver function (LFT)
- Loewe
- long-acting thyroid stimulating hormone (LATS)
- Lowenthal
- Lücke
- lupus band

test *(continued)*
    lupus erythematosus (LE) cell
    luteinizing hormone (LH)
    Luttke
    Lyle and Curtman
    lymphocyte proliferation
    lymphocyte transformation
    lysozyme
    Macdonald
    Machado
    Machado-Guerreiro
    Maclagan thymol turbidity
    MacLean
    MacLean-de Wesselow urea
      concentration
    MacMunn
    macrophage migration inhibition
    MacWilliam
    magnesionitric
    magnesium
    magnetic susceptibility
    Magpie
    Malot
    maltose
    Mann-Whitney
    Mann-Whitney-Wilcoxon
    Mantoux intracutaneous tuberculin
    Mantoux skin
    Maréchal
    Marquis
    Masset
    Mathews
    Maumené
    Mayerhofer
    Mayer
    Mazzotti (for onchocerciasis)
    McNemer ascites
    Meigs
    melanin
    Meltzer-Lyon
    Mendel
    mercury

test *(continued)*
    Mester
    metabisulfite (for sickle cell
      hemoglobin)
    metanephrine, total
    methanol
    methionine
    methyl red
    methylphenylhydrazine
    metratrophic
    Mett
    metyrapone stimulation
    MHA-TP (microhemagglutination-
      Treponema pallidum)
    Michailow
    Micral urine dipstick
    Microflow
    microhemagglutination
    microprecipitation
    microsomal antibodies, thyroid
    migration inhibitory factor (MIF)
    Millard
    Miller-Kurzrok
    Millon
    Millon-Nasse (for protein)
    Mitscherlich
    mixed agglutination
    mixed lymphocyte culture (MLC)
    Mohr
    Molisch
    Moloney
    Mono-Diff
    Monoscreen
    Monospot
    Monosticon Dri-Dot
    Montenegro
    Moore
    Morelli (exudate vs. transudate)
    Moretti (typhoid fever)
    Moritz
    Mörner
    Mosenthal

test *(continued)*

 motility
 Motulsky dye reduction
 mucin clot
 Mulder
 multiple-puncture intracutaneous
  tuberculin
 mumps sensitivity
 Murayama
 MycoAKT latex bead agglutination
 mycologic
 myelin basic protein
 Myers and Fine
 Mylius
 myoglobin
 Nakayama
 Nencki
 Neukomm
 neutralization
 niacin (for *Mycobacterium*
  tuberculosis)
 Nickerson-Kveim
 ninhydrin
 Nippe
 nitrate reduction
 Nitrazine
 nitric acid
 nitric acid–magnesium sulfate
 nitrites
 nitroblue tetrazolium (NBT)
 nitrogenous compound
 nitrogen partition
 nitrogen, total
 nitropropiol
 nitroprusside
 nitroso-indole-nitrate
 Nobel
 Noguchi
 nontreponemal antigen
 normetanephrine, total
 Northern blot
 Nyiri

test *(continued)*

 Obermayer
 Obermueller cholesterol
 occult blood
 OCT (oxytocin challenge)
 oleic acid-^{131}I absorption
 Oliver
 optochin sensitivity
 Oral Fluid Vironostika HIV-1
  Microelisa System
 oral lactose tolerance
 orosomucoid
 OraSure HIV-1 Oral Specimen
  Collection Device
 Osgood-Haskins
 osmolality
 osmolality ratio, urine/serum
 osmotic fragility
 Osterberg
 Ouchterlony
 ova and parasites (O&P)
 OvuGen
 OvuKIT
 OvuQUICK
 oxalate
 ox cell hemolysin
 oxidase
 oxygen, partial pressure (PO_2)
 oxygen saturation
 oxytocin
 Palmer acid (for peptic ulcer)
 palmin
 pancreatic function
 pancreozymin-secretin
 PAP (Papanicolaou)
 PAP (peroxidase-antiperoxidase)
 Papnet
 parathyroid hormone (PTH)
 partial thromboplastin time
 passive cutaneous anaphylaxis
 passive protection
 patch

test *(continued)*
 paternity
 Patterson
 Paul-Bunnell
 Paul-Bunnell-Davidsohn
 Pavy
 PBI (protein-bound iodine)
 peak and trough levels
 peak secretory flow rate (PSFR)
 penicillinase
 pentagastrin
 pentagastrin gastric secretory
 pentagastrin infusion
 pentagastrin provocative
 pentagastrin stimulated analysis
 pentoses
 Penzoldt
 Penzoldt-Fischer
 pepsin
 pepsinogen (PG I)
 peptide
 peptone
 Peria
 periodic acid-Schiff (PAS)
 Perls hemosiderin
 peroxidase
 peroxidase-antiperoxidase (PAP)
 Petri
 Pettenkofer
 Petzetaki
 pH
 PharmChek sweat patch drug
   detection
 phenacetin
 phenol
 phenolphthalein
 phenolsulfonphthalein
 phenoltetrachlorophthalein
 phentolamine (for pheochromocytoma)
 phenylalanine
 phenylhydrazine

test *(continued)*
 phenylpyruvic acid, qualitative
 phosphatase
   acid
   alkaline
 phospholipids, total
 phosphoric acid
 phosphorus, inorganic
 Pincus
 pine wood
 pineapple
 Piria
 Pirquet cutaneous tuberculin
 placental lactogen (hPL)
 plasmacrit
 platelet adhesion
 platelet aggregation
 Plugge
 POA (pancreatic oncofetal antigen)
 Pohl
 Pollacci
 polyuria
 Porges-Meier flocculation
   (for syphilis)
 porphobilinogen (PBG)
 Porter
 positive whiff
 Posner
 postcoital
 post-heparin lipolytic activity
 postprandial
 potassium
 potassium iodide
 PPD skin
 precipitation
 precipitin
 Precision-G handheld blood glucose
 Precision Q-I-D handheld blood
   glucose
 pregnancy
 pregnanediol
 pregnanetriol

test *(continued)*
  pregnenolone
  Preyer
  progesterone
  progesterone receptor assay (PRA)
  proinsulin
  prolactin (PRL)
  prolactin–insulin stimulation
  properdin
  prostaglandins
  protection
  protein-bound iodine
  protein, total
  proteose
  prothrombin
  prothrombin consumption
  prothrombin-proconvertin
  Protocult
  protoporphyrin
  provocative
  pseudocholinesterase (PCHE)
  Purdy
  Pyramidon
  pyruvic acid
  quantitative fecal fat
  Quick prothrombin
  QuickVue Chlamydia
  quinine carbacrylic resin (for gastric anacidity)
  Quinlan
  Raabe
  Rabuteau
  radioactive iodide uptake
  radioactive iodinated serum albumin (RISA)
  radioallergosorbent (RAST)
  radioimmunosorbent (RIST)
  Raji cell assay
  Ralfe
  Ramon flocculation
  Randolph
  Rantzman

test *(continued)*
  rapid plasma reagin (RPR)
  rapid serum amylase
  Rapoport differential ureteral catheterization
  RAST (radioallergosorbent)
  Rebuck skin window
  red cell adherence
  red phenolsulfonphthalein
  reducing substances
  Rees
  Rehberg
  Reichl
  Reinsch
  Reiter complement fixation (for syphilis)
  renal function
  renal plasma flow (RPF)
  renin
  rennin
  reptilase
  resorcinol–hydrochloric acid
  Response GM (for granulocyte count)
  Reuss
  reverse triiodothyronine (rT_3)
  Reynolds
  Rh blocking
  rheumatoid arthritis
  rhubarb
  riboflavin (vitamin B_2)
  rice-flour breath
  Riegler
  Rimini
  ring
  ring precipitin
  RISA (radioactive iodinated serum albumin)
  RIST (radioimmunosorbent)
  Roberts
  Robinson-Kepler
  Ronchese

test *(continued)*
  rose bengal
  rose bengal radioactive (^{131}I)
  Rosenbach (for bile in urine)
  Rosenbach-Gmelin
  Rosenthal
  Rose-Waaler agglutination
  Rosin
  rosette
  Ross-Jones
  Rotazyme
  Rothera
  Rothera nitroprusside (for ketone
    bodies)
  Rous
  Roussin
  Rowntree and Geraghty
  RPR (rapid plasma reagin)
  rubella HI (hemagglutination
    inhibition)
  Rubner
  Ruhemann
  Rumpel-Leede
  Ruttan and Hardisty
  Saathoff
  Sabin-Feldman dye
  saccharimeter
  Sachs-Georgi
  Sachsse
  Sahli-Nencki
  Sakaguchi
  salicylic acid
  saline continence
  Salkowski
  Salkowski and Schipper
  Salkowski-Ludwig
  sand
  Sandrock
  santonin
  SART (standard acid reflux)
  Saundby (for blood in stool)
  scarification

test *(continued)*
  S-CCK-Pz (secretin, cholecysto-
    kinin, pancreatozymin)
  Schaffer
  Schalfijew
  Scherer
  Schick
  Schiller
  Schilling
  Schivoletto
  Schlesinger
  Schlichter
  Schönbein
  Schroeder
  Schulte
  Schultze
  Schumm
  scratch
  screening
  secretin
  secretin-CCK stimulation
  secretin-pancreozymin
  secretin provocation
  secretin stimulation
  sediment
  sedimentation rate (sed rate)
  Seidel
  SeHCAT (selenium-labeled
    homocholic acid conjugated
    with taurine)
  selenium
  Selivanoff
  semen analysis (sperm count)
  semiquantitative
  senna
  Sereny
  serial cardiac isoenzymes
  serologic (for syphilis) (STS)
  serotonin
  serum amylase
  serum bactericidal activity
  serum iron

test *(continued)*
  serum protein
  serum protein electrophoresis
  serum neutralization
  Sgambati reaction
  SGOT (now AST)
  SGPT (now ALT)
  shake
  sheep cell agglutination (SCAT)
  Sia
  Sicard-Cantelouble
  sickle cell
  Sickledex
  Sicklequik
  sickling
  Siebold and Bradbury
  silver
  Sims
  skin
  skin puncture (for Behçet
    syndrome)
  skin window
  slide
  slide clumping factor
  slide coagulase
  SMAC
  SMA-6
  SMA-12
  SMA-20
  small increment sensitivity index
    (SISI)
  smear
  Smith
  sodium
  Soldaini
  Solera
  solubility screening (for sickle cell
    hemoglobin)
  somatomedin C
  Sonnenschein
  Southern blot
  soybean

test *(continued)*
  specific gravity
  spectrophotometric
  sperm penetration assay
  Spiegler
  Spiro
  spironolactone
  split renal function
  spot (for infectious mononucleosis)
  standard acid reflux (SART)
  standard serologic (for syphilis)
    (STS for syphilis)
  standing plasma
  starch
  starch-iodine
  stat
  Sterneedle tuberculin
  stimulated gastric secretion
  Stock
  Stokvis
  Stoll
  stool cytotoxin
  stool electrolyte
  stool osmolality
  stool osmotic gap
  Strassburg
  Struve
  Stypven time
  sucrose
  sucrose hemolysis
  sucrose lysis
  SUDS (Single Use Diagnostic
    System)
  sulfosalicylic acid turbidity
  sulfur
  Sullivan
  susceptibility
  sweat
  swordfish
  syphilis
  Szabo
  Tanret

test *(continued)*
  taurine
  Taylor
  TCPI Rapid (for HIV)
  Teichmann
  Tensilon
  Test-Tape urine glucose
  testosterone
    free
    total
  TestPackChlamydia
  tetrahydrocortisol (THF)
  tetrahydrodeoxycortisol
  thalleioquin
  thermostable opsonin
  thiocyanate
  Thompson
  Thormählen
  Thorn
  thromboplastin generation
  Thudichum
  thymol turbidity
  thyroglobulin (Tg)
  thyroid antibodies
  thyroid function (TFT)
  thyroid hemagglutination
  thyroid microsomal antibodies
  thyroid-stimulating hormone (TSH)
  thyroid suppression
  thyroid uptake of radioactive iodine
  thyrotropin-releasing hormone (TRH) stimulation
  thyroxine
    free (FT$_4$)
    free (index)
    total
  thyroxine-binding globulin (TBG)
  thyroxine ratio, effective (ETR)
  thyroxine/TBG ratio
  TIBC (total iron-binding capacity)
  Tidy

test *(continued)*
  tilt
  tine
  tine tuberculin
  titratable acidity
  Tizzoni
  tolbutamide
  Tollens, Neuberg, and Schwket
  Torquay
  total catecholamine
  total fecal weight
  total iron-binding capacity (TIBC)
  toxigenicity
  TPHA (*Treponema pallidum* hemagglutination)
  TPI (*Treponema pallidum* immobilization)
  transcortin
  transferrin
  transketolase
  Treponema pallidum complement fixation
  Tretop
  trichophytin
  triglycerides (TG)
  triiodothyronine (T$_3$) resin uptake
  triiodothyronine (T$_3$) uptake
  triketohydrindene hydrate
  triolein-^{131}I absorption
  Trommer
  Trousseau
  tryptophan load
  TSH (thyroid stimulating hormone)
  tube coagulase
  tuberculin
  tuberculosis
  tubular reabsorption of phosphate (TRP)
  T$_3$ uptake
  two-stage prothrombin
  two-stage triolein
  typhoid fever

test *(continued)*
   tyramine
   tyrosine
   Tyson
   Tzanck
   Udranszky
   Uffelmann
   Ulrich
   Ultzmann
   Umber
   unheated serum reagin (USR)
   urea
   urea clearance
   urea concentration
   urea nitrogen
   urea nitrogen/creatinine ratio
   urease
   Urecholine supersensitivity
   uric acid
   Uricult dipslide
   urine (see Table, pp. 561-563)
   urine concentration
   urine sediment
   urine volume
   urobilin
   urobilinogen
   uroporphyrin
   urorosein
   USR (unheated serum reagin)
   vaginal cornification
   vaginal mucification
   Vagitest
   valine
   van Deen (for blood)
   van den Bergh
   van der Velden
   vanillylmandelic acid
   Van Slyke
   vasoactive intestinal polypeptide
     (VIP)
   VDRL (for syphilis)
   ViraPap

test *(continued)*
   Vironostika Mixt ELISA HIV
     antibody
   viscosity
   Vitali
   vitamin A
   vitamin A tolerance
   vitamin B_2
   vitamin B_6
   vitamin B_{12} absorption
   vitamin B_{12} intrinsic factor
   vitamin C
   vitamin C saturation
   vitamin D
   Vitamin D assay
   vitamin E
   Voelcker and Joseph
   Vogel and Lee
   Voges-Proskauer
   Volhard (for renal function)
   Vollmer tuberculin patch
   von Aldor
   von Jaksch
   von Kossa calcium
   von Maschke
   von Pirquet
   von Zeynek and Mencki
   Waaler-Rose
   Wagner
   Waldenström (for porphyrin
     in urine)
   Wang
   Warburg
   Wassermann
   water
   water-gurgle
   water-sipping
   water-soluble contrast esophageal
     swallow
   Watson-Schwartz
   Webster
   Weichbrodt

test *(continued)*
  Weidel
  Weil-Felix
  Weisz
  Welcozyme HIV 1+2 ELISA
    antibody
  Wender
  Wenzell
  Weppen
  Werner thyroid suppression
  Westergren sedimentation rate
  Western immunoblot
  Wetzel
  Weyl
  Wheeler–Johnson
  whiff
  Widal
  Widal agglutination
  Widal serum
  Wideroe
  Widmark
  Wijs
  Wilcoxon
  Williamson blood
  Winckler
  Wishart
  Witz
  Woldman
  Woodbury
  Wood's light
  Worm-Mueller
  Wormley (for alkaloids)
  Wurster (for tyrosine)
  xylose
  xylose absorption
  Yvon (for alkaloids)
  Zaleski
  Zimmermann
  zona-free hamster egg penetration
  Zsigmondy
Tes-Tape urine glucose test
test meal

test on venous blood for:
  bile pigments
  carbohydrates
  electrolytes
  hormones
  lipids
  nitrogenous wastes
  prescribed drugs
  proteins (including enzymes)
  toxic substances
  vitamins
Tes-Tape
test panel
test profile
test result
  abnormal
  high normal
  low normal
  normal
testicles, undescended
testicular artery
testicular atrophy
testicular cyst
testicular degeneration
testicular feminization syndrome
testicular hormone
testicular nerve
testicular tumor
testicular vein
testing
  antibiotic sensitivity
  compatibility (cross-match)
testing antibody
testing antigen
testing electrolyte
testis (pl. testes)
  appendix
  ectopic
  efferent ductules of
  rete
  undescended
testis-determining factor (TDF)

testis teratocarcinoma
testis teratoma
testosterone hormone
testosterone test
  free
  total
TestPackChlamydia (no spaces)
Testut, ligament of
tetanus
tetanus bacillus
tetany
tetrachrome stain
tetrahydrocortisol (THF) test
tetrahydrodeoxycortisol test
tetraiodothyronine (thyroxine, T_4)
tetralogy of Fallot
tetroxide, osmium
Teutleben ligament
Texas fever
texture
  beefy
  bumpy
  buttery
  fleshy
  grainy
  granular
  greasy
  meaty
  nodular
  rough
  rubbery
  smooth
T_4 (thyroxine)
T_4/TBG ratio (thyroxine/thyroxine-
  binding globulin)
TFT (thyroid function test)
T4/T8 ratio
T-4 helper/inducer cell
T-4 lymphocyte
T-4 lymphocyte count
T-8 suppressor/cytotoxic cell
Thai hemorrhagic fever

thalassemia
thalassemia major
thalassemia minor
thalleioquin test for quinine
thallium poisoning
Thayer-Martin culture medium
Thayer-Martin medium
theca (pl. thecae)
  externa
  interna
theca cell of stomach
theca-lutein cell
theca-lutein cyst
thecal abscess
thecal sac
Theile canal
Theile gland
Theiler virus
thelarche
T helper cell
thenar eminence
Theobald Smith phenomenon
therapeutic abortion
therapeutic level of drug
therapeutic malaria
therapeutic range of a drug
therapy
  radiation
  steroid
thermal capacity
thermal energy
Thermoactinomyces sacchari
thermocoagulation change
Thermomax microplate reader
thermostable opsonin test
thiamine
thiazide diabetes
thickened material
thickened plaque
thickening of skin
thick-walled gallbladder
thigh

thigh muscle
thin bone cortex
thin-layer chromatography
thin skin
thin-walled cyst
thin-walled gallbladder
thin-walled hemangiomatous nodule
thin-walled venous sinuses
thiocyanate test
thioflavine T stain
thionin
third-trimester placenta
thixotropy
Thoma fixative
Thoma-Zeiss counting chamber
Thompson ligament
Thompson test
thoracentesis fluid
thoracic aorta
thoracic aorta artery
thoracic aperture
thoracic artery
thoracic bones
thoracic cage
    bony
    osseocartilaginous
thoracic cavity
thoracic duct
thoracic inlet
thoracic kidney
thoracic outlet
thoracic stomach
thoracic vertebra
thoracic wall
thoracic wall bone
thoracoabdominal diaphragm
thoracoabdominal incision
thoracoabdominal nerve
thoracocentesis
thoracolumbar fascia
thorax (pl. thoraces)
thorax, floor of

Thormählen test for melanin in urine
Thorn test
thornlike intercellular bridges
thornlike projections
threadlike
threatened abortion
three-cornered bone
three-vessel umbilical cord
threshold
    convulsant
    galvanic
threshold sugar
throat culture
throat swab
thrombasthenia
thrombin-antithrombin III complex
    (TAT)
thrombin time
thromboangiitis obliterans
thrombocyte
thrombocytopenia
thromboembolic disease
thromboembolism
thrombomodulin
thrombophlebitis
thromboplastin
thromboplastin generation test
thrombosed hemorrhoid
thrombosis
    arterial stenosis without
    intravascular
    recurrent intravascular
    widespread intravascular
thrombosis in arteriosclerotic vessel
thrombosis of a venous sinus
Thrombosphere synthetic platelets
thrombotic infarct
thrombotic thrombocytopenic purpura
    (TTP)
thrombus
    antemortem
    fibrin

thrombus *(continued)*
  lamellated
  laminated
  mural
  organization of
  organized
  postmortem
  traumatic
thrombus embolus
thrush of oral cavity
Thudichum test for creatinine
thumb, principal artery of
thymic abscess
thymic atrophy
thymic dysplasia
thymic lymphopoietic
thymidine, uptake of isotopically
  tagged
thymol turbidity test
thymoma
thymus-dependent lymphocyte
thymus-derived lymphocyte
thymus gland
thymus hyperplasia of
thymus, medulla of
Thy-1 antigen
thyrocervical trunk
thyrocyte
thyroepiglottic ligament
thyroglobulin antibody
thyroglobulin (Tg) test
thyroglossal duct cyst
thyrohyoid ligament
thyroid, accessory
thyroidal clearance
thyroid antibodies test
thyroid artery
thyroid atrophy
thyroid capsule
thyroid carcinoma
thyroid crisis
thyroidectomy

thyroid degeneration
thyroid eminence
thyroid follicle
thyroid function test (TFT)
thyroid gland
  accessory
  enlarged
  hyperplasia of
  indurated
  tender
  woody hard
thyroid goiter
thyroid hemagglutination test
thyroid hormone
  T_3 (triiodothyronine)
  T_4 (tetraiodothyronine, thyroxine)
thyroiditis
  acute
  autoimmune
  chronic fibrous
  de Quervain
  fibrous
  Hashimoto
  invasive fibrous
  ligneous
  lymphocytic
  Riedel
  subacute
  subacute granulomatous
thyroid microsomal antibody
thyroid panel
thyroid profile
thyroid scan (fluorescent scan)
thyroid-stimulating hormone (TSH)
thyroid-stimulating hormone-releasing
  factor (TSH-RF)
thyroid suppression test for hyperthyroidism
thyroid tumor
thyroid uptake tests
  perchlorate discharge test
  RAI (radioactive iodine) uptake test

thyroid *(continued)*
  radioimmunoassay for TSH
  ^{99m}Tc-pertechnetate uptake test
  thyroxine ^{125}I uptake test
  thyroxine ^{131}I uptake test
  TSH stimulation test
  TRH stimulation test
  T_3 suppression test
thyroid uptake of radioactive iodine test
thyrotoxic complement-fixation factor
thyrotoxicosis
thyrotropic hormone
thyrotropin
thyrotropin receptor antibody
thyrotropin-releasing factor (TRF)
thyrotropin-releasing hormone (TRH)
thyrotropin-releasing hormone stimulation test
thyroxine (T_4, tetraiodothyronine)
  free
  total
thyroxine assays
  free thyroxine (FT_4)
  free thyroxine index (FT_4 index)
  protein bound iodine (PBI)
  serum thyroxine by column
    chromatography: T_4(C)
  total serum T_4
thyroxine-binding albumin
thyroxine-binding globulin (TBG)
thyroxine-binding globulin assays
thyroxine-binding prealbumin (TBPA)
thyroxine-binding protein (TBP)
thyroxine hormone
thyroxine I 125 (^{125}I) radioactive agent
thyroxine I 131 (^{131}I) radioactive agent
thyroxine index, free (FT_4 index)
  total T_4
  T_3 resin uptake test
thyroxine ratio, effective (ETR)
thyroxine/TBG ratio
thyroxine test, free (FT_4)

TIBC (total iron-binding capacity)
tibia bone, nutrient artery of
tibial artery, posterior
tibial collateral ligament
tibial nerve, anterior
tibiocalcaneal ligament
tibiofibular articulation
tibiofibular joint
tibiofibular ligament, anterior inferior
tibionavicular ligament
tibiotarsal articulation
tibiotarsal joint
tick bite
tickborne (or tick-borne)
tickborne encephalitis
tickborne fever
tickborne illness
tickborne viruses
Tidy test for albumin in urine
Tiedemann gland
tigering
tightly packed round cell
"tigroid" appearance from fat deposit
tigroid mass
tigroid retina
Tilden stain
tilted sacrum
time
  activated coagulation
  activated thromboplastin
  bleeding
  clotting
  coagulation
  dextrinizing
  euglobulin clot lysis (ECLT)
  fixed interval of
  Mielke bleeding
  one-stage prothrombin
  partial thromboplastin (PTT)
  prothrombin (PT)
  reptilase
  turnaround

time-of-flight measurement
timothy bacillus
T-independent antigen
tinea barbae
tinea capitis
tinea circinata
tinea corporis (ringworm)
tinea cruris (jock itch)
tinea faciei
tinea favosa
tinea glabrosa
tinea imbricata
tinea manuum
tinea nigra palmaris
tinea pedis (athlete's foot)
tinea unguium (dermatophytic
   onychomycosis)
tinea versicolor
tine test
tine tuberculin test
tip of coccyx
tip of spleen
Tiselius apparatus
Tiselius electrophoresis cell
tissue
   aberrant
   abnormal formation of connective
   absence of germinal centers in
     lymphoid
   acinar
   adenoid
   adipose
   aerated lung
   archival
   areolar
   areolar connective
   basement
   blood-forming
   bony
   brain
   breakdown of muscle
   brown adipose

tissue *(continued)*
   cancellous
   cardiac muscle
   cartilaginous
   cavernous
   cellular
   cerebral
   chondroid
   chorionic
   chromaffin
   cicatricial
   clear
   collagenous
   connective
   cortical
   crushed
   damaged
   dartoic
   dead
   debridement
   degenerated
   dense connective
   dermal
   destruction of
   devitalized
   disorganization of connective
   ectopic
   elastic
   endothelial
   epidermal
   epithelial
   erectile
   exocervical
   extracellular
   extraperitoneal
   exuberant granulation
   exuberant hypertrophic granulation
   fatty
   fatty connective
   fibroadipose
   fibroareolar
   fibrocartilaginous

tissue *(continued)*
  fibrofatty
  fibrofatty connective
  fibrohyaline
  fibromuscular
  fibrosing granulation
  fibrous
  fibrous connective
  fibrous scar
  fibrovascular
  flabby
  gelatiginous
  gelatinous
  glandular
  glial
  granulation
  gross examination of
  grumous
  gut-associated lymphoid (GALT)
  healing
  hematopoietic
  hemolymphatic
  hepatic
  heterotopic
  hyperplastic
  infected
  inflamed
  intercellular
  interlobular
  interstitial
  intertrabecular
  joint
  lacerated
  lipomatous-like
  living
  loose connective
  lymphatic
  lymph node
  lymphoid
  lymphoreticular
  mature scar
  mesenchymal

tissue *(continued)*
  mesenteric
  mesocolonic fat
  microscopic examination
  muscle
  muscular
  myeloid
  necrosis
  necrotic
  neoplastic
  nerve
  nervous
  nidus of inflamed
  nidus of necrotic
  nodal
  nonfunctioning
  nongerminal
  nonviable
  normal bone
  osseous
  osteoid
  parafollicular lymphoid
  parenchymal
  periappendiceal adipose
  periarticular
  peribronchial connective
  pericolic adipose
  periorbital
  perisplenic soft
  pliable
  preparation of
  proliferation of fibrous
  regeneration of
  regular connective
  repair of damaged
  representative
  reticular connective
  reticulated
  scar
  septal
  soft
  somatic

tissue *(continued)*
  spinal cord
  splenic
  subcutaneous
  subcutancous connective
  subperitoneal fatty areolar
  synovial
  taenia
  tendon
  underlying
tissue antigen
tissue block
tissue change
tissue culture
tissue death due to
  abnormal antibodies
  circulatory impairment
  malignant tumor
tissue differentiation
tissue equivalent material
tissue factor
tissue fluid
tissue hormone
tissue lymph
tissue metamorphosis
tissue polypeptide antigen (TPA)
tissue section
  mounting of
  staining of
tissue space
tissue specimen
tissue typing
titer
  agglutination
  anti-deoxyribonuclease-B
  antibody
  antihyaluronidase
  ASO (antistreptolysin O)
  heterophile
  serologic
titratable acidity test
titration

Tizzoni stain
Tizzoni test for iron in tissues
T lymphocyte
Tm cell
T method of staining
TNM (tumor size, nodal involvement, metastatic progress) classification
TNM classification
TNM node
TNTC (too numerous to count)
tobacco nodule
Todaro tendon
Todd cirrhosis
Todd units
toe tag
toe, webbed
togavirus
Toison solution
Toison stain
tolbutamide test
Toldt, line of
Tollens, Neuberg, and Schwket test
toluene
toluidine blue
toluidine blue stain
toluol
tones, bowel
T1–T12 (thoracic vertebrae)
tongue
tongue bone
tongue gland
tongue, strawberry
tonofibril
tonofilament
tonsil
  eustachian
  faucial
  lingual
  Luschka
  palatine
  pharyngeal
tonsillar artery

tonsillar crypt
tonsillitis, follicular
tonsil of auditory tube
too numerous to count (TNTC)
tooth (pl. teeth)
Tooth atrophy
tophus (pl. tophi)
TORCH infections (toxoplasmosis,
   rubella, cytomegalovirus,
   herpes simplex)
Tornwaldt abscess
Torquay test for bile
torr (1 millimeter of mercury, mm Hg)
Torrance and Bothwell method
torsional deformity
torsion of spermatic cord
torso crease
tortuous aorta
tortuous tubule
Torulopsis candida
Torulopsis glabrata
torulopsosis
torulosis
torulus
torus
torus tubarius auditory tube
Toscana virus
total catecholamine test
total hematuria
total iron-binding capacity (TIBC)
total knee replacement
total lesion
total lung capacity (TLC)
total necrosis
total protein
total protein concentration of spinal
   fluid
totipotent cell
totipotential cell
toto, in
touch cell
touch prep

tough capsule
tourniquet test for capillary fragility
Tourtual canal
Touton giant cell
Towbin method of immunoblotting
toxemia, bacterial
toxemia of pregnancy
toxemic pneumonia
toxic atrophy
toxic cirrhosis
toxic goiter
toxic granulation
toxic granule
toxic hepatitis
toxic inflammation
toxic insult
toxic level
toxic myocarditis
toxic nephrosis
toxic neuritis
toxic pneumonia
toxic shock syndrome
toxic substances test on venous blood
toxic vacuolization
toxicologic
toxicology screen
toxicosis, Frank capillary
toxigenic
toxigenicity test
toxin
Toxocara canis
Toxoplasma body
Toxoplasma gondii
toxoplasmosis, congenital
toxoplasmotic myocarditis
TPA (tissue plasminogen activator)
TPA (tissue polypeptide antigen)
TP53 tumor suppressor gene
TPHA (*Treponema pallidum*
   hemagglutination) test
TPI (*Treponema pallidum* immobilization) test

trabecula (pl. trabeculae)
trabecular adenocarcinoma
trabecular bone
trabecular degeneration in bronchial
   walls
trabecular endoplasmic reticulum
trabecula, septomarginal
trabeculated
trachea
   annular ligament of
   carina of
   scabbard
tracheal artery
tracheal gland
tracheitis
tracheobronchial lavage
tracheobronchial lymph node
tracheobronchial mucosal inflammation
tracheobronchial mucosal necrosis
tracheobronchial tree
tracheoesophageal (TE)
tracheoesophageal junction
tracheoesophageal fistula
trachoma
trachoma gland
tract
   alimentary
   ascending nerve
   auditory
   biliary
   central tegmental
   cerebellorubral
   cerebellothalamic
   comma
   corticobulbar
   corticopontine
   corticospinal
   crossed pyramidal
   cuneocerebellar
   dead
   deiterospinal
   dentatothalamic

tract *(continued)*
   descending
   digestive
   direct pyramidal
   dorsolateral
   fastigiobulbar
   fistulous
   frontopontine
   frontotemporal
   gastrointestinal (GI)
   geniculocalcarine
   genital
   hepatic outflow
   ileal inflow
   Maissiat
   pancreaticobiliary
   pyramidal
   spinothalamic
   upper gastrointestinal (UGI)
   uveal
traction alopecia
traction artifact
traction diverticulum
traction epiphysis
trait
   dominant
   sickle cell
transaminase
   glutamic oxaloacetic (GOT)
   glutamic pyruvic (GPT)
   serum glutamic-oxaloacetic (SGOT)
   serum glutamic-pyruvic (SGPT)
transbronchial
transcobalamin 2 deficiency
transcortin test
transdermal patch for glucose
   monitoring
transducer cell
transect
transepithelial migration
transepithelial migration of chronic
   inflammatory cells

transferase
  gamma-glutamyl (GGT)
  glucuronyl
  terminal deoxynucleotidyl (TdT)
transfer factor
transferrin test
transformation zone
transforming factor
transforming gene
transforming growth factor
transfusion
  arterial
  autologous
  blood
  direct
  exchange
  exsanguination
  fetomaterial
  immediate
  indirect
  intraperitoneal
  intrauterine
  mediate
  mismatched blood
  packed red blood cell
  placental
  reciprocal
  twin-to-twin
transfusion hepatitis
transfusion malaria
transfusion nephritis
transfusion of incompatible blood
transfusion reaction
transfusion recipient
transient acantholytic dermatosis
transient hyperphenylalaninemia
transient neonatal systemic lupus
  erythematosus
transient phenylketonuria
transient proteinuria
transilluminate
transillumination

transitional cell
transitional cell carcinoma
transitional cell papilloma
transitional epithelial cell
transitional epithelium
transitional meningioma
transition zone
transitory gastroenteritis
transitory loss of consciousness
transitory papule
transketolase test
translocation
  chromosomal abnormality of
  reciprocal
  robertsonian
transmission electron microscope
transmural myocardial infarction
transneuronal atrophy
transneuronal degeneration
transparency
transparent
transpeptidase
  gamma-glutamyl (GGTP)
  serum gamma-glutamyl (SGGT)
transplant (or transplantation)
  allogeneic
  bone marrow
  cadaveric
  corneal
  heart
  heart-lung
  hematopoietic stem cell (HSC)
  heterotopic
  homotopic
  kidney
  liver
  living related donor
  living unrelated donor
  orthotopic
  pancreas
  renal
  syngeneic

transplant *(continued)*
  syngenesioplastic
  tendon
  tooth
transport medium
transport protein
transport vesicle
transposition of great vessels
transpyloric plane (TPP)
transseptal needle
transtubercular plane (TTP)
transudate
transudative
transumbilical plane (TUP)
transurethral resection of prostate
  (TURP)
transverse aorta
transverse artery of neck
transverse atlantal ligament
transverse band
transverse carpal ligament
transverse cerebral fissure
transverse cervical artery
transverse colon
transverse colon loop
transverse crural ligament
transverse facial artery
transverse genicular ligament
transverse humeral ligament
transverse ligament
transverse mesocolon
transverse metacarpal ligament
transverse metatarsal ligament
transverse muscle of tongue
transverse myelitis
transverse oval pelvis
transverse palatine folds
transverse pericardial sinus
transverse perineal artery
transverse perineal muscle
transverse process
transverse rectal fold

transverse scapular artery
transverse section
transverse sinus
transverse tarsal articulation
transverse tarsal joint
transverse tibiofibular ligament
transversus abdominis muscle
trapezium bone
trapezoid bone
trapezoid ligament
Traube semilunar space
trauma
  acoustic
  birth
  blunt
  multiple
  penetrating
  physical
traumatic alopecia
traumatic aneurysm
traumatic degeneration
traumatic herpes
traumatic inflammation
traumatic meningocele
traumatic neuritis
traumatic orchitis
traumatic pneumonia
traumatic scar
traumatic thrombus
traumatopneic wound
trauma to spinal cord
Trautmann triangular space
TRC (tanned red cell)
Treacher Collins syndrome
treatment, acid-wash
tree
  biliary
  hepatobiliary
  tracheobronchial
trefoil dermatitis
trefoil tendon
Treitz arch

Treitz, ligament of
trematode (fluke)
trench mouth
Treponema
Treponema buccale
Treponema carateum
Treponema pallidum
Treponema pallidum complement
   fixation test
Treponema pallidum immobilization
   (TPI) test
Treponema pallidum pertenue
Treponema pertenue
Treponema vincentii
treponematosis
Tretop test
triad
   acute compression
   Charcot
   Dieulafoy
   hepatic
   portal
   Saint
   Whipple
triangle
   anal
   auricular
   axillary
   Calot
   cardiohepatic
   carotid
   cephalic
   cervical
   clavipectoral
   crural
   cystohepatic
   deltoideopectoral
   digastric
   facial
   femoral
   Grynfeltt
   Henke

triangle *(continued)*
   Hesselbach
   inguinal
   Labbe
   Lesgaft
   Livingston
   lumbocostoabdominal
   mesenteric
   Pawlik
   Scarpa
   urogenital
   vertebrocostal
triangular bone
triangular fibrocartilage
triangular fibrocartilage complex
triangular fontanelle
triangular ligaments of liver
triangular muscle
triangular suprarenal gland
tributary
trichilemmoma
Trichinella myocarditis
Trichinella spiralis
trichinosis
trichinous embolism
trichinous myositis
trichocyst
trichoma
trichomonal vaginitis
Trichomonas tenax
Trichomonas vaginalis
trichomoniasis, vaginal
trichophytic granuloma
trichophytin test
Trichophyton
Trichophyton ajelloi
Trichophyton concentricum
Trichophyton equinum
Trichophyton fisheri
Trichophyton flavescens
Trichophyton floccosum
Trichophyton georgiae

Trichophyton gloriae
Trichophyton gourvilii
Trichophyton longifusum
Trichophyton mariatii
Trichophyton megninii
Trichophyton mentagrophytes
Trichophyton phaseoliforme
Trichophyton rubrum
Trichophyton schoenleinii
Trichophyton simii
Trichophyton soudanense
Trichophyton terrestre
Trichophyton tonsurans
Trichophyton vanbreuseghemii
Trichophyton verrucosum
Trichophyton violaceum
Trichosporon beigelii
trichosporosis
trichrome stain
trichuriasis (whipworm)
Trichuris trichiura
trick knee
tricuspid orifice
tricuspid valve
tricuspid valvular leaflet
trifid stomach
trigeminal cave
trigeminal impression
trigeminal nerve
trigger finger
triglyceride enzyme deficiency
triglyceride level, normal fasting
triglycerides (TG)
   long chain (LCT)
   medium chain (MCT)
   serum
trigone
   angles of
   collateral
   deltoideopectoral
   Henke
   hypoglossal

trigone *(continued)*
   Lieutaud
   Müller
   Pawlik
   vertebrocostal
trigone of bladder
trihexosidase, ceramide
triiodothyronine (T_3) hormone
triiodothyronine resin uptake test
triiodothyronine uptake test
triketohydrindene hydrate test
trimellitic anhydritic pneumonitis
triolein–^{131}I absorption test
triple phosphate
triquetral bone
triquetrohamate joint
triquetrum
Tris-HCl
trisomy
Triton X-100 buffer solution
trocar, aspiration
trocar plug
trochanter
   greater
   lesser
trochanteric bursitis
trochlea
trochlear
trochoid joint
trochoidal articulation
Trommer test for glucose in urine
trophic lesion
trophoblast
trophoblastic
trophozoite
tropical abscess
tropical ear
tropical eczema
tropical stomatitis
tropical swelling
tropic hormone
troponin T protein in cardiac muscle

trough, gingival
trough level
Trousseau test for bile in urine
Truant auramine–rhodamine stain
Trucut cutting biopsy needle
true aneurysm
true back muscles
true mole
true pelvis
true plasma
true proteinuria
true rib
truncus arteriosus
   embryonic
   persistent
trunk
   articulations of
   atrioventricular (AV)
   bifurcation of pulmonary
   brachiocephalic
   bronchomediastinal
   bronchomediastinal lymph
   celiac
   cordlike
   costocervical
   joints of
   lumbosacral
   lymph
   nerve
   posterior vagal
   thyrocervial
   vagal
trunk artery
trypan blue
Trypanosoma cruzi
Trypanosoma gambiense
Trypanosoma rhodesiense
trypanosome
trypticase soy agar
trypticase soy broth
tryptic soy agar with sRBC
trypsin G-banding stain

tryptophan load test
T_3 (triiodothyronine)
T_3 resin uptake (triiodothyronine
   uptake)
TSH (thyroid stimulating hormone)
TTP (thrombotic thrombocytopenic
   purpura)
tubal abortion
tubal air cell
tubal canal
tubal ligation
tubal mole
tubal nephritis
tubal pregnancy
tube
   auditory
   bronchial
   calices (calyces)
   capillary
   corneal
   digestive
   endotracheal (ET)
   Eppendorf
   eustachian
   fallopian
   muscular
   nasogastric (NG)
   neural
   separator
   solid-phase extraction
   uterine
tube coagulase test
tubercle
   accessory
   acoustic
   adductor
   amygdaloid
   articular
   ashen
   auricular
   calcaneal
   carotid

tubercle *(continued)*
  conoid
  corniculate
  crown
  cuneiform
  darwinian
  dental
  dissection
  epiglottic
  fibrous
  genital
  Ghon
  greater
  iliac
  lesser
  Lister
  postmortem
  prominent scalene
  pubic
  scalene
  sella turcica
tubercle bacillus
tubercle of Darwin, auricular
tubercle of rib, facet for
tubercle of temporal bone, articular
tuberculin test
tuberculoid leprosy
tuberculoid lesion
tuberculoid myocarditis
tuberculosis
  avian
  bone
  disseminated
  exudative
  fulminant
  genitourinary
  hematogenous
  inhalation
  meningeal
  miliary
  postprimary
  primary

tuberculosis *(continued)*
  pulmonary
  renal
tuberculosis of bone
tuberculosis test
tuberculous abscess
tuberculous arthritis
tuberculous gumma
tuberculous infiltration
tuberculous meningitis
tuberculous myocarditis
tuberculous nephritis
tuberculous nodule
tuberculous pericarditis
tuberculous pneumonia
tuberculous salpingitis
tuberculous spondylitis
tuberculum
tuberosity (pl. tuberosities)
  bicipital
  calcaneal
  coracoid
  costal
  deltoid
  ischial
  omental
tuberous sclerosis
tuboabdominal pregnancy
tuboligamentary pregnancy
tubo-ovarian abscess
tubo-ovarian pregnancy
tubotympanic canal
tubouterine pregnancy
tubular aneurysm
tubular gland
tubular reabsorption of phosphate
  (TRP) test
tubule
  collecting
  connecting
  convoluted
  convoluted seminiferous

tubule *(continued)*
 dental
 dentinal
 discharging
 distal convoluted
 proximal convoluted
 renal
 seminiferous
 straight
 tortuous
tubulitis
tubuloacinar gland
tubuloalveolar gland
Tuffier inferior ligament
tufted cell
tuft, vascular
tularemia
tularemic pneumonia
tumor
 adrenal
 anaplastic
 Askin
 benign epidermal
 bladder
 bone
 breast
 Brenner
 brown
 carcinoid
 CNS (central nervous system)
 cutaneous
 dental
 discrete
 embryonal
 endocardial
 Ewing
 focal
 gastrin-secreting non-beta islet cell
 gastrointestinal
 giant cell
 globular
 grading

tumor *(continued)*
 granular cell
 granulosa cell
 gray
 gritty
 gross
 highly vascular
 intracranial
 invasive
 islet cell
 kidney
 Krukenberg
 liver
 lobulated
 locally invasive
 lung
 lymphoid
 main
 malignant
 malignant mesenchymal
 metastatic
 myxomatous
 ovarian
 pancreatic
 pancreatic islet cell
 paraffin
 parathyroid
 periampullary
 pituitary
 reddish
 retinal
 salivary gland
 scirrhous
 small cell
 submucosal
 subserosal
 testicular
 thyroid
 urinary
 uterine
 vascular cutaneous and hepatic
 virilizing adrenal

tumor *(continued)*
   Warthin (adenolymphoma)
   Wharton (cystadenoma)
   white
   Wilms
tumoral calcinosis
tumor angiogenic factor (TAF)
tumor antigen
tumor capsule
tumor embolism
tumor erosion
tumor marker
   AFP (alpha-fetoprotein)
   CA 15-2 RIA
   CA 15-3 antigen
   CA 15-3 breast cancer
   CA 19-9 antigenic
   CA 19-9 carbohydrate antigen
   CA 27.29
   CA 50
   CA 72-4 antigen
   CA 125 antigen
   CA 125 cross-reactivity
   CA 125 ovarian
   CA 125-11
   CA 195
   CA 549 breast cancer
   CA M26
   CA M29
   CEA (carcinoembryonic antigen)
   PSA (prostate-specific antigen)
tumor mass
tumor necrosis factor (TNF)
tumor registry
tumor-specific antigen
tumor staging
tumor suppressor gene
   APC (adenomatous polyposis coli)
   DCC (deleted in colon carcinoma)
   mutant
   NF (neurofibromatosis)
   NF1

tumor suppressor gene *(continued)*
   NF2
   p53
   RB1
   TP53
   VHL
   WT1
tumor virus
tunica adventitia
tunica albuginea
tunica fibrosa
tunica intima
tunica media
tunica mucosa
tunica muscularis
tunica propria
tunica serosa
tunica vaginalis
tunnel
   carpal
   cubital
   retropancreatic
   tarsal
tunnel cell
turbid fluid
turbidity
turbinate(d) bones
Turbo TMB colorimetric reader
turcica, sella
Türck degeneration
Türk cell
Türk irritation leukocyte
turnaround time
Turnbull blue
Turner biopsy needle
Turner syndrome
TURP (transurethral resection of
   prostate)
Tween-albumin broth culture
Tween-20
20-channel chemistry profile
24-hour urine specimen

twig
   cutaneous
   muscular
twigs to pelvic diaphragm
twigs to piriformis muscle
twin pregnancy
twin-to-twin transfusion
twisted
2060 virus
two-hour postprandial blood-sugar
   level
two-hour postprandial sugar
Twort-d'Herelle bacteriophagia
   phenomenon
two-stage prothrombin test
two-step indirect immunoperoxidase
   method
two-vessel umbilical cord
tympanic air cell
tympanic artery
tympanic bone
tympanic canal
tympanic cell
tympanic gland
tympanic membrane, perforated
tympanitic abscess
tympanocervical abscess
tympanohyal bone
tympanomastoid abscess
tympanostapedial junction
Tyndall light
type and crossmatch (T&C)
type, blood (blood group)
type I cell

type I diabetes mellitus
type 1 hereditary orotic aciduria
type I insulin-dependent diabetes
type II cell
type II diabetes mellitus
type II non-insulin-dependent diabetes
typhoid bacillus
typhoid fever
typhoid fever test
typhoid nodule
typhoid osteomyelitis
typhoid pleurisy
typhoid pneumonia
typhus
   endemic
   epidemic
   flea-borne
   louse-borne
   scrub
typhus nodule
typical rib
typing
   blood
   column
   tissue
typing and crossmatching of blood
   for transfusion
tyramine test
tyrosine test
Tyson gland
Tyson test for bile acids in urine
Tzanck cell
Tzanck smear of vagina
Tzanck test

U, u

ubiquinone
ubiquitin
U-cell lymphoma
UCHL1 monoclonal antibody
Udranszky test for bile acids
U echovirus
Uffelmann test
Uganda S virus
ulcer
    acute peptic
    anastomotic
    aphthous
    buccal
    cervical
    chiclero
    chronic
    chronic peptic
    corneal
    Curling
    Cushing
    cutaneous
    decubitus
    duodenal
    flask-shaped
    gastric
    genital
    granulomatous

ulcer *(continued)*
    healing
    herpes
    Hunner
    incised
    intestinal
    mucosal
    oral
    painless indurated
    penetrating
    peptic
    puncture
    rodent
    shallow mucosal
    urinary
    venereal
ulceration
    corneal
    gastrointestinal
ulcerative colitis
ulcerative dermatosis
ulcerative inflammation
ulcerative stomatitis
Ulex europaeus agglutinin 1
ulnar artery
ulnar bone
ulnar carpal artery

ulnar collateral artery
ulnar collateral ligament of elbow
ulnar collateral ligament of wrist
ulnar head
ulnocarpal ligament
ulnolunate ligament
ulnotriquetral ligament
Ulrich test for albumin
ultimobranchial gland
ultimobranchial pouch
ultracentrifugation
ultracentrifuge
ultramicrotome
ultrasound diagnosis
ultrathin section
ultraviolet light
ultraviolet radiation
ultravirus
Ultzmann test for bile pigments
Umber test for scarlet fever
umbilical artery in fetus
umbilical canal
umbilical cord
   three-vessel
   two-vessel
umbilical fold
umbilical hernia
umbilical ligament
umbilical region
umbilical vein
umbilicated
umbilicus
umbilicus granuloma
umbrella cell
unattended death
unciform bone
uncinarial dermatitis
uncinate process of pancreas
uncircumcised
unconjugated bilirubin, deposition of
uncontrolled diabetes
uncontused

unconventional virus
uncoupling protein
uncovertebral joint
uncus
undegenerated nerve cell
underlying tissue
undersurface of liver
undescended testicle
undescended testis
undifferentiated adenocarcinoma
undifferentiated carcinoma
undifferentiated carcinoma of thyroid
undifferentiated cell
undifferentiated columnar epithelial
   cell
undifferentiated leukemia
undifferentiated lymphoma
undigested food in stool
undilated
undulant fever
unencapsulated
unequivocal
unesterified free fatty acid
unformed stool
unheated serum reagin (USR) test
uniaxial joint
unicellular gland
unicellular microorganism
unicellular organism
unicornis, uterus
unilateral facial atrophy
unilobular cirrhosis
unilocular cyst
unilocular joint
unilocular pustule
un-ionized acid
unipennate muscle
unipolar cell
unit
   arbitrary
   Bessey-Lowry
   Bodansky

unit *(continued)*
 IU (international)
 King-Armstrong
 mIU (milli-international)
 motor
 pilosebaceous
 SI (Système International)
 Todd
uniting canal
units per volume
unmyelinated postganglionic fibers
Unna disease
Unna mark
Unna nevus
Unna-Pappenheim stain
Unna stain
Unna-Taenzer stain
unobstructed
unpaired visceral branches
unremarkable
unresolved pneumonia
unruptured follicles
unsaturated fatty acid
unsegmented neutrophils
unstable hemoglobin
unsuspected cause of death
unwinding protein
upper esophageal sphincter (UES)
upper extremity
upper gastrointestinal tract (UGI)
upper jaw bone
upper limb
upper lip
upper motor neuron lesion
Uppsala virus
uptake of isotopically tagged thymidine
urachal adenocarcinoma
urachal ligament
urachus
uranium nitrate
uranoschisis
uranyl acetate

uranyl acetate stain
urate, amorphous
urate calculus
urate crystals
urate crystals stain
urea (urea nitrogen)
urea clearance test
urea concentration test for renal
 efficiency
urea nitrogen (BUN, blood urea
 nitrogen)
urea nitrogen/creatinine ratio
urea nitrogen test
urea, urinary
Ureaplasma urealyticum
urease-producing organism
urease test
Urecholine supersensitivity test
uremia
uremic acidosis
uremic coma
uremic pneumonitis
uremic pruritus
uremic stomatitis
ureter
 circumcaval
 ectopic
 kinked
 postcaval
 retrocaval
 retroiliac
ureteral colic
ureteral meatus
ureteral opening
ureteral orifice
ureteric artery
ureteric calculus
ureteric pelvis
ureteric stone
ureteropelvic junction (UPJ)
ureterovesical junction (UVJ)
ureterovesical obstruction

urethra
  bulb of
  membranous
  prostatic
  spongy
urethral abscess
urethral artery
urethral bulb artery
urethral calculus
urethral crest
urethral discharge
urethral diverticulum
urethral gland
urethral groove
urethral hematuria
urethral orifice, external
urethral pressure profile
urethritis
  gonococcal
  gonorrheal
  gouty
  granular casts in
  nongonococcal
  nonspecific
  prophylactic
  simple
  specific
urethrovaginal fistula
uric acid
uric acid crystals in gout
uric acid infarct
uric acid test
Uricult dipslide test
urinalysis
urinary (see *urine*)
urinary abscess
urinary aldosterone
urinary amylase
urinary arsenic
urinary bladder
urinary bladder fundus
urinary calculus

urinary catecholamines
urinary creatinine
urinary excretion of coproporphyrin
urinary excretion of 5-hydroxy-
  indolcacetic acid (5-HIAA)
urinary excretion of 17-ketosteroid
urinary hemoglobin
urinary 17-ketosteroid excretion
urinary lead level
urinary leukocyte esterase test (LET)
urinary metanephrines
urinary mucosa
urinary obstruction
urinary osmolality
urinary oxalate
urinary protein
urinary protein electrophoresis
urinary red blood cell (RBC)
urinary sediment
urinary smear
urinary specific gravity
urinary stone
urinary tract infection (UTI)
urinary tumor
urinary ulcer
urinary urea
urinary urobilinogen
urinary urobilinogen excretion
urine
  abnormal casts in
  acetone in
  albumin in
  amber color
  amorphous sediment in
  Bence Jones protein in
  bilirubin in
  black
  calcareous material in
  cells in sediment of
  chorionic gonadotropin in
  chylous
  clarity of

urine *(continued)*
  clean-catch
  clear
  cloudiness of
  cloudy
  Coca-Cola
  color of
  crude
  crystals in
  dark concentrated
  diabetic
  dried smears of
  dyspeptic
  febrile
  fragments of tissue in
  freshly voided
  gouty
  granular casts in
  high-colored
  homogeneous casts in
  honey
  hyaline casts in
  ketones in
  leakage of
  light-colored
  maple syrup odor in
  milky
  mucus shreds in
  myoglobin in
  nebulous
  odorous
  pink
  pregnancy
  protein in
  residual
  scanty
  smoky brown
  specific gravity of
  straw-colored
  turbidity of
  watery
  yellow

urine, abnormalities in
  bile
  bilirubin
  blood
  color changes due to
      abnormal waste products
      drugs
      pigments from foods
  crystals of sulfanilamide derivatives
  cystine
  epithelial cells
  fat
  glucose
  granular casts
  hemoglobin
  hyaline casts
  ketone bodies
  mucous casts
  occult blood
  proteins
  proteoses
  pus
  spermatozoa
  waxy casts
urine androgen level
urine bacilli
urine chloride
urine colony count
urine concentration test
urine culture
urine cytology
urine dip slide
urine electrolyte
urine estrogen level
urine glucose
urine leakage
urine osmolality
urine pH
urine/plasma ratio (U/P)
urine reaction
urine sediment test
urine smear

urine specimen
   catheterized
   clean catch
   clean-voided
   first-voided
   freshly voided
   midstream
   twenty-four hour
urine sediment test
urine specific gravity
urine stagnation
urine sugar
urine tests (see Table, pp. 561-563)
urine volume
uriniparous
urinocryoscopy
urinogenital
urinogenous
urinoglucosometer
urinoma
urinometer
urinophilous
urinosexual
urinous infiltration
uriposia
Uristix
uroacidimeter
uroammoniac
uroazotometer
urobilin
urobilinemia
urobilinogen
   fecal
   stool
   urinary
urobilinogen excretion
urobilinogen test
urobilin test
urobilinuria
urocanase deficiency
urocele
urochezia

urocystitis
Urocyte diagnostic cytometry system
uroerythrin
urofuscin
urofuscohematin
urogenital canal
urogenital diaphragm
urogenital region
urogenital triangle
urolithiasis
uropathy, obstructive
uroporphyrinogen-1-synthetase enzyme
uroporphyrin test
uropygial gland
urorosein test
urothelial cell
urothelium
urticaria
urticarial eruption
urticaria pigmentosa with systemic
   mastocytosis
urushiol (skin-sensitizing agent)
USR (unheated serum reagin) test
uta (leishmaniasis)
uteri, fundus
uterine artery
uterine calculus
uterine canal
uterine cavity
uterine cervical ganglion
uterine cervix
uterine didelphia
uterine dysfunctional bleeding
uterine fibroid
uterine fibromyoma
uterine fundus
uterine gland
uterine horn
uterine leiomyoma (leiomyomata)
uterine myometrium
uterine ostium
uterine polyp

uterine relaxing factor (URF)
uterine tube, ampulla of
uterine tumor
uteroabdominal pregnancy
uterocervical canal
uterosacral ligament
uterotubal junction
uterotubal pregnancy
uterovaginal canal
uterovaginal plexus
uterovesical junction
uterovesical ligament
uterovesical pouch
uterus
    adhesions of
    anteflexed
    anteverted
    aplastic
    bicameral
    bicornuate
    bilocular
    bipartite
    bleeding, dysfunctional
    boggy
    broad ligament of
    cervix of
    cochleate
    cornu of
    Couvelaire
    didelphic
    double
    double-mouthed
    duplex
    fetal
    fibroid
    gravid
    heart-shaped
    horn of
    hypoplastic
    infantile
    isthmus of
    pear-shaped

uterus *(continued)*
    pregnant
    pubescent
    retroflexed
    retroverted
    ribbon
    round ligament of
    saddle-shaped
    septate
uterus arcuatus
uterus bicameratus vetularum
uterus bicornis
uterus bicornis bicollis
uterus bicornis unicollis
uterus biforis
uterus bilocularis
uterus bipartitus
uterus cordiformis
uterus didelphys
uterus incudiformis
uterus masculinus
uterus parvicollis
uterus planifundalis
uterus rudimentarius
uterus septus
uterus simplex
uterus subseptus
uterus triangularis
uterus unicornis
UTI (urinary tract infection)
utricle
    prostatic
    urethral
utricular gland
utriculosaccular canal
uveal melanoma
uveal nevus
uveal tract
uveitis (pl. uveitides)
    anterior
    Förster
    granulomatous

uveitis *(continued)*
   lens-induced
   nongranulomatous
   phacoantigenic
   phacotoxic
   posterior

uveoparotid fever
U virus
UVJ (ureterovesical junction)
uvula of bladder

V, v

Vabra aspiration
vaccinia virus
vacuolar degeneration of adrenal and
   thyroid glands
vacuolar degeneration of sarcoplasm
vacuolar nephrosis
vacuolated cells
vacuolating virus
vacuolation of cells
vacuole
   autophagic
   contractile
   cytoplasmic
   fatty
vacuoles in stratum granulosum
vacuolization, toxic
Vacutainer
vagal trunk
vagina
   anterior fornix of
   azygos artery of
   Candida albicans infection of
   double
   fornix of
   genital warts of
   gonorrheal infection of
   herpes simplex lesions of

vagina *(continued)*
   Neisseria gonorrhoeae infection of
   squamous cell carcinoma of
   syphilitic chancres of
   Trichomonas vaginalis infection of
   vestibule of
vagina, ectocervix, endocervix (VCE)
   smear
vagina fundus
vaginal adenocarcinoma
vaginal adenosis
vaginal artery
vaginal atrophy
vaginal bands, transverse
vaginal canal
vaginal candidiasis
vaginal carcinoma
vaginal clear cell adenocarcinoma
vaginal cornification
vaginal cyst
vaginal cytology
vaginal epithelial abnormality
vaginal flora
vaginal fornix
vaginal gland
vaginal hypertrophy
vaginal intraepithelial neoplasia (VIN)

vaginal introitus, complete closure of
vaginal irrigation smear
vaginalis
  Candida
  Gardnerella
  Neisseria
  Trichomonas
vaginal microflora
vaginal mucification test
vaginal mucosa
vaginal opening
vaginal orifice
vaginal pH
vaginal plexus
vaginal secretion
vaginal smear
vaginal trichomoniasis
vaginal wall
vaginitis
  adhesive
  atrophic
  chlamydial
  desquamative inflammatory
  diphtheritic
  emphysematous
  Gardnerella
  monilial
  nonspecific
  senile
  trichomonal
  yeast
vaginomycosis
vaginosis, bacterial
Vagitest
vagus, auricular nerve of
vagus nerve
vagus pneumonia
valgus, cubitus
valine test
vallate papillae
vallecula (pl. valleculae)
vallecular pooling

valley fever
valproic acid
Valsalva antrum
Valsalva ligaments
valve
  anal
  aortic
  aortic semilunar
  atrioventricular
  ball
  bicuspid
  capillary
  cardiac
  caval
  coronary
  eustachian
  frenulum of
  globular
  ileocecal
  incompetent
  leaky mitral
  mitral
  pulmonary
  pulmonic
  rectal
  semilunar
  tricuspid
  venous
valve cusp
valve leaflet
valve of Bauhin
valve of coronary sinus
valve of Houston
valve of Kerckring
valve of navicular fossa
valvula (pl. valvulae)
valvular leaflet
valvular ring
valvular sclerosis
van Deen test for blood
van den Bergh test
van der Velden test

van Ermengen stain
van Gieson stain
van Heuven anatomic classification of
    diabetic retinopathy
van Horne canal
vanillylmandelic acid (VMA)
Vanox fluorescence microscope
Vanox-T microscope
Van Slyke apparatus
Van Slyke test
variant, clear cell
variation, alpha-beta
variceal column
variceal wall
varicella (chickenpox)
varicella pneumonia
Varicellavirus
varicella-zoster virus
varices (pl. of varix), esophageal
varicocele
varicose aneurysm
varicose eczema
varicose vein
varicosity (pl. varicosities)
variegated
variegate porphyria (VP)
variola (smallpox)
variola virus (now extinct)
varix (pl. varices)
    cirsoid
    conjunctival
    esophageal
vascular apron
vascular atrophy
vascular birthmark
vascular cirrhosis
vascular collapse
vascular congestion
vascular cutaneous and hepatic tumors
vascular disease of retina
vascular engorgement
vascular gland

vascular goiter
vascular hemophilia
vascular hypertension
vascularization in cornea
vascularization, patches of
vascular myxoma
vascular nephritis
vascular nevus
vascular osteitis
vascular plexus
vascular polyp
vascular sclerosis
vascular tuft
vascular wall
vasculitic rejection
vasculitis
    granulomatous
    obliterative
    systemic necrotizing
vas deferens, artery of
vasoactive cell
vasoactive intestinal peptide (VIP)
vasoactive intestinal polypeptide (VIP)
vasoconstriction
vasodilation
vasoformative cell
vasomotor nerve
vasopressin hormone
vasopressin-resistant diabetes
vasorum, vasa
Vater
    ampulla of
    papilla of
vaterian segment
vault
    cranial
    rectal
VCE (vagina, ectocervix, endocervix)
    smear
VDRL (Venereal Disease Research
    Laboratory)
VDRL antigen

VDRL test for syphilis
veal infusion
vector
  arthropod
  biological
  mechanical
vector-borne infection
vegetation, destructive
vegetations of cardiac valve
vegetative form
veil (or veiled) cell
Veillonella
Veillonella parvula
vein (see Table of Veins)
  accessory cephalic
  accessory hemiazygos
  accessory saphenous
  accessory vertebral
  accompanying
  anal
  anastomosing
  anastomotic
  angular
  anonymous
  antebrachial
  anterior cardiac
  anterior jugular
  appendicular
  aqueous
  arciform
  arcuate
  arterial
  ascending lumbar
  auditory
  auricular
  axillary
  azygos
  basal
  basilic
  basivertebral
  brachial
  brachiocephalic

vein *(continued)*
  bronchial
  capillary
  cardiac
  cardinal
  cavernous
  central
  cephalic
  cerebral
  cervical
  choroid
  ciliary
  circumflex
  colic
  common basal
  common cardinal
  common facial
  companion
  condylar emissary
  conjunctival
  coronary
  costoaxillary
  cutaneous
  cystic
  digital
  diploic
  dorsispinal
  duodenal
  embryonic umbilical
  emissary
  epigastric
  episcleral
  esophageal
  ethmoidal
  external pudendal
  facial
  femoral
  fibular
  frontal
  gastric
  gastroepiploic
  great cardiac

vein *(continued)*
  great saphenous
  hemiazygos
  hepatic
  ileocolic
  inferior pulmonary
  inferior rectal
  intercostal
  jugular
  labial
  left hepatic
  median antebrachial
  mesenteric
  middle cardiac
  middle rectal
  oblique
  pancreatic
  paraumbilical
  pericardial
  portal
  posterior auricular
  prepyloric
  pudendal
  pulmonary
  renal
  Retzius
  saphenous
  scrotal
  small cardiac
  splenic
  subclavian
  superior mesenteric
  superior pulmonary
  superior rectal
  systemic
  testicular
  varicose
vein stripper
velamentous insertion
velamentous placenta
vellus hair
Velpeau canal

velvetlike
velvety
vena cava
  inferior
  infrahepatic
  superior
  suprahepatic
Venereal Disease Research Laboratory
  (VDRL)
venereal ulcer
venereal warts
venereum, lymphogranuloma
venipuncture
venosum, ligamentum
venosus, sinus
venous angioma
venous blood
venous capillary
venous congestion
venous dorsal arch
venous embolism
venous groove
venous lake
venous ligament
venous network
venous obstruction
venous plexus
  prostatic
  vertebral
  vesical
venous sinus of brain
venous stasis
venous system, portal
venous valves
venous web
ventilation pneumonitis
ventral aorta
ventral hernia
ventral horn
ventral mesentery
ventral pancreatic bud
ventral primary ramus

ventral root
ventral sacrococcygeal ligament
ventral sacroiliac ligament
ventricle
  Arantius
  auxiliary
  cephalic
  cerebral
  double-inlet left
  double-inlet right
    associated with pulmonary
      stenosis
    doubly committed
    subaortic
    subpulmonic
    uncommitted
  double-outlet left
  double-outlet right
  Duncan (fifth)
  fifth
  fourth
  Galen
  laryngeal
  lateral
  left
  Morgagni
  pineal
  right (of heart)
  single
  sixth (Verga)
  Sylvius
  terminal
  third
  Verga
ventricles of brain
  fourth
  lateral (two)
  third
ventricular aneurysm
ventricular canal
ventricular free wall
ventricular ligament

ventricular loop
ventricular papillary muscle
ventricular septal defect
venule
vera, polycythemia
Verga lacrimal groove
Verga ventricle
verge, anal
Verhoeff elastic stain
vermian fossa
vermiform appendix
vermiform body
vermiform granule
vermilion border
verminous abscess
verminous dermatitis
vermis
vernal conjunctivitis
Verneuil canal
Vero cell culture
verruca vulgaris
verrucous carcinoma
verrucous hemangioma
verrucous nevus
verruga peruana
versicolor, tinea
vertebra (pl. vertebrae)
  articular process of
  basilar
  caudal
  cervical (C1 through C7)
  coccygeal
  codfish
  cranial
  dorsal (D)
  false
  lumbar (L1 through L5)
  sacral (S1 through S5)
  thoracic (T1 through T12)
  true
vertebral arch
vertebral artery

vertebral body
vertebral canal
vertebral column
vertebral foramen
vertebral fracture
vertebral groove
vertebral part of medial surface
vertebral pleural reflection
vertebral spinous process
vertebral venous plexus
vertebra prominens
vertebrocostal rib
vertebrocostal triangle
vertebrocostal trigone
vertebropelvic ligament
vertebrosternal rib
vertical cleft
vertical heart
vertical muscle of tongue
verumontanum
very low density lipoprotein (VLDL)
Vesalius bone
vesical artery
vesical calculus
vesical fistula
vesical hematuria
vesical plexus
vesical scrapings
vesical venous plexus
vesication
vesicle
   acoustic
   acrosomal
   air
   allantoic
   auditory
   blastodermic
   cerebral
   cervical
   cutaneous
   encephalic
   germinal

vesicle *(continued)*
   seminal
   transport
vesicle of endoplasmic reticulum
vesicoprostatic calculus
vesicoumbilical ligament
vesicourethral canal
vesicouterine fistula
vesicouterine ligament
vesicouterine pouch
vesicovaginal space
vesicular dermatitis
vesicular eruption
vesicular mole
vesicular nuclei
vesicular pharyngitis
vesicular stomatitis virus
vesiculation
Vesiculovirus
vessel
   afferent
   afferent lymph
   arcuate
   blood
   capillary
   chyle
   collateral
   collecting
   deep lymph
   efferent
   efferent lymph
   gastroepiploic
   intercostal
   internal pudendal
   kidney
   lymph
   musculophrenic
   pole of
   renal
   splenic
   superficial lymph
   superior gluteal

vessel leak
vestibular canal
vestibular ganglion
vestibular gland
vestibular hair cells
vestibular labyrinth
vestibular ligament
vestibular neuritis
vestibular schwannoma
vestibule
  aortic
  bulb of
  esophagogastric
  gastroesophageal
vestibule of vagina
vestigial fold
vestigial organ
Vetastain Elite kit
veto cell
V gene
VHDL (very high density lipoprotein)
VHL tumor suppressor gene
viable fetus
Vibrio alginolyticus
Vibrio cholerae
Vibrio damsela
Vibrio fetus
Vibrio fluvialis
Vibrio hollisae
Vibrio jejuni
Vibrio metschnikovii
Vibrio mimicus
vibrissae
Vidas image analyzer
vidian artery
vidian canal
Vieussens ansa
Vieussens loop
villi (pl. of villus)
villonodular synovitis
villous adenoma
villous atrophy

villous carcinoma
villous hypertrophy of synovial
  membrane
villous papilloma
villous placenta
villus (pl. villi)
  anchoring
  chorionic
  duodenal
  floating
  gallbladder
  intestinal
  placental
vimentin
Vim-Silverman needle
VIN (vaginal intraepithelial neoplasia)
Vincent infection
Vincent stomatitis
vinegar stain
violaceous
violet
  crystal
  gentian
  methyl
violet rash
violin-string adhesions
VIP (vasoactive intestinal polypeptide)
viral culture
viral encephalitis
viral exanthem
viral gastroenteritis
viral hemorrhagic fever
viral hepatitis
viral infection
viral inflammatory conditions
viral meningitis
viral myelitis
viral myocarditis
viral pericarditis
viral pneumonia
viral respiratory infection
viral septicemia

ViraPap test
ViraType
Virchow bone-splitting chisel
Virchow cells
Virchow gland
Virchow hydatid
Virchow-Robin space
viremia
Viridans streptococci
virilization
virilization of genitalia
virilizing adrenal tumor
virion
Virocult
virocyte
virology
Vironostika Mixt ELISA HIV
　antibody test
virulence
virus (pl. viruses) (see *pathogen* for
　　names of viruses)
　adeno-associated
　animal
　arthropod-borne
　avian leukosis
　bacterial
　BK (BKV)
　bluetongue
　border disease
　cancer-inducing
　chikungunya
　common cold
　croup-associated (CA v.)
　cytomegalic inclusion disease
　defective
　dengue
　dermotropic
　DNA
　DNA tumor
　encephalomyocarditis
　enteric
　enteric orphan

virus *(continued)*
　enveloped
　epidemic keratoconjunctivitis
　helper
　hemadsorption
　herpangina
　infectious pancreatic necrosis
　infectious wart
　influenza
　iridescent
　latent
　lymphocyte-associated
　lytic
　masked
　measles
　milker's node
　molluscum contagiosum
　mosquito-borne
　mucosal disease
　mumps
　naked
　negative strand
　neurotropic
　newborn pneumonitis
　nonenveloped
　nonoccluded
　nononcogenic
　oncogenic
　orphan
　papilloma
　poliomyelitis
　polyoma
　rabies
　respiratory
　rubella
　satellite
　slow
　temperate
　tickborne or tick-borne
　unconventional
　vacuolating
　vesicular stomatitis

virusemia
virustatic
virus-transformed cell
viscera (pl. of viscus)
  abdominal
  abdominopelvic
  hollow
  intraperitoneal
  pelvic
visceral arch
visceral artery
visceral branches
visceral cleft, first
visceral edema
visceral embolism
visceral larva migrans
visceral layer
visceral leishmaniasis
visceral lymph node
visceral pelvic fascia
visceral pericardium
visceral peritoneum
visceral pleura
visceral skeleton
visceral surface of liver
viscerocranium, cartilaginous
viscid bile
viscosity
viscous (adj.)
viscous bile
viscous fluid
viscous greenish exudate
viscous lubricant
viscous metamorphosis
viscus (pl. viscera)
visual cell
visual field
visual impairment, progressive
visual pigment
visual receptor cells
visual zone
vital capacity (VC)

Vitali test for alkaloids
vital stain
vitamin
  antineuritic
  test on venous blood for
vitamin A (retinol, dehydroretinol)
vitamin A tolerance test
vitamin B_1 (thiamine)
vitamin B_6 (pyridoxine)
vitamin B_{12} (cobalamin)
vitamin B_{12} intrinsic factor test
vitamin B_{12} tagged with radioactive
  cobalt, oral administration of
vitamin C (ascorbic acid)
vitamin C saturation test
vitamin D (calciferol)
vitamin D_3 (calciferol, cholecalciferol)
vitamin D-binding protein (DBP)
vitamin D intoxication
vitamin deficiencies due to inherited
    metabolic disorders
  malabsorption
  malnutrition
vitamin D test
vitamin E (tocopherol)
vitamin E test
vitamin K (phytonadione,
  menaquinone, menadione)
Vitek
vitelline duct
vitelline fistula
vitelline gland
vitiligo
vitreous abscess
vitreous body
vitreous cell
vitreous chamber
vitreous humor
vitreous membrane
vitro, in
vivax fever
vivax malaria

vivo, in
VLDL (very low density lipoprotein)
VMA (vanillylmandelic acid)
vocal cord
  pachyderma of
  papilloma of
vocal ligament
Voelcker and Joseph test
Vogel and Lee test for mercury
Voges-Proskauer test
volar arch artery, superficial
volar artery, superficial
volar capitate
volar carpal artery
volar carpal ligament
volar interosseous artery
volar ligament
volar sling
volar ulnar sling
vole bacillus
Volhard test for renal function
Volkmann canal
Volkmann contracture
Vollmer tuberculin patch
volume
  blood
  plasma
  mean corpuscular (MCV)
  mean platelet (MPV)
  red cell
  vertebral
volume-corrected mitotic index
volume of packed cells
volumetric analysis
voluntary muscle
volvulus, cecal
vomer, alae of
vomer bone

vomerine canal
vomerobasilar canal
vomerorostral canal
vomerovaginal canal
vomiting
vomiting blood
vomitus
von Aldor test
von Bezold abscess
von Gierke disease
von Jaksch test
von Kossa calcium stain
von Kossa stain
von Kupffer cell
von Maschke test for creatinine
von Meyenburg complex
von Pirquet test
von Recklinghausen disease of bone
von Recklinghausen disease of skin
von Willebrand disease
von Willebrand factor (vWF)
von Willebrand factor antigen
von Zeynek and Mencki test
voodoo death
vortex mixed
VP (variegate porphyria)
vulgaris, pemphigus verruca
Vulpian atrophy
vulva, labial artery of
vulvar canal
vulvar dystrophy
vulvitis
vulvouterine canal
vulvovaginal gland
vulvovaginitis
vWF (von Willebrand factor) antigen
VZV (varicella-zoster virus)

W, w

Waaler-Rose test
Wagner test for occult blood
waist of scaphoid
Waldenström macroglobulinemia
Waldenström purpura
Waldenström test for urine porphyrin
Waldeyer fascia
Waldeyer gland
Waldeyer ring
Waldeyer space
wall
  abdominal
  anterior abdominal
  axial
  body
  bowel
  carotid
  cavity
  cell
  chest
  gallbladder
  midabdominal
  nasal cavity
  posterior abdominal
  thoracic
  vaginal
  variceal

wall akinesis
wallerian degeneration
Walther canal
Walther oblique ligament
wandering abscess
wandering cell
wandering gallbladder
wandering goiter
wandering histiocyte
wandering kidney
wandering pneumonia
Wangiella dermatitidis
Wang test
Warburg apparatus
wart (verruca vulgaris)
  dermal
  epidermal
  flat genital
  genital
  Hassall-Henle
  keratotic
  mosaic
  pitch
  plantar
  postmortem
  precancerous
  venereal

Warthin cell
Warthin-Finkeldey cell
Warthin-Finkeldey giant cell
Warthin-Finkeldey giant cell in
  lymphoid tissue and skin
Warthin sign
Warthin-Starry silver stain
Warthin-Starry tissue-staining method
Warthin tumor (adenolymphoma)
wartlike
wart virus, infectious
warty
warty papilloma
washed clot
washed sperm
washerman's mark dermatitis
washing
  bladder
  bronchial
  gastric
  sperm
washings and brushings
Wasmann gland
wasserhelle (water-clear) cells
Wassermann test
wastes
  creatinine
  urea
  nitrogen
wasting, muscle
water balance
water-borne gastroenteritis
water-borne infection
water-buffalo leprosy
water-clear cell of parathyroid
watered-silk retina
water-filled pouch
Waterhouse-Friderichsen syndrome
water itch
Waters Nova-Pak C18 reversed-phase
  column
water-soluble

water-soluble proteins
water test
watery diarrhea
watery stool
watery urine
Watson-Schwartz test
wave
  A
  B
  brain
  C
  cannon
  delta
  dicrotic
  fluid
  peristaltic
wax
  bone
  paraffin
  tubercle bacillus
wax block
waxy casts in urine
waxy degeneration of skeletal muscle
waxy kidney
Wayson stain
WB (Western blot)
WBC (white blood cell) count
    consisting of:
  bands
  basos (basophils)
  blasts
  differential
  eos (eosinophils)
  immature forms
  leukocytes
  lymphs (lymphocytes)
  monos (monocytes)
  neutrophils
  polys or PMNs (polymorpho-
    nuclear leukocytes)
  segs (segmented neutrophils)
  stabs

WBC/hpf (white blood cells per
   high-power field)
weakness of peripheral pulses
weal (wheal)
wear and tear pigments
web
   digital
   duodenal
   esophageal
   fibrous
   hepatic
   intestinal
   laryngeal
   postcricoid
   terminal
   venous
webbed digit
webbed finger
webbed neck
webbed penis
webbed toe
Weber-Christian panniculitis
Weber gland
Weber-Rendu-Osler disease
Weber staining method
weblike fold
wedge-and-groove joint
wedge bone
wedge-shaped
Weeks bacillus
weeping eczema
Wegener granulomatosis
Weibel-Palade body
Weibel-Palade granule
Weichbrodt test for globulin
Weidel test for uric acid
Weigert-Gram stain
Weigert iron hematoxylin
Weigert-Pal method
Weigert stain
weightbearing bone
weightbearing joints

weight-per-volume concentration
Weil disease
Weil-Felix agglutinins
Weil-Felix test
Weil myelin sheath stain
Weil stain
Weiss-Mallory syndrome
Weisz test
Weitbrecht ligament
Welch abscess
Welch bacillus
Welcozyme HIV 1+2 ELISA antibody
   test
well-differentiated adenocarcinoma
well-differentiated carcinoma
well-healed surgical incision
Wender test for glucose
Wenzell test for strychnine
Wepfer gland
Weppen test for morphine
Werdnig-Hoffmann spinal muscular
   atrophy
Werner thyroid suppression test
Wernicke encephalopathy
Wernicke field
Wesselsbron virus
Westberg space
Westcott cutting biopsy needle
Westergren method
Westergren sedimentation rate
Western blot (WB) analysis
Western blot procedure
Western blotting
western equine encephalitis antibody
Western immunoblot test
West Nile virus
Westphal zone
wet brain
wet gangrene
wet pleurisy with effusion
wet preparation
wet smear

Wetzel test
Weyl test for creatinine
Wharton jelly
Wharton tumor (cystadenoma)
wheal (also weal)
Wheeler and Johnson test
whettle bones
whiff test
whiplike cilia
whiplike process
Whipple triad
whipworm (trichuriasis)
whistling deformity
white atrophy
white bile
white blood cell (WBC)
white blood cell count
white blood cells per high-power field
   (WBC/hpf)
"white cell" (slang for white blood cell)
white cell casts
white corpuscle
"white count" (slang for white blood
   cell count)
white fatty stool
white gangrene
Whitehead deformity
white light
white line
white matter
white piedra
white plague
white pulp
white pulp of spleen
white ramus communicans
white sponge nevus
white thrombus
white tissue
white tumor
whitlow, herpetic
Whitmore bacillus
whole blood

whole protein
whooping cough (pertussis)
whorl
   coccygeal
   digital
   fingerprint
   keratin
whorled cell formation
whorled mass
WI-38 cells (Wistar Institute)
Wiberg classification of patellar types
Widal agglutination test
Widal serum test
wide-angle glaucoma
wide-mouth sac
Wideroe test
widespread bleeding
widespread intravascular thrombosis
widespread metastasis
Widmark test
width
   platelet distribution (PDW)
   red cell distribution
Wijsman method of end-labeling
Wijs test
Wilcoxon test
Wilder reticulum stain
wild-type DNA
Wilkie artery
Williams factor
Williamson blood test
Williams stain
Willis
   antrum of
   artery of
   circle of
Willis pancreas
Wilms tumor
Wilson disease
Wilson-Kimmelstiel disease
Winckler test for alkaloids
winding

windows of jejunum
windpipe
wing, ashen
wing cell
Winslow, foramen of
Winslow pancreas
Winslow ligament
Winterbottom sign
winter eczema
winter itch
wire-loop appearance
wire-loop lesion
wire, pacemaker
Wirsung canal
Wirsung duct
Wirtz-Conklin spore stain
wisdom teeth
Wishart test for acetonemia
Wiskott-Aldrich syndrome
within normal limits (WNL)
without irreversible injury
Witz test
WNL (within normal limits)
Woldman test
Wolfe breast carcinoma classification
Wolfer gland
wolffian cyst
Wolfring gland
Wolinella
Woodbury test
Wood's light test
woodworker's lung disease
woody
woolly-hair nevus
woolsorter's disease
woolsorter's pneumonia
work, blood
working diagnosis
worm (pl. worms) (see also *pathogen*)
    appendiceal
    bladder
    cecal

worm *(continued)*
    fluke
    guinea
    mucosal
    parasitic
    rectal
worm abscess
Wormley test for alkaloids
Worm-Mueller test
worms in appendix
worms in cecum
worms in mucosa of cecum and
    appendix
worms in rectum
wound
    abraded
    aseptic
    avulsed
    ballistic
    blowing
    clean
    closed
    contaminated
    contused
    craniocerebral penetrating
    crease
    cross-irrigation of
    cutaneous
    depths of
    exit
    gaping
    glancing
    gunshot (GSW)
    gutter
    high-energy gunshot
    high-velocity gunshot
    incised
    lacerated
    nonpenetrating
    open
    penetrating
    perforating

wound *(continued)*
   plantar puncture
   puncture
   septic
   seton
   stab
   subcutaneous
   sucking
   tangential
   tetanus-prone
   traumatopneic
wound hematoma
wound infection
wound repair
woven bone

wrenched knee
Wright stain
wrinkle
Wrisberg ligament
wrist
wrist joint
wrist tag
wrongful death suit
wry neck (torticollis)
WT1 tumor suppressor gene
Wucheraria bancrofti
Wu method
Wurster test
Wyeomyia melanocephala mosquito
Wyeomyia virus

X, x

xanthelasma
xanthemia
xanthochromia of cerebrospinal fluid
xanthochromic spinal fluid
xanthogranuloma, juvenile
xanthogranulomatous pyelonephritis
xanthoma
  disseminated
  eruptive
  malignant fibrous
  planar
  tendinous
  tuberoeruptive
  verruciform
xanthoma cell
xanthomatosis, cerebrotendinous
xanthomatous granuloma
xanthoma tuberosum
Xanthomonas
xanthosarcoma
xanthosis
xenobiotics

xenogenous
xenon skin clearance test
xenon washout technique measurement
xeroderma
xerosis
xerotic eczema
Xg blood group
xiphicostal ligaments of Macalister
xiphisternal articulation
xiphisternal joint
xiphoid appendix
xiphoid bone
xiphoid ligament
xiphoid process
X-linked gene
X-linked infantile agammaglobulinemia
x-ray dermatitis
xylene
xylose absorption test
xylose test
Xylohypha bantiana

Y, y

Yale SK virus
Yatapoxvirus
yaws (frambesia)
Y body
yeast
yeast fungus
yeast infection
yeastlike fungus
yellow
   acid
   fast
   alizarin
   brilliant
   butter
   corallin
   imperial
   Manchester
   metanil
   methyl
   naphthol
   Philadelphia
yellow atrophy
yellow cartilage
yellow crusted patches
yellow elastic fiber
yellow fever

yellow fever virus
yellowish-gray plaques
yellow jaundice
yellow marrow
yellow plaque, fibrofatty
yellow tissue
yellow urine
Yersinia
Yersinia enterocolitica (formerly
    Pasteurella enterocolitica)
Yersinia frederiksenii
Yersinia intermedia
Yersinia kristensenii
Yersinia pestis (formerly *Pasteurella
    pestis*)
Yersinia pseudotuberculosis (formerly
    Pasteurella pseudotuberculosis)
Y-linked gene
yoke, alveolar
yoke bone
yolk cell
Young diabetes
Y-shaped incision
Y-shaped ligament
Yvon test for alkaloids

Z, z

Zaleski test
Zenker fixative
Zenker fluid
Zenker solution
Ziemann dots
Zika fever
Zimmermann test
zona-free hamster egg penetration
zone
  abdominal
  apical
  border
  cervical
  cervical transformation
  ciliary
  contact area
  coronal
  cutaneous
  dentofacial
  dolorogenic
  entry
  ependymal
  epileptogenic
  erogenous
  fetal
  Flechsig primordial
  gingival

zone *(continued)*
  Golgi
  grenz
  His
  keratogenous
  medullary
  nephrogenic
  neutral
  occlusal
  peripheral
  periventricular
  placental
  portal
  pupillary
  Rolando
  segmental
  T
  thymus-dependent
  thymus-independent
  transition
  transitional
  transformation
  visual
  Westphal
zone of antibody excess
zone of antigen excess
zone of discontinuity

zonula adherens
zonula occludens
zonular space
zonule, ciliary
zoo blot analysis
zoster, herpes
Zsigmondy test
Zubrod scale
zuckergussleber
Zuckerkandl gland
zygapophyseal articulation
zygapophyseal joint
zygogenic cell
zygoma
zygomatic arch

zygomatic artery
zygomatic bone
zygomatic nerve
zygomaticofacial canal
zygomatico-orbital artery
zygomaticotemporal canal
zygomaticotemporal nerve
zygomatic process
zygomycetous fungus
zygomycosis
zygote
zymogen cell
zymogen granule
zymogenic cell
zymoid

Appendix

Table of Arteries

artery	arteria (pl. arteriae)
Abbott's artery	
abdominal aorta artery	arteria aorta abdominalis
aberrant artery	
aberrant obturator artery	
accessory meningeal artery	arteria meningea accessoria
accessory obturator artery	arteria obturatoria accessoria
accessory pudendal artery	arteria pudenda accessoria
accompanying artery of ischiadic nerve	arteria comitans nervi ischiadici
accompanying artery of median nerve	arteria comitans nervi mediani
acetabular artery	ramus acetabularis arteriae circumflexae femoris medialis
acromial artery	
acromiothoracic artery	
Adamkiewicz, artery of	arteria radicularis magna
adipose arteries of kidney	rami capsulares arteriae renis
adrenal artery, middle	arteria suprarenalis media
afferent artery of glomerulus	vas afferens glomeruli
alar artery of nose	
alveolar artery, inferior	arteria alveolaris inferior
alveolar arteries, superior, anterior	arteriae alveolares superiores anteriores
alveolar artery, superior, posterior	arteria alveolaris superior posterior
anastomotic atrial artery	ramus atrialis anastomoticus arteriae coronariae sinistrae
angular artery	arteria angularis
angular gyrus artery	arteria gyri angularis
anonymous artery	
anterior auricular artery	arteria auricularis anterior
anterior cecal artery	arteria cecalis anterior
anterior cerebellar artery	arteria cerebelli anterior
anterior cerebral artery	arteria cerebri anterior
anterior choroidal artery	arteria choroidea anterior
anterior ciliary artery	arteria ciliaris anterior

artery	arteria (pl. arteriae)
anterior circumflex humeral artery	arteria circumflexa humeri anterior
anterior communicating artery	arteria communicans anterior
anterior conjunctival artery	arteria conjunctivalis anterior
anterior descending artery	
anterior ethmoidal artery	arteria ethmoidalis anterior
anterior humeral circumflex artery	
anterior inferior cerebellar artery	arteria cerebelli inferior anterior
anterior inferior segmental artery of kidney	arteria segmenti anterioris inferioris renis
anterior intercostal arteries	rami intercostales anteriores
anterior interosseous artery	arteria interossea anterior
anterior interventricular artery	ramus interventricularis anterior arteriae coronariae sinistrae
anterior labial arteries	arteriae labiales anteriores
anterior lateral malleolar artery	arteria malleolaris anterior lateralis
anterior medial malleolar artery	arteria malleolaris anterior medialis
anterior mediastinal arteries	rami mediastinales arteriae thoracicae internae
anterior meningeal artery	arteria meningea anterior
anterior parietal artery	arteria parietales anterior
anterior peroneal artery	ramus arteriae fibularis anterior
anterior radial carpal artery	arteria radialis carpalis
anterior spinal artery	arteria spinalis anterior
anterior superior alveolar arteries	arteriae alveolares superiores anteriores
anterior superior dental artery	arteria alveolaris anterior superior
anterior superior segmental artery of kidney	arteria segmenti anterioris superioris renis
anterior temporal artery	arteria temporalis anterior
anterior tibial artery	arteria tibialis anterior
anterior tibial recurrent artery	arteria recurrens tibialis anterior
anterior tympanic artery	arteria tympanica anterior
anterolateral central arteries	arteriae centrales anterolaterales
anterolateral striate arteries	arteriae centrales anterolaterales
anterolateral thalamostriate arteries	arteriae centrales anterolaterales
apicoposterior artery	
appendicular artery	arteria appendicularis
arch of aorta	arteria arcus aortae

artery	arteria (pl. arteriae)
arciform arteries	arteriae arcuatae renis
arcuate artery of foot	arteria arcuata pedis
arcuate arteries of kidney	arteriae arcuatae renis
articular artery, proper, of little head of fibula	ramus circumflexus fibulae arteriae tibialis posterioris
ascending artery	arteria ascendens
ascending aorta	arteria aorta ascendens
ascending cervical artery	arteria cervicalis ascendens
ascending palatine artery	arteria palatina ascendens
ascending pharyngeal artery	arteria pharyngea ascendens
atrial anastomotic artery	ramus atrialis anastomoticus arteriae coronariae sinistrae
atrial arteries	arteriae atriales
atrioventricular node, artery to	ramus nodi atrioventricularis
atrioventricular nodal artery	ramus nodi atrioventricularis arteriae coronariae dextrae
auditory artery, internal	arteria labyrinthina
auricular arteries, anterior	rami auriculares anteriores arteriae temporalis superficialis
auricular artery	arteria auricularis
axillary artery	arteria axillaris
axis thoracic artery	arteria thoracica axillaris
azygos arteries of vagina	vaginales arteriae uterinae
basilar artery	arteria basilaris
brachial artery	arteria brachialis
brachiocephalic artery	truncus brachiocephalicus
bronchial arteries	rami bronchiales
buccal artery, buccinator artery	arteria buccalis
bulbourethral artery	arteria bulbi urethrae
bulb of penis, artery of	arteria bulbi penis
bulb of vestibule of vagina, artery of	arteria bulbi vestibuli vaginae
calcaneal arteries	rami calcanei
calcarine artery	
calf, artery of	arteria sural
callosomarginal artery	arteria callosomarginalis
capsular artery	arteria suprarenalis
caroticotympanic arteries	arteriae caroticotympanicae
carotid artery	
caudal artery	arteria sacralis mediana

artery	arteria (pl. arteriae)
caudate lobe, artery of	arteria lobi caudati
cavernous artery	
cecal artery	arteria caecalis
celiac artery	
central arteries	arteriae centrales
central artery of retina, Zinn's artery	arteria centralis retinae
central sulcus artery	arteria sulci centralis
cephalic artery	arteria carotis communis
cerebellar artery	arteria cerebelli
cerebral artery, cerebral arteries	arteria cerebri, arteriae cerebrales
cervical artery	arteria cervicalis
cervicovaginal artery	arteria cervicovaginalis
Charcot's artery	
chief artery of thumb	arteria princeps pollicis
choroid artery, anterior	arteria choroidea anterior
ciliary arteries	arteriae cilliares
circle of Willis	
circumflex artery	ramus circumflexus arteriae coronariae sinistrae
circumflex artery, deep, internal	ramus profundus arteriae circumflexae femoris medialis
circumflex femoral artery, lateral	arteria circumflexa femoris lateralis
circumflex femoral artery, medial	arteria circumflexa femoris medialis
circumflex humeral artery, anterior	arteria circumflexa anterior humeri
circumflex humeral artery, posterior	arteria circumflexa posterior humeri
circumflex iliac artery, deep	arteria circumflexa iliaca profunda
circumflex iliac artery, superficial	arteria circumflexa iliaca superficialis
circumflex scapular artery	arteria circumflexa scapulae
clavicular artery	
clitoris, artery of, deep	arteria profunda clitoridis
clitoris, artery of, dorsal	arteria dorsalis clitoridis
coccygeal artery	arteria sacralis mediana
cochlear artery	ramus cochlearis arteriae labyrinthi
Cohnheim's artery	arteria terminalis
coiled artery	
colic artery	arteria colica
collateral artery	arteria collateralis
common carotid artery	arteria carotis communis
common hepatic artery	arteria hepatica communis

artery	arteria (pl. arteriae)
common iliac artery	arteria iliaca communis
common interosseous artery	arteria interossea communis
common palmar digital artery	arteria digitalis palmaris communis
common plantar digital artery	arteria digitalis plantaris communis
communicating artery of cerebrum	arteria communicans cerebri
companion artery	
conducting artery	
conjunctival artery	arteria conjunctivalis
conus artery	ramus coni arteriosi arteriae coronariae
copper-wire artery	
corkscrew artery	
coronary artery of heart	arteria coronaria
coronary artery of stomach	arteria gastrica
corpus cavernosum	
cortical artery	
costocervical trunk artery	
cremasteric artery	arteria cremasterica
cricothyroid artery	ramus cricothyroideus
crural artery	
cystic artery	arteria cystica
deep artery of clitoris	arteria profunda clitoridis
deep artery of penis	arteria profunda penis
deep artery of thigh	arteria profunda femoris
deep auricular artery	arteria auricularis profunda
deep brachial artery	arteria profunda brachii
deep cervical artery	arteria cervicalis profunda
deep circumflex iliac artery	arteria circumflexa iliaca profunda
deep epigastric artery	arteria epigastrica profunda
deep external pudendal artery	arteria pudenda profunda externa
deep femoral artery	arteria femoralis profunda
deep iliac circumflex artery	arteria circumflexa iliaca superficialis
deep lingual artery	arteria profunda linguae
deep palmar arch	arcus palmaris profundus
deep penis artery	arteria profunda penis
deep plantar artery	ramus plantaris profundus
deep temporal artery	arteria temporalis profunda
deep volar branch of ulnar artery	arteria ulnaris
deferential artery	arteria ductus deferentis
deltoid artery	ramus deltoideus arteriae profundae brachii

artery	arteria (pl. arteriae)
dental artery	arteria alveolaris
descending branch of occipital artery	arteria occipitalis descendens
descending genicular artery	arteria anastomotica magna
descending palatine artery	arteria palatina descendens
descending scapular artery	arteria scapularis descendens
diaphragmatic arteries	arteriae phrenicae inferiores
digital arteries	arteriae digitales
digital collateral artery	arteria digitalis palmaris propria
distributing artery	
dorsal artery of clitoris	arteria dorsalis clitoridis
dorsal artery of foot	arteria dorsalis pedis
dorsal artery of great toe	arteria dorsalis hallucis
dorsal artery of nose	arteria dorsalis nasi
dorsal artery of penis	arteria dorsalis penis
dorsal carpal artery	arteria dorsalis carpal
dorsal digital artery	arteria digitalis dorsalis
dorsal interosseous artery	arteria interossea dorsalis
dorsal metacarpal artery	arteria metacarpalis dorsalis
dorsal nasal artery	arteria dorsalis nasi
dorsalis pedis artery	arteria dorsalis pedis
dorsalis penis artery	arteria dorsalis penis
dorsal metacarpal artery	arteria metacarpea dorsalis
dorsal metatarsal artery	arteria metatarsea dorsalis
dorsal nasal artery	arteria nasi externa
dorsal pancreatic artery	arteria pancreatica dorsalis
dorsal scapular artery	arteria dorsalis scapulae
Drummond, artery of (marginal artery of colon)	
ductus deferens, artery of	arteria ductus deferentis
duodenal arteries	arteriae pancreaticoduodenales inferiores
efferent artery of glomerulus	vas efferens glomeruli
elastic artery	
emulgent artery	arteria renalis
end artery (terminal artery)	
epigastric artery	arteria circumflexa iliaca
epiphyseal artery	
episcleral arteries	arteriae episclerales
esophageal arteries	rami esophagei arteriae gastricae

artery	arteria (pl. arteriae)
ethmoidal artery	arteria ethmoidalis
external carotid artery	arteria carotis externa
external iliac artery	arteria iliaca externa
external mammary artery	arteria thoracica lateralis
(lateral thoracic artery)	
external maxillary artery (facial artery)	arteria maxillaris externa
external pudendal arteries	arteriae pudendae externae
external spermatic artery	
(cremasteric artery)	
facial artery	arteria facialis
fallopian artery	areria uterina
femoral artery	arteria femoralis
fibular artery (peroneal artery)	arteria fibularis
foot, artery of, dorsal	arteria dorsalis pedis
frontal artery (supratrochlear artery)	arteria supratrochlearis
frontobasal artery, lateral	arteria frontobasalis lateralis
funicular artery	arteria testicularis
gastric artery	arteria gastrica
gastroduodenal artery	arteria gastroduodenalis
gastroepiploic artery	arteria gastro-omentalis
gastro-omental artery	arteria gastro-omentalis
genicular artery	arteria genicularis
glaserian artery (anterior tympanic)	arteria tympanica anterior
glomerular artery	
gluteal artery	arteria glutealis
great anastomotic artery	arteria radicularis magna
greater palatine artery	arteria palatina major
great pancreatic artery	arteria pancreatica magna
great radicular artery	arteria radicularis magna
great superior pancreatic artery (dorsal)	arteria pancreatica magna superior
helicine arteries of penis	arteriae helicinae penis
hemorrhoidal artery	arteria rectalis
hepatic artery	arteria hepatica
Heubner, artery of (medial striate artery)	
highest intercostal artery (superior)	rami intercostales superiores
highest thoracic artery (superor)	arteria thoracica superior
humeral artery (brachial artery)	arteria humeri
hyaloid artery	arteria hyaloidea
hyoid artery	ramus suprahyoideus arteriae lingualis

artery	arteria (pl. arteriae)
hypogastric artery (internal iliac artery)	arteria iliaca interna
hypophysial artery	arteria hypophysialis
ileal arteries	arteriae ileales
ileocolic artery	arteria ileocolica
iliac artery	arteria iliaca
iliolumbar artery	arteria iliolumbalis
inferior alveolar artery	arteria alveolaris inferior
inferior cerebellar artery	arteria cerebelli inferior
inferior dental artery	arteria alveolaris inferior
inferior epigastric artery	arteria epigastrica inferior
inferior gastroduodenal artery	arteria gastroduodenalis inferior
inferior genicular artery	arteria genicularis inferior
inferior gluteal artery	arteria glutea inferior
inferior hemorrhoidal artery	arteria rectalis inferior
inferior hypophysial artery	arteria hypophysialis inferior
inferior labial artery	arteria labialis inferior
inferior laryngeal artery	arteria laryngea inferior
inferior lateral genicular artery	arteria genus inferior lateralis
inferior medial genicular artery	arteria genus inferior medialis
inferior mesenteric artery	arteria mesenterica inferior
inferior pancreatic artery	arteria pancreatica inferior
inferior pancreaticoduodenal artery	arteria pancreaticoduodenalis inferior
inferior phrenic artery	arteria phrenica inferior
inferior profunda artery	arteria profunda inferior
inferior rectal artery	arteria rectalis inferior
inferior segmental artery of kidney	arteria segmenti inferioris renis
inferior suprarenal artery	arteria suprarenalis inferior
inferior thyroid artery	arteria thyroidea inferior
inferior tympanic artery	arteria tympanica inferior
inferior ulnar collateral artery	arteria collateralis ulnaris inferior
inferior vesical artery	arteria vesicalis inferior
infracostal artery	ramus costalis lateralis arteriae thoracicae internae
infrahyoid artery	arteria infrahyoideus
infraorbital artery	arteria infraorbitalis
infrascapular artery	arteria infrascapularis
innominate artery	truncus brachiocephalicus
inguinal arteries	rami inguinales arteriae femoralis
innominate artery	truncus brachiocephalicus

artery	arteria (pl. arteriae)
insular arteries	arteriae insulares
intercostal arteries	rami intercostales arteriae thoracicae
interlobar arteries of kidney	arteriae interlobares renis
interlobular arteries of kidney	arteriae interlobulares renis
interlobular arteries of liver	arteriae interlobulares hepatis
intermediate atrial artery	ramus atrialis intermedius
intermediate temporal artery	arteria temporalis intermedia
intermetacarpal arteries	arteriae metacarpales palmares
internal auditory artery (labyrinthine)	arteria labyrinthi
internal carotid artery	arteria carotis interna
internal iliac artery	arteria iliaca interna
internal malleolar artery	arteria malleolaris interna
internal mammary artery (thoracic)	arteria thoracica interna
internal maxillary artery	arteria maxillaris interna
internal palpebral artery	arteria palpebralis interna
internal plantar artery	arteria plantaris interna
internal pubic artery	arteria pubicus interna
internal pudendal artery	arteria pudenda interna
internal spermatic artery (testicular)	arteria testicularis interna
internal thoracic artery	arteria thoracica interna
interosseous artery	arteria interossea
interosseous palmar artery	arteria palmaris interossea
intersegmental artery	
interventricular artery	ramus interventricularis
intestinal arteries (ileal or jejunal)	arteriae intestinales
jejunal arteries	arteriae jejunales
kidney, arteries of (segmental arteries of kidney)	arteriae renis
Kugel's anastomotic artery	arteria anastomotica auricularis magna
labial arteries of vulva	rami labiales arteriae femoralis
labyrinthine artery	arteria labyrinthi
lacrimal artery	arteria lacrimalis
laryngeal artery	arteria laryngea
lateral calcaneal artery	arteria calcanei lateralis
lateral circumflex femoral artery	arteria circumflexa femoris lateralis
lateral circumflex artery of thigh	arteria circumflexa femoris lateralis
lateral costal artery	
lateral frontobasal artery	arteria frontobasalis lateralis
lateral inferior genicular artery	arteria genicularis lateralis inferior

artery	arteria (pl. arteriae)
lateral malleolar arteries	rami malleolares laterales
lateral nasal artery	arteria nasi lateralis
lateral occipital artery	arteria occipitalis lateralis
lateral palpebral artery	arteria palpebralis lateralis
lateral plantar artery	arteria plantaris lateralis
lateral sacral artery	arteria sacralis lateralis
lateral striate arteries	arteriae centrales anterolaterales
lateral tarsal artery	arteria tarsea lateralis
lateral thoracic artery	arteria thoracica lateralis
left anterior descending coronary artery	ramus interventricularis anterior arteriae coronariae sinistrae
left colic artery	arteria colica sinistra
left coronary artery	arteria coronaria sinistra
left gastric artery	arteria gastrica sinistra
left gastroepiploic artery	arteria gastro-omentalis sinistra
left gastro-omental artery (left gastroepiploic artery)	
left hepatic artery	ramus sinister arteriae hepaticae propriae
left pulmonary artery	arteria pulmonalis sinistra
lenticulostriate arteries (Charcot's artery) (lateral striate arteries)	
lesser palatine artery	arteria palatina minor
lienal artery (splenic artery)	
lingual artery	arteria lingualis
lingual artery, dorsal	arteria lingualis dorsalis
lobar artery	
long central artery (medial striate artery)	
long ciliary artery	arteria ciliaris longa
long posterior ciliary artery	arteria ciliaris posterior longa
long thoracic artery (lateral)	arteria thoracica lateralis
lowest lumbar arteries	arteriae lumbales imae
lowest thyroid artery	arteria thyroidea ima
lumbar artery	arteria lumbalis
macular arteries	
malleolar artery	arteria malleolaris
mammary artery	arteria thoracica
mandibular artery	arteria alveolaris inferior
marginal artery	ramus marginalis

artery	arteria (pl. arteriae)
marginal artery of colon (artery of Drummond, Riolan's arc)	arteria marginalis coli
masseteric artery	arteria masseterica
mastoid artery	rami mastoidei arteriae auricularis posterioris
maxillary artery	arteria maxillaris
medial artery of foot, superficial	ramus superior arteriae plantaris medialis
medial circumflex femoral artery	arteria circumflexa femoris medialis
medial frontobasal artery	arteria frontobasalis medialis
medial malleolar arteries	arteriae malleolares posteriores mediales
medial palpebral artery	
medial striate artery	
medial tarsal artery	
median artery	arteria comitans nervi mediani
median sacral artery	arteria sacralis mediana
mediastinal arteries, anterior	rami mediastinales arteriae thoracicae internae
mediastinal arteries, posterior	rami mediastinales aortae thoracicae
medullary artery	arteria nutriens
meningeal artery, accessory	ramus meningeus accessorius arteriae meningeae mediae
meningeal artery, anterior	ramus meningeus anterior arteriae ethmoidalis anterioris
meningeal artery, middle	arteria meningea media
meningeal artery, posterior	arteria meningea posterior
mental artery	arteria mentalis
mesencephalic arteries	arteriae mesencephalicae
mesenteric artery	arteria mesenterica
metacarpal arteries	arteriae metacarpales
metaphyseal artery	
metatarsal artery	arteria metatarsae
middle capsular artery	arteria suprarenalis media
middle cerebral artery	arteria cerebri media
middle colic artery	arteria colica media
middle collateral artery	arteria collateralis media
middle genicular artry	arteria articularis azygos
middle hemorrhoidal artery	

artery	arteria (pl. arteriae)
middle meningeal artery	arteria meningea media
middle rectal artery	arteria rectalis media
middle sacral artery	arteria sacralis media
middle suprarenal artery	arteria suprarenalis media
middle temporal artery	arteria temporalis media
middle vesical artery	arteria vesicalis media
Mueller, arteries of	arteriae helicinae penis
musculophrenic artery	arteria musculophrenica
mylohyoid artery	ramus mylohyoideus arteriae alveolaris inferioris
myomastoid artery	ramus occipitalis arteriae auricularis posterioris
nasal artery, dorsal	arteria dorsalis nasi
nasopalatine artery	arteria sphenopalatina
Neubauer's artery	arteria thyroidea ima
nodal artery	
nose, dorsal artery of	arteria dorsalis nasi
nutrient artery	arteria nutricia
obliterated hypogastric artery	
obliterated umbilical artery	
obturator artery	arteria obturatoria
occipital artery	arteria occipitalis
omental artery	
omphalomesenteric artery	
ophthalmic artery	arteria ophthalmica
orbital artery	
orbitofrontal artery (lateral frontobasal)	
ovarian artery	arteria ovarica
palatine artery	arteria palatina
palmar metacarpal artery	arteria metacarpea palmaris
palpebral arteries	arteriae palpebrales
pancreatic artery	arteria pancreatica
pancreaticoduodenal artery	arteria pancreaticoduodenalis
paracentral artery	arteria paracentralis
parietal arteries, anterior and posterior	arteriae parietales anterior et posterior
parieto-occipital artery	arteria parieto-occipitalis
parieto-temporal artery	
pectoral artery	
pelvic artery, posterior	arteria iliaca interna

artery	arteria (pl. arteriae)
penis, deep artery of	arteria profunda penis
penis, dorsal artery of	arteria dorsalis penis
perforating arteries	arteriae perforantes
pericallosal artery	arteria pericallosa
pericardiac arteries, posterior	rami pericardiaci aortae thoracicae
pericardiacophrenic artery	arteria pericardiacophrenica
perineal artery	arteria perinealis
periosteal artery	
peroneal artery, fibular artery	arteria peronea, arteria fibularis
pharyngeal artery, ascending	arteria pharyngea ascendens
phrenic arteries	arteriae phrenicae
plantar artery	arteria plantaris
plantar metatarsal artery	arteria metatarsea plantaris
pontine arteries	arteriae pontis
popliteal artery	arteria poplitea
postcentral sulcal artery	arteria sulci postcentralis
posterior alveolar artery	arteria alveolaris posterior
posterior auricular artery	arteria auricularis posterior
posterior cecal artery	arteria cecalis posterior
posterior cerebral artery	arteria cerebri posterior
posterior choroidal artery	arteria choroidea posterior
posterior circumflex humeral artery	arteria circumflexa humeri posterior
posterior communicating artery	
posterior descending coronary artery	ramus interventricularis posterior arteriae coronariae dextrae
posterior humeral circumflex	artria circumflexa humeri posterior
posterior inferior cerebellar artery	arteria cerebelli posterior inferior
posterior intercostal artery	
posterior interosseous artery	arteria interossea posterior
posterior pancreaticoduodenal artery	arteria pancreaticoduodenalis posterior
posterior scapular artery	arteria scapulae posterior
posterior scrotal artery	arteria scrotalis posterior
posterior septal artery of nose	arteria nasalis posterior septi
posterior spinal artery	arteria spinalis posterior
posterior superior alveolar artery	arteria alveolaris superior posterior
posterior temporal artery	arteria temporalis posterior
posterior tibial artery	arteria tibialis posterior
posterior tibial recurrent artery	arteria recurrens tibialis posterior
posterior tympanic artery	arteria tympanica posterior

artery	**arteria** (pl. **arteriae**)
posterolateral central artery	arteriae centrales posterolaterales
posteromedial central arteries	arteriae centrales posteromediales
precentral sulcal artery	arteria sulci precentralis
princeps pollicis artery	arteria princeps pollicis
precuneal artery	arteria precunealis
prepancreatic artery	arteria prepancreatica
presegmental artery	arteria presegmenti
prevertebral artery	arteria prevertebralis
principal artery of thumb	arteria princeps pollicis
profunda brachii artery	arteria profunda brachii
profunda femoris artery	arteria profunda femoris
proper hepatic artery	arteria hepatica propria
proper palmar digital artery	arteria digitalis palmaris propria
proper plantar digital artery	arteria digitalis plantaris propria
pterygoid arteries	rami pterygoidei
pterygoid canal, artery of	arteria canalis pterygoidei
pubic artery	ramus pubicus arteriae epigastricae inferioris
pudendal arteries	arteriae pudendae externae
pulmonary artery	truncus pulmonalis
pyloric artery	arteria gastrica dextra
quadriceps artery of femur	ramus descendens arteriae circumflexae femoris lateralis
radial artery	arteria radialis
radial artery of index finger	arteria volaris radialis indicis
radial carpal artery	
radial collateral artery	arteria collateralis radialis
radial recurrent artery	arteria recurrens radialis
radiate arteries of kidney	arteriae interlobulares renis
radicular arteries	rami spinales arteriae vertebralis
ranine artery	arteria profunda linguae
rectal artery	arteria rectalis
recurrent artery	arteria centralis longa
recurrent artery, radial	arteria recurrens radialis
recurrent artery, tibial, anterior	arteria recurrens tibialis anterior
recurrent artery, tibial, posterior	arteria recurrens tibialis posterior
recurrent artery, ulnar	arteria recurrens ulnaris
recurrent interosseous artery	arteria interossea recurrens
recurrent radial artery	arteria recurrens radialis

artery	arteria (pl. arteriae)
recurrent ulnar artery	arteria recurrens ulnaris
renal artery, renal arteries	arteria renalis, arteriae renales
retinal artery	
retrocostal artery	ramus costalis lateralis arteriae thoracicae internae
retroduodenal artery	arteria retroduodenalis
retroesophageal subclavian artery	artery subclavia retroesophagei
revehent artery	vas efferens glomeruli
right colic artery	arteria colica dextra
right coronary artery	arteria coronaria dextra
right gastric artery	arteria gastrica dextra
right gastroepiploic artery	arteria gastro-omentalis dextra
right hepatic artery	ramus dexter arteriae hepaticae propriae
right pulmonary artery	arteria pulmonalis dextra
round ligament of uterus, artery of	arteria ligamenti teretis uteri
sacral arteries	arteriae sacrales
sacrococcygeal artery	arteria sacralis mediana
saphenous artery	
scapular artery	arteria scapulare
sciatic artery	arteria comitans nervi ischiadici
scrotal arteries, anterior	rami scrotales anteriores arteriae femoralis
scrotal arteries, posterior	rami scrotales posteriores arteriae pudendae internae
segmental artery	arteria segmenti
semilunar ganglion artery	
septal arteries, anterior	rami interventriculares septales
septal arteries, posterior	rami interventricularis posterioris
short central artery	arteria centralis brevis
short ciliary artery	arteria ciliaris brevis
short gastric artery	arteriae gastricae breves
short posterior ciliary artery	arteria ciliaris posterior brevis
sigmoid arteries	arteriae sigmoideae
sinoatrial nodal artery, sinuatrial (S-A) node artery	ramus nodi sinuatrialis arteriae coronaria dextra
somatic artery	
spermatic artery, external	arteria cremasterica
spermatic artery, internal	arteria testicularis
sphenopalatine artery	arteria sphenopalatina

artery	arteria (pl. arteriae)
spinal arteries	rami spinales arteriae vertebralis
spiral artery	
splanchnic artery	
splenic artery	arteria splenica
stapedial artery	
sternal arteries, posterior	rami sternales arteriae thoracicae internae
sternocleidomastoid artery, superior	ramus sternocleidomastoideus arteriae thyroideae superioris
straight arteries of kidney	arteriolae rectae renis
striate arteries	arteriae centrales anterolaterales
stylomastoid artery	arteria stylomastoidea
subclavian artery	arteria subclavia
subcostal artery	arteria subcostalis
sublingual artery	arteria sublingualis
submaxillary glandular artery	
submental artery	arteria submentalis
subscapular artery	arteria subscapularis
sulcal artery	
superficial brachial artery	arteria brachialis superficialis
superficial cervical artery	arteria cervicalis superficialis
superficial circumflex iliac artery	arteria circumflexa iliaca superficialis
superficial epigastric artery	arteria epigastrica superficialis
superficial external pudendal artery	arteria pudenda superficialis externa
superficial iliac circumflex artery	arteria circumflexa iliaca superficialis
superficial palmar arch artery	arteria arcus palmaris superficialis
superficial perineal artery	arteria perinealis superficialis
superficial petrosal artery	
superficial temporal artery	arteria temporalis superficialis
superficial volar artery	
superficial volar arch artery	
superior cerebellar artery	arteria cerebelli superior
superior epigastric artery	arteria epigastrica superior
superior gluteal artery	arteria glutea superior
superior hemorrhoidal artery	arteria rectalis superior
superior hypophysial artery	arteria hypophysialis superior
superior intercostal artery	arteria intercostalis suprema
superior labial artery	arteria labialis superior
superior laryngeal artery	arteria laryngea superior
superior lateral genicular artery	arteria genus superior lateralis

artery	arteria (pl. arteriae)
superior medial genicular artery	arteria genus superior medialis
superior mesenteric artery	arteria mesenterica superior
superior pancreaticoduodenal artery	arteria pancreaticoduodenalis superior
superior phrenic artery	arteria phrenica superior
superior profunda artery	arteria profunda superior
superior rectal artery	arteria rectalis superior
superior segmental artery of kidney	arteria segmenti superioris renis
superior suprarenal arteries	arteriae suprarenales superiores
superior thoracic artery	arteria thoracica superior
superior thyroid artery	arteria thyroidea superior
superior tympanic artery	arteria tympanica superior
superior ulnar collateral artery	arteria collateralis ulnaris superior
superior vesical artery	arteria vesicalis superior
supraduodenal artery	arteria supraduodenalis
suprahyoid artery	arteria superhyoideus
supraorbital artery	arteria supraorbitalis
suprarenal artery, aortic	arteria suprarenalis media
suprascapular artery	arteria suprascapularis
supratrochlear artery	arteria supratrochlearis
sural artery	arteria suralis
sylvian artery	arteria cerebri media
tarsal artery	arteria tarsalis
temporal artery	arteria temporalis
terminal artery (Cohnheim's artery)	
testicular artery	arteria testicularis
thalamostriate arteries, anterolateral	arteriae centrales anterolaterales
thoracic artery	arteria thoracica
thoracicoacromial artery	arteria thoracoacromialis
thoracodorsal artery	arteria thoracodorsalis
thymic arteries	rami thymici arteriae thoracicae internae
thyroid artery	arteria thyroidea
thyroid artery, inferior, of Cruveilhier	ramus cricothyroideus arteriae thyroideae superioris
thyroid ima artery	arteria thyroidea ima
tibial artery	arteria tibialis
tonsillar artery	ramus tonsillaris arteriae facialis
tracheal artery	
transverse artery of neck	arteria transversa cervicis
transverse cervical artery	arteria transversa cervicis

artery	arteria (pl. arteriae)
transverse facial artery	arteria transversa faciei
transverse perineal artery	arteria transversa perinealis
transverse scapular artery	arteria transversa scapulae
trunk artery	
tubo-ovarian artery	arteria ovarica
tympanic artery	arteria tympanica
ulnar artery	arteria ulnaris
ulnar carpal artery	
ulnar collateral artery, inferior	arteria collateralis ulnaris inferior
ulnar collateral artery, superior	arteria collateralis ulnaris superior
umbilical artery	arteria umbilicalis
upper limb, arteries of	arteriae membri superioris
ureteric artery	
urethral artery	arteria urethralis
urethral bulb artery	
uterine artery	arteria uterina
uterine artery, aortic	arteria ovarica
vaginal artery	arteria vaginalis
venous arteries	venae pulmonales
ventricular arteries	arteriae ventriculares
vermiform artery	arteria appendicularis
vertebral artery	arteria vertebralis
vesical artery, inferior	arteria vesicalis inferior
vesical arteries, superior	arteriae vesicales superiores
vestibular arteries	rami vestibulares arteriae labyrinthi
vidian artery	arteria canalis pterygoidei
visceral artery	
vitelline artery	arteria vitellina
volar carpal artery	
volar interosseous artery	arteria interossea volaris
Zinn, artery of	arteria centralis retinae
zygomatic artery	
zygomatico-orbital artery	arteria zygomatico-orbitalis

Table of Bones

bone (region)	os (pl. ossa)
acetabulum	os acetabuli
acromial bone	os acromiale
	os acromiale secondarium
ankle bone	talus
atlas (neck)	atlas
axis (neck)	axis
basilar bone	os basilare
Bertin's bone	
blade bone	scapula
breast bone	sternum
Breschet's bone	os suprasternale
calcaneus (foot)	calcaneus; os calcis; os tarsi fibulare
capitate bone (wrist)	os capitatum; os carpale distale tertium
carpal bones (wrist)	ossa carpi; ossa carpalia
central bone (wrist)	os centrale
clavicle (shoulder)	clavicula
coccyx (lower back)	os coccygis
compact bone	substantia compacta
concha, inferior nasal (skull)	concha nasalis inferior
cortical bone	substantia corticalis
cranial bones	ossa cranii; ossa cranialia
cuboid bone (foot)	os cuboideum
cuneiform bone, intermediate (foot)	os cuneiforme intermedium
cuneiform bone, lateral (foot)	os cuneiforme laterale
cuneiform bone, medial (foot)	os cuneiforme mediale
digits, bones of	ossa digitorum
elbow bone (olecranon process of ulna)	cubitus
epipteric bone (Flower's bone)	
ethmoid bone	os ethmoidale
fabella (knee)	
facial bones	ossa facialia; ossa faciei
femur (thigh)	femur

bone (region)	os (pl. ossa)
fibula (leg)	fibula
flat bone	os planum
Flower's bone (epipteric bone)	
foot, bones of	ossa pedis
frontal bone (skull)	os frontale
digits of hand	ossa digitorum manus
digits of foot	ossa digitorum pedis
Goethe's bone (preinterparietal bone)	
greater multangular bone	trapezium
hamate bone (wrist)	os hamatum; os carpale distale quartum
hand, bones of (carpals, metacarpals, phalanges)	ossa manus
heel bone	calcaneus
hip bone (pelvis and hip)	os coxae
hollow bone (pneumatic bone)	
hooked bone (hamate bone)	
humerus (arm)	humerus
hyoid bone (neck)	os hyoideum
iliac bone; ilium (pelvis)	os ilii; os ilium
incisive bone	os incisivum
incus (ear)	incus
inferior limb, bones of (os coxae, pelvis, patella, tibia, fibula, tarsus metatarsus, digits of foot)	ossa membri inferioris
innominate bone (hip bone)	os coxae
intermaxillary bone	os incisivum
interparietal bone	os interparietale
irregular bone	os irregulare
ischial bone; ischium (pelvis)	os ischii
jaw bone (mandible)	mandibula
jugal bone (zygomatic bone)	os zygomaticum
Krause's bone (small bone)	
lacrimal bone (skull)	os lacrimale
lamellar bone	
lesser multangular bone (trapezoid)	os trapezoideum
lingual bone (hyoid bone)	
long bone (pipe bone)	os longum
lunate bone (wrist)	os lunatum
malar bone	os zygomaticum

bone (region)	os (pl. ossa)
malleus (ear)	malleus
mandible (lower jaw)	mandibula
mastoid bone of occipital bone	margo mastoideus squamae occipitalis
maxilla (skull, upper jaw)	maxilla
metacarpal bones (hand)	ossa metacarpalia
metacarpal bone, third or middle	os metacarpale tertium
metatarsal bones (foot)	ossa metatarsalia
nasal bone (nose)	os nasale
navicular bone of foot	os naviculare; os centrale tarsi
navicular bone of hand	os scaphoideum
nonlamellar bone (woven bone)	
occipital bone (skull)	os occipitale
palatine bone (skull)	os palatinum
parietal bone (skull)	os parietale
patella (knee)	patella
pelvis	os pelvicum
penis bone	os penis
perichondral bone (periosteal bone)	
periosteal bone (perichondral bone)	
peroneal bone (fibula)	
petrosal bone	
phalanges (pl. of phalanx) (fingers, toes)	ossa digitorum
phalanx, proximal	os phalanx proximalis
phalanx, middle	os phalanx media
phalanx, distal	os phalanx distalis
ping-pong bone	
pipe bone (long bone)	
Pirie's bone (dorsal talonavicular bone)	
pisiform bone (wrist)	os pisiforme
pneumatic bone	os pneumaticum
postsphenoid bone	
preinterparietal bone (Goethe's bone)	
premaxillary bone	os incisivum
presphenoid bone	
pubic bone (pelvis)	os pubis; mons pubis
pyramidal bone (triquetral bone)	os triquetrum
radius (forearm)	radius
replacement bone (endochondral bone)	
reticulated bone (woven bone)	

bone (region)	os (pl. ossa)
rib, ribs	os costae, os costale; ossa costalis
rider's bone (cavalry bone, exercise bone)	
Riolan's bone	
sacrum (lower back)	os sacrum
scaphoid bone (wrist)	os scaphoideum
scapula (shoulder)	scapula
scroll bones	
septal bone (interalveolar septum)	
sesamoid bones of hand	ossa sesamoidea manus
sesamoid bones of foot	ossa sesamoidea pedis
shank bone (cannon bone; tibia)	
shin bone (tibia)	
short bone	os breve
sieve bone	
skull, bones of	ossa cranii
sphenoid bone (base of skull)	os sphenoidale
splint bone (fibula)	
spongy bone	
stapes (ear)	stapes
sternum (chest)	sternum
superior limb, bones of (humerus, radius, ulna, carpus, metacarpus, digits of hand)	ossa membri superioris
suprainterparietal bone	
suprasternal bones	ossa suprasternalia
sutural bones	ossa suturalia; ossa fonticulorum
tail bone (coccyx)	os coccygis
talus (ankle)	talus; os tarsi tibiale
tarsal bones (ankle and foot)	ossa tarsi
temporal bone (skull)	os temporale
thigh bone (femur)	
thoracic bones	ossa thoracis
three-cornered bone (triquetral bone)	os triquetrum
tibia (leg)	tibia
tongue bone (hyoid bone)	
trabecular bone	
trapezium bone (wrist)	os trapezium; os carpale distale primum
trapezoid bone (wrist)	os trapezoideum; os carpale distale secundum

bone (region)	os (pl. ossa)
triangular bone	os trigonum
triquetral bone (wrist)	os triquetrum
turbinate bone, inferior	
(inferior nasal concha)	
tympanic bone	
ulna (forearm)	ulna
unciform bone (hamate bone)	
upper jaw bone (maxilla)	
vertebrae (back)	
vertebrae, cervical	vertebrae cervicales
vertebrae, thoracic (dorsal)	vertebrae thoracicae
vertebrae, lumbar	vertebrae lumbales
vertebrae, sacral	vertebrae sacrales
vertebrae, coccygeal	vertebrae coccygeae
Vesalius' bone; vesalian bone	os vesalianum pedis
vomer (skull)	vomer
wedge bone (intermediate cuneiform)	
woven bone (nonlamellar; reticulated)	
yoke bone (zygomatic bone)	
zygomatic bone (skull)	os zygomaticum

Table of Normal Laboratory Values

All are adult values, unless otherwise specified.

Abbreviations and symbols used in these tables:

±	plus or minus
≤	less than or equal to
≥	greater than or equal to
/	per
%	percent
<	less than
>	greater than
μ	micron
μ^3	cubic micron
μg	microgram
μmol	micromole
μU	microunit
d	day
dL	deciliter
EU	Ehrlich units
g	gram
Hb	hemoglobin
hr.	hour
IU	international unit
kg	kilogram
L	liter
mEq	milliequivalent
mg	milligram
mIU	international milliunit
mL	milliliter
mmol	millimole
mOsm	milliosmole
mU	milliunit
ng	nanogram
pg	picogram
s	seconds
U	unit

Blood

acetaldehyde	<0.2 mg/L
acetoacetate	negative
acid hemolysis test (Ham's test)	<5% lysis
acetone	negative
acid phosphatase	0 to 7 mU/mL, or less than 3 ng/mL
acidified serum test (Ham's test)	<5% lysis
ACT (activated coagulation time)	107 ± 13 s
ACTH (adrenocorticotropic hormone)	25 to 100 pg/mL
activated coagulation time (ACT)	107 ± 13 s
activated partial thromboplastin time (APTT)	25 to 35 s
adrenocorticotropic hormone (ACTH)	25 to 100 pg/mL
AFP (alpha-fetoprotein) tumor marker	0 to 10 ng/mL
A/G (albumin/globulin) ratio	1.1 to 2.3
alanine aminotransferase—see *ALT*.	
albumin	3 to 5 g/dL
albumin/globulin (A/G) ratio	1.1 to 2.3
aldolase	1 to 8 U/L
aldosterone	supine, 3 to 10 ng/dL
	upright, 5 to 30 ng/dL
alkaline phosphatase	10 to 32 mU/mL, or 30 to 120 U/L
alpha$_1$-antitrypsin	105 to 200 mg/dL
alpha-1-fetoprotein, serum (AFP)	<40 ng/mL
ALT (alanine aminotransferase) (formerly SGPT)	0 to 17 mU/mL
aminotransferase—see *ALT* and *AST*.	
ammonia	0 to 50 μmol/L
ammonia nitrogen	15 to 45 μg N/dL
amylase	0-88 U/L
ANA (antinuclear antibody)	negative
angiotensin I	11 to 88 pg/mL
angiotensin II	arterial, 2.4 ± 1.2 ng/dL
	venous, 50% to 75% of arterial
anion gap	7 to 16 mmol/L
anti-centromere screen and titer	negative
alpha$_1$-antichymotrypsin	30 to 60 mg/dL
antideoxyribonuclease B titer (anti-DNAse titer)	≤ 170 units

Blood

antidiuretic hormone (ADH)
  (vasopressin) mOsmol/kg

270-280:	<1.5 pg/mL
280-285:	<2.5 pg/mL
285-290:	1 to 5 pg/mL
290-295:	2 to 7 pg/mL
295-300:	4 to 12 pg/mL

anti-DNA antibodies
  indirect fluorescence   negative in 1:10 dilution
  Farr method   <20% of DNA bound
  Ginsberg/Keiser $\leq 1\mu g/mL$
antihyaluronidase (AH) titer ≤ 128 units
antinuclear antibody (ANA)   negative
antistreptolysin-O (ASO) titer ≤ 166 Todd units
alpha$_1$-antitrypsin   105 to 200 mg/dL
antithrombin III (AT-III)
  radioimmunodiffusion   plasma, 21 to 30 mg/dL
     serum, 17 to 25 mg/dL

  amidolytic   plasma, 85 to 115% of standard
     serum, 55 to 80% of standard

APTT (activated partial
  thromboplastin time)   25 to 35 s
arterial blood gases—see *blood gases.*
ascorbic acid   0.6 to 2.0 mg/dL
ASO (antistreptolysin-O) titer ≤ 166 Todd units
aspartate aminotransferase—see *AST.*
AST (aspartate aminotransferase)   0 to 19 mU/mL
  (formerly SGOT)
bands (banded neutrophils)   3% to 5%
  on WBC differential
base excess   -3 to +3
basos (basophils) on WBC
  differential   0 to 0.75%
beta carotene   60 to 200 $\mu g/dL$
bicarbonate (CO_2), arterial   23 to 29 mEq/L
bile acids, total
  fasting   0.3 to 2.3 $\mu g/mL$
  2-hr. postprandial   1.8 to 3.2 $\mu g/mL$

Blood

bilirubin	
direct (conjugated)	0.1 to 0.4 mg/dL
indirect (unconjugated)	0.2 to 0.7 mg/dL
total	0.3 to 1.2 mg/dL
bleeding time	
Duke	1 to 5 minutes
Ivy	2 to 7 minutes
Simplate	2.75 to 8 minutes
blood factors—see *factors*.	
blood gases, arterial	
calculated bicarbonate	18 to 23 mmol/L
PCO_2	35-45 mm Hg
pH	7.35-7.45
PO_2	75-100 mm Hg
oxygen (O_2) saturation	96-100%
blood volume	8.5 to 9.0% of body weight
	females, 50 to 75 mL/kg
	males, 52 to 83 mL/kg
bone marrow differential (%)	
myeloblasts	0.3 to 5.0
promyelocytes	1 to 8
myelocytes	
neutrophilic	5 to 19
eosinophilic	0.5 to 3.0
basophilic	0 to 0.5
metamyelocytes	13 to 32
polymorphonuclear neutrophils	7 to 30
polymorphonuclear eosinophils	0.5 to 4.0
polymorphonuclear basophils	0.0 to 0.7
lymphocytes	3 to 17
plasma cells	0 to 2
monocytes	0.5 to 5.0
reticulum cells	0.1 to 2.0
megakaryocytes	0.03 to 3.0
pronormoblasts	1 to 8
normoblasts	7 to 32
BUN (blood urea nitrogen)	10 to 26 mg/dL
calcitonin (hCT)	<100 pg/mL

Blood

calcium	
ionized	4.25 to 5.25 mg/dL or
	1/13 to 1.32 mmol/L
total	9.2 to 11 mg/dL
cancer antigen (CA-125)	0 to 35 U/mL
capillary fragility test	<5 to 10 petechiae on forearm
	halfway between systolic and
	diastolic pressures
carbon dioxide	
partial pressure (PCO_2)	35 to 45 mm Hg
total	23 to 31 mmol/L
carbon monoxide	nonsmokers, <2% total Hb
	smokers, <10% total Hb
carcinoembryonic antigen (CEA)	nonsmokers, <3 ng/mL
	smokers, <5 ng/mL
cardiac isoenzymes (CK, creatine kinase)	
CK-BB	absent
CK-MB	absent
CK-MM	present
carotenoids	0.5 to 3.0 μg/mL
catecholamines, serum (random)	
norepinephrine	104 to 548 pg/mL
epinephrine	<88 pg/mL
dopamine	<136 pg/mL
CBC (complete blood count)	
hematocrit	females, 35 to 46%
	males, 41 to 53%
hemoglobin	females, 12 to 16 g/dL
	males, 13.5 to 17.5 g/dL
MCH (mean corpuscular hemoglobin)	25.4 to 34.6 pg/cell
MCHC (mean corpuscular hemoglobin concentration)	32 to 36 g/dL
MCV (mean corpuscular volume)	80 to 105 μ^3
RBC (red blood cell) count	3.5 to 6.0 million
WBC (white blood cell) count	4,500 to 10,000
(see also *white blood cell differential*)	
CD2 (T11) total T cells	70 to 94%
CD3 (T3) mature T cells	57 to 91%
CD4/CD3 lymphocyte ratio	CD4 = 32 to 68%
	CD3 = 57 to 91%

Blood

CD4/CD8 lymphocyte ratio	CD4 = 32 to 68%
	CD3 = 57 to 91%
	CD8 = 10 to 36%
cell count—see *white count differential.*	
ceruloplasmin	14 to 40 mg/dL
C (complement components or inhibitor proteins, C1–C9, not subscripts)	
$C1_s$ esterase inhibitor immuno-differential	2.1 to 4.1 mg/dL
C1q, serum	5.1 to 7.9 mg/dL
C2, serum	1.9 to 2.5 mg/dL
C3, serum	83 to 177 mg/dL
C4, serum	12 to 36 mg/dL
C5, serum	3.8 to 9.0 mg/dL
C6, serum	4.0 to 7.2 mg/dL
C7, serum	4.9 to 7.0 mg/dL
C8, serum	4.3 to 6.3 mg/dL
C9, serum	4.7 to 6.9 mg/dL
chloride (Cl), serum	96 to 106 mEq/L
cholesterol	
HDL (high-density lipoprotein)	>35 mg/dL recommended
LDL (low-density lipoprotein)	<130 mg/dL recommended
total	<200 mg/dL recommended
cholic acid	0.20 ± 0.17 µg/mL
cholinesterase II	
RID	0.5 to 1.5 mg/dL
DuPont ACA	7 to 19 U/mL
chorionic gonadotropin	nondetectable unless pregnant
7-10 days	>5.0 mIU/mL
30 days	>100 mIU/mL
40 days	>2000 mIU/mL
10 weeks	50,000 to 100,000 mIU/mL
14 weeks	10,000 to 20,000 mIU/mL
trophoblastic disease	>100,000 mIU/mL
citrulline, serum	12 to 55 µmol/L
CK (creatine kinase)	females, 0 to 150 IU/L
	males, 0 to 175 IU/L
CK (creatine kinase) isoenzymes—see *cardiac isoenzymes.*	
coagulation (clotting) time	5 to 15 minutes

Blood

coagulation factors—see *Factors*.

cold hemolysin test (Donath-Landsteiner)	negative
Coombs test, direct and indirect	negative
copper	70 to 155 μg/dL
corticosterone	0.13 to 2.3 μg/dL
cortisol, serum	8:00 AM, 5 to 23 μg/dL
	4:00 PM, 3 to 15 μg/dL
	10:00 PM, $\leq$50% of 8:00 AM value
C-peptide	$\leq$5.0 ng/mL
C-reactive protein (CRP)	68 to 820 ng/mL

creatine kinase—see *cardiac isoenzymes*.

creatinine, serum	0.7 to 1.5 mg/dL
creatinine clearance	88 to 137 mL/minute
CRP (C-reactive protein)	68 to 820 ng/mL
cryoglobulin screen	negative
cyanide, serum	nonsmokers, 0.004 mg/L
	smokers, 0.006 mg/L
dehydroepiandrosterone (DHEA)	1.7 to 5.2 ng/mL
dehydroepiandrosterone sulfate	females, 0.11 to 3.38 μg/mL
(DHEA-SO$_4$)	males, 1.99 to 3.34 μg/mL
deoxycholic acid, total	0.22$\pm$0.13 μg/mL
dihydrotestosterone (DHT)	adult females, 10 to 40 ng/dL
	adult males, 60 to 300 ng/dL
2,3 diphosphoglycerate	
(2,3 DPG)	12.27 $\pm$1.87 μmol/g Hb
electrolytes	
bicarbonate (CO$_2$)	23 to 29 mEq/L
chlorides (Cl)	96 to 106 mEq/L
potassium (K)	3.5 to 5.0 mEq/L
magnesium (Mg)	1.3 to 2.5 mEq/L
sodium (Na)	136 to 146 mEq/L
electrophoresis	
globulin	0.1 to 0.4 g/dL
alpha-1	0.4 to 1.1 g/dL
alpha-2	0.5 to 1.6 g/dL
beta	0.5 to 1.4 g/dL
gamma	0.7 to 1.2 g/dL
hemoglobin	HbA >95%
	HbA2 1.5% to 3.5%
	HbF <2%

Blood

eosinophils (eos) on WBC differential	1% to 3%
eosinophil count	50 to 350 cells/mL
erythrocyte count (RBC)	3.5 million to 5.5 million/mL
erythrocyte sedimentation rate (ESR or sed rate)	Wintrobe: 0 to 15 mm/hr. Westergren: 0 to 20 mm/hr.
erythropoietin	
hemagglutination	25 to 125 mIU/mL
RIA	<5 to 20 mIU/mL
bioassay	5 to 18 mU/mL
ESR (erythrocyte sedimentation rate)	Wintrobe: 0 to 15 mm/hr. Westergren: 0 to 20 mm/hr.
estradiol, serum	females, 10 to 500 pg/mL (varies with menstrual cycle) males, 8 to 36 pg/mL
estriol	
free	positive with pregnancy, 3.5 to 34.0 μg/L
total serum	males and nonpregnant females, <2 mg/mL positive with pregnancy, 30 to 350 ng/mL
estrogens, total	menstruating, 61 to 437 pg/mL prepubertal/postmenopausal females, ≤40 pg/mL males, 40 to 115 pg/mL
estrogen receptor assay (ERA)	>10 fmol/mg protein
estrone (E1)	female pubertal, 0 to 80 pg/mL female adult, 20 to 150 pg/mL male pubertal, 11 to 21 pg/mL male adult, 30 to 170 pg/mL
factors, blood coagulation	
factor I (fibrinogen)	200 to 400 mg/dL
factor II (prothrombin)	0.5 to 1.5 U/mL
factor II antigen	75% to 125% of normal
factor V	0.5 to 2.0 U/mL
factor VII	65% to 135% of normal
factor VIII (antihemophiliac)	55% to 145% of normal
factor VIII antigen	50% to 200% of normal
factor IX	60% to 140% of normal
factor X	60% to 130% of normal

Blood

factors, blood coagulation *(continued)*

factor XI	65% to 135% of normal
factor XII (Hageman)	65% to 150% of normal
factor XIII (fibrin stabilizing)	0.02 to 0.05 U/mL

fatty acid profile

oleic	26 to 45%
palmitic	23 to 25%
stearic	10 to 14%
linoleic	8 to 16%
fatty acids, total	190 to 420 mg/dL
ferritin	females, 12 to 150 ng/mL
	males, 15 to 200 ng/mL
fibrin lysis time	>60 minutes
fibrinogen	200 to 400 mg/dL
5'-nucleotidase	1 to 12 U/L
fluoride	0.01 to 0.2 μg/mL

folate

serum	3 to 12 ng/mL
red blood cell	153 to 605 ng/mL
follicle stimulating hormone (FSH)	menstruating females,
	4 to 90 mIU/mL
	pregnant females, low to undetectable
	postmenopausal females,
	40 to 250 mIU/mL
	males, 4 to 25 mIU/mL

free thyroxine index—see *thyroxine index.*

fructose	1 to 6 mg/dL
FTA-IgM, serum (fluorescent treponemal antibody)	nonreactive
galactose	<5 mg/dL

gamma-glutamyl transpeptidase—older name for GGT *(gamma-glutamyl-transferase)*

gastrin, serum	<60 years old, <100 pg/mL
	>60 years old, 100 to 800 pg/mL

GGT (gamma-glutamyltransferase) (formerly gamma-glutamyl transpeptidase or GGTP)   5 to 40 U/L

GGTP (gamma-glutamyl transpeptidase)— see *GGT.*

Blood

glucose	fasting, 70 to 110 mg/dL
	2 hr. postprandial, < 120 mg/dL
glucose tolerance test (GTT)	fasting, 70 to 110 mg/dL
	at 1 hr., 120 to 170 mg/dL
	at 1-1/2 hr., 100 to 140 mg/dL
	at 2 hr., 70 to 120 mg/dL
glycerol, free	0.29 to 1.72 mg/dL
glycosylated hemoglobin (Hgb Al$_c$)	5.6 to 7.5%
gold	< 10 μg/dL (therapeutic, 38-50)
growth hormone (hGH or GH)	females, < 10 ng/mL
	males, < 2 ng/mL
Ham's acidified serum test	< 5% lysis
haptoglobin	
RID	30 to 175 mg/dL
nephelometry	25 to 175 mg/dL
haptoglobin/hemopexin (under two years)	
haptoglobin	100 to 300 mg/dL
hemopexin	40 to 100 mg/dL
HCG, hCG (human chorionic	< 2 mIU/mL
gonadotropin) tumor marker	
HDL (high density lipoprotein) cholesterol	> 35 mg/dL recommended
hematocrit (HCT, Hct)	females, 35 to 46%
	males, 41 to 53%
hemoglobin (Hb)	females, 12 to 16 g/dL
	males, 13.5 to 17.5 g/dL
hemoglobin A	> 95%
hemoglobin A2 (HbA2)	1.5% to 3.5%
hemoglobin A1C (HbA$_{1C}$)	
electrophoresis	5.6 to 7.5%
column	6 to 9%
hemoglobin electrophoresis	HbA > 95%
	HbA2 1.5% to 3.5%
	HbF < 2%
hemoglobin F	< 2.0
hemoglobin H (HbH)	No precipitation at 40 minutes
high-density liproprotein (HDL) cholesterol	> 35 mg/dL recommended
human chorionic gonadotropin	< 2 mIU/mL
(HCG, hCG) tumor marker	
hydroxyproline	females, 0 to 34 μmol/L
	males, 0 to 42 μmol/L

Blood

immunoglobulins
  IgA   60 to 383 mg/dL
  IgD   0 to 8 mg/dL
  IgE   0 to 230 IU/mL
  IgG   600 to 1900 mg/dL
  IgM   40 to 345 mg/dL

immunoglobulins	
IgA	60 to 383 mg/dL
IgD	0 to 8 mg/dL
IgE	0 to 230 IU/mL
IgG	600 to 1900 mg/dL
IgM	40 to 345 mg/dL
insulin, 12-hr. fasting	<60 years old, 7 to 24 μU/mL
	>60 years old, 6 to 35 μU/mL
ionized calcium	4.25 to 5.25 mg/dL
iron	newborn, 100 to 250 μg/dL
	infant, 40 to 100 μg/dL
	child, 50 to 120 μg/dL
	adult females, 40 to 150 μg/dL
	adult males, 50 to 160 μg/dL
iron-binding capacity, total (TIBC)	250 to 410 μg/dL
iron saturation	20 to 55%
isocitrate dehydrogenase (ICD)	1.2 to 7.0 U/L
isoenzymes, serum by agarose gel	
electrophoresis	
Fraction 1	14 to 26% of total
Fraction 2	29 to 39% of total
Fraction 3	20 to 26% of total
Fraction 4	8 to 16% of total
Fraction 5	6 to 16% of total
ketone bodies	
qualitative	negative
quantitative	0.5 to 3.0 mg/dL
lactate	venous, 4.5 to 20 mg/dL
	arterial, 4.5 to 14.4 mg/dL
lactate dehydrogenase (LDH)	50 to 220 U/L
lactose	<0.5 mg/dL
LDH (lactate dehydrogenase)	50 to 220 U/L
LDL (low-density lipoprotein) cholesterol	<130 mg/dL recommended
lead	0 to 50 μ/dL
leucine	75 to 175 μmol/L
lipase	
Cherry-Crandall	0 to 1.5 units
Tietz	0.1 to 1.0 U/mL
lipase, BMD	<180 U/L
lipoprotein electrophoresis	distinct beta band

Blood

liver functions
    acid phosphatase   0 to 7 mU/mL
    alkaline phosphatase   10 to 32 mU/mL
    ALT (formerly SGPT)   0 to 17 mU/mL
    AST (formerly SGOT)   0 to 19 mU/mL
    bilirubin
        direct (conjugated)   0.1 to 0.4 mg/dL
        indirect (unconjugated) 0.2 to 0.7 mg/dL
        total   0.3 to 1.1 mg/dL
low-density lipoprotein (LDL) cholesterol   <130 mg/dL recommended
luteinizing hormone (LH)
    females:
        follicular   follicular phase, 5-30 mIU/mL
        midcycle   75 to 150 mIU/mL
        luteal   3 to 40 mIU/mL
        postmenopausal   30 to 200 mIU/mL
    males   6 to 23 mIU/mL
lymphs (lymphocytes)   25% to 33%
lysozyme (muramidase)   5 to 15 μg/mL
magnesium (Mg)   1.3 to 2.5 mEq/L
MB isoenzyme, bands, or fraction   <5%
MCH (mean corpuscular hemoglobin)   25.4 to 34.6 pg/cell
MCHC (mean corpuscular hemoglobin   32 to 36 g/dL
    concentration)
MCV (mean corpuscular volume)   80 to 105 microns
mercury   <5 μg/dL
methanol   <0.15 mg/dL
methemalbumin   negative
methionine   6 to 40 μmol/L
methemoglobin (MetHb)   0.06 to 0.24 g/dL or
                        0 to 1.5% of total hemoglobin
monos (monocytes) on WBC differential   3% to 7%
myoglobin   6 to 85 ng/mL
5'-nucleotidase   1 to 12 U/L
orosomucoid   55 to 140 mg/dL
osmolality
    serum   275 to 295 mOsmol/kg
    urine/serum ratio   1 to 3; >3 after 12 hr. fluid restriction
oxygen (O_2) saturation   96-100%
oxytocin   <3.2 μU/mL

Blood

partial thromboplastin time (PTT)	35 to 40 s
PCO$_2$ (partial pressure of carbon dioxide)	35-45 mm Hg
pH (measures acidity)	7.35-7.45
phosphatase	
acid	0 to 7 mU/mL, or less than 3 ng/mL
alkaline	10 to 32 mU/mL, or 30 to 120 U/L
phosphate, serum	3.0 to 4.5 mEq/L
phospholipids, total	<65 years old, 125 to 275 mg/dL
	>65 years old, 196 to 366 mg/dL
phosphorus, inorganic	3 to 4.5 mg/dL (or 1 to 1.5 mEq/L)
plasma volume	females, 28 to 45 mL/kg
	males, 25 to 43 mL/kg
phenylalanine	0.8 to 1.8 mg/dL
platelets	150,000 to 400,000/mL
PMNs or polys (polymorphonuclear neutrophils) on WBC differential	54 to 62%
prealbumin, serum	8 to 31 mg/dL
potassium (K)	3.5 to 5.0 mEq/L
PO$_2$ (partial pressure of oxygen)	75-100 mm Hg
progesterone	
pubertal females	0 to 13 ng/mL
adult females	0.02 to 0.9 ng/mL follicular phase
adult females	6 to 30 ng/mL luteal phase
pubertal males	0.11 to 0.26 ng/mL
adult males	0.12 to 0.3 ng/mL
prolactin	
nonpregnant females	5 to 40 ng/mL
pregnant females	<80 to <400 ng/mL
adult males	up to 20 ng/mL
protein	
albumin	3 to 5 g/dL
globulin	1.5 to 3.7 g/dL
total	6 to 8 g/dL
prostaglandins	
E	25 to 200 pg/mL
F	25 to 150 pg/mL
prostate specific antigen (PSA)	
healthy men	0 to 2.8 ng/mL
post prostatectomy	<0.2 ng/mL
prothrombin time (PT, pro time)	12 to 14 s

Blood

protoporphyrin	$<50~\mu g/dL$
PSA (prostate specific antigen)	
healthy men	0 to 2.8 ng/mL
post prostatectomy	<0.2 ng/mL
pseudocholinesterase	
RID	0.5 to 1.5 mg/dL
DuPont ACA	7 to 19 U/mL
PTH-intact (parathyroid hormone)	10 to 65 pg/mL
PT (pro time, prothrombin time)	12 to 14 s
PTT (partial thromboplastin time)	35 to 40 s
pyruvic acid	0.3 to 0.9 mg/dL
sulfhemoglobin (SHb)	$\leq 1.0\%$ of total hemoglobin
RA latex (rheumatoid arthritis)	negative
red blood cells	3.5-6.0 million
red blood cell indices—see *CBC*.	
red cell distribution width (RDW)	$<15\%$
red cell volume	females, 19 to 31 mL/kg
	males, 20 to 36 mL/kg
renin	supine, 1.6 ± 1.5; standing, 4.5 ± 2.9
reticulocyte count	
range	0.5 to 1.5%
absolute count	25,000 to 75,000/mL
reverse triiodothyronine (rT_3)	30 to 80 ng/dL
riboflavin (vitamin B_2)	See *Urine* section below.
RPR (rapid plasma reagin)	negative
secretin	37 ± 8 pg/mL
sedimentation rate	Wintrobe: 0 to 15 mm/hr.
	Westergren 0 to 20 mm/hr.
segs (segmented neutrophils) on WBC	54 to 62%
differential; also *polys* and *PMNs*	
selenium	10 to 34 $\mu g/dL$
serotonin	whole blood, 39 to 361 ng/mL
SGOT (serum glutamic oxalo-acetic	
transaminase)—see *AST*.	
SGPT (serum glutamic pyruvic	
transaminase)—see *ALT*.	
sodium (Na)	136 to 146 mEq/L
somatomedin C	0.4 to 2.0 U/mL
somatotropin (growth hormone)	females, <10 ng/mL
	males, <2 ng/mL

Blood

stab (also "band," banded neutrophil)	3% to 5%
sucrose	mean, 0.06 mg/dL
sulfate	2.9 to 3.5 mg/dL
testosterone, free	
prepubertal females	0.04 ±0.01 ng/dL
adult females	0.31±0.07 ng/dL
prepubertal males	0.04±0.01 ng/dL
adult males	7.9±2.3 ng/dL
testosterone, total	
prepubertal females	6.6±2.5 ng/dL
adult females	37±10 ng/dL
prepubertal males	6.6±2.5 ng/dL
adult males	572±135 ng/dL
thrombin time	±2 s when control is 9 to 13 s, or 14.5 to 18.9 s
thyroid function tests	
T_3 (triiodothyronine) uptake	25% to 38%
T_4 (thyroxine)	4.4 to 9.9 μg/dL
TSH (thyroid stimulating hormone)	2 to 10 μU/mL
thyroid antibodies	≤1:10 dilution
thyroid microsomal antibodies	nondetectable
thyroid stimulating hormone (TSH)	2 to 10 μU/mL
thyroid uptake of radioactive iodine	2 hr.: <6%
	6 hr.: 3 to 20%
	24 hr.: 8 to 30%
thyrotropin-releasing hormone (TRH)	5 to 60 pg/mL
thyroxine (T_4)	
free	0.8 to 2.4 ng/dL
serum (total)	4.4 to 9.9 μg/dL
	pregnant females, 6.1 to 17.6 μg/dL
thyroxine-binding globulin (TBG)	15 to 34 μg/mL
thyroxine index, free (FT_4I)	5.5 to 10
TIBC (total iron-binding capacity)	250 to 410 μg/dL
tourniquet test	<5 to 10 petechiae on forearm halfway between systolic and diastolic pressures
transcortin	females, 1.6 to 2.5 mg/dL
	pregnant females, 4.7 to 7.0 mg/dL
	males, 1.5 to 2.0 mg/dL
transferrin	200 to 400 mg/dL
transketolase	9 to 12 μmol/hr./mL whole blood

Blood

triglycerides	35 to 160 mg/dL
triiodothyronine	
T_3-RIA	115 to 190 ng/dL
free	230 to 660 pg/dL
total	150 to 250 ng/dL
reverse (rT_3)	30 to 80 ng/dL
2,3 diphosphoglycerate (2,3 DPG)	12.27 $\pm$1.87 μmol/g Hb
tyrosine	0.8 to 1.3 mg/dL
urea nitrogen	8 to 23 mg/dL
urea nitrogen/creatinine ratio	12:1 to 20:1
uric acid	2.2 to 7.7 mg/dL
valine	141 to 317 μmol/L
vasoactive intestinal polypeptide (VIP)	20 to 53 pg/mL
VDRL (Venereal Disease Research Lab)	nonreactive
viscosity, serum	1.10 to 1.22 Centipoise
vitamin	
A	30 to 65 μg/dL
B_2 (riboflavin)	See *Urine* section below.
B_6	3.6 to 18 ng/mL
B_{12}	110 to 800 pg/mL
C	0.6 to 2.0 mg/dL
D	1,25-dihydroxy: 20 to 45 pg/mL
	25-hydroxy: 15 to 18 ng/mL
E	5.0 to 20 μg/mL
white blood cells	4,500 to 10,000
white blood cell differential	
polys or PMNs (polymorphonuclear neutrophils [or leukocytes], also known as segmented neutrophils)	54% to 62%
bands (banded [immature] neutrophils, also called "stabs")	3% to 5%
lymphs (lymphocytes)	25% to 33%
eos (eosinophils)	1% to 3%
monos (monocytes)	3% to 7%
basos (basophils)	0 to 0.75%
xylose absorption test	child, 1 hr.: >30 mg/dL
	adult, 2 hr.: >25 mg/dL
zinc	70 to 150 μg/dL

Urine

acetoacetate	negative
acetone	negative
alanine (24-hr. urine)	8 to 48 mg/d
albumin	negative (less than 80 mg/d)
ammonia nitrogen	500 to 1200 mg/d
ammonium chloride loading test	pH should fall to ≤ 5.2 two to eight hours after dosing
amorphous	few
amylase	1 to 17 U/hr.
bacteria	few or moderate
bilirubin	negative
blood	negative
calcium, 24-hr.	< 300 mg/d
casts	negative
catecholamines, 24-hr.	
epinephrine	< 15 μg/d
norepinephrine	< 100 μg/d
chloride, 24-hr.	110 to 250 mEq/d
citrulline, 24-hr.	0.4 to 8 mg/d
color	yellow, straw, or colorless
copper, 24-hr.	0 to 50 μg/d
coproporphyrin, 24-hr.	30 to 250 μg/d
cortisol, free, 24-hr.	10 to 100 μg/d
creatine	females, < 100 mg/d
	males, < 40 mg/d
creatinine, 24-hr.	14 to 26 mg/kg/d
crystals	few
cystine or cysteine	random, negative
	24-hr., 10 to 100 mg/d
DHEA (dehydroepiandrosterone), 24-hr.	0 to 2.3 ng/mL
endothelial cells	few or moderate
estrogen, 24-hr.	menstruating females, 4 to 100 μg/d
	postmenopausal females, < 10 μg/d
	pregnant females, $< 45,000$ μg/d
	males, 5 to 25 μg/d
estradiol, 24-hr.	females, 0 to 14 μg/d
	males, 0 to 6 μg/d
estriol, total, 24-hr.	6 to 42 mg/d with pregnancy
FIGLU, 24 hr. after dose of histidine	< 35 mg/d
5-HIAA (5-hydroxyindoleacetic acid)	random, negative; 24-hr., 2 to 8 mg/d

Urine

fluoride	0.2 to 1.1 μg/mL
folate absorption test, 24-hr.	45$\pm$7% of dose
glucose	negative
glycine, 24-hr.	59 to 294 mg/d
glycolic acid, 24-hr.	15 to 60 mg/d
hemoglobin/myoglobin	negative
homocystine, random	negative
homovanillic acid (HVAA), 24-hr.	child, 3 to 16 μg/mg creatinine
	adult, <15 mg/d
17-hydroxycorticosteroids, 24-hr.	children, 1 to 5.6 mg/d
	females, 2 to 8 mg/d
	males, 3 to 10 mg/d
5-HIAA (5-hydroxyindoleacetic acid)	random, negative; 24-hr., 2 to 8 mg/d
ketones	negative
17-ketosteroids, 24-hr.	4 to 18 mg/d
lactose	12 to 40 mg/dL
lead	<80 μg/d
leucine, 24-hr.	3 to 70 mg/d
magnesium, 24-hr.	6 to 10 mEq/d
mercury, 24-hr.	<20 μg/L (toxic >150 μg/L)
metanephrine, total, 24-hr.	0.05 to 1.20 μg/mg creatinine
microscopic	
amorphous	few
bacteria	few or moderate
epithelial cells/hpf	few or moderate
hyaline casts/hpf	negative or occasional (0 to 1)
crystals	few
mucus	few
RBC/hpf (red blood cells per high-power field)	negative
WBC/hpf (white blood cells per high-power field)	negative
mucus	few or moderate
nitrite	negative
occult blood	negative
pH	4.5 to 8.0
phenylalanine, 24-hr.	trace to 17 mg/d
phosphorus, inorganic, 24-hr.	0.4 to 1.3 g/d
porphobilinogen	random, negative; 24-hr., 0 to 2 mg/d

Urine

protein, 24-hr.	<150 mg/d
red blood cells	negative
riboflavin (vitamin B2)	80 to 269 μg/g creatinine
sediment	clear or cloudy
selenium, 24-hr.	10 to 100 μg/L
17-hydroxycorticosteroids, 24-hr.	children, 1 to 5.6 mg/d
	females, 2 to 8 mg/d
	males, 3 to 10 mg/d
17-ketosteroids, 24-hr.	4 to 18 mg/d
specific gravity	1.002 to 1.030 random;
	24-hr., 1.015 to 1.025
sucrose	mean, 2.2 mg/dL
tetrahydrocortisol (THF), 24-hr.	0.5 to 1.5 mg/d
tetrahydrodeoxycortisol, 24-hr.	<1000 μg/d
urobilinogen, 24-hr.	0.5 to 4.0 EU/d
uroporphyrin, 24-hr.	<50 μg/d
vanillylmandelic acid (VMA), 24-hr.	1 to 9 mg/d
volume	females, 600 to 1600 mL/d
	males, 800 to 1800 mL/d
white blood cells	negative
xylose absorption test (5-hr.)	child, 16 to 33% of ingested dose
	adult, 5 g dose at 5 hr. >1.2
	adult, 25 g dose at 5 hr., >4.0

Miscellaneous Body Fluids

cerebrospinal fluid (CSF)
    chloride   118 to 132 mEq/L
    electrophoresis   mostly albumin
    glutamine   6 to 16 mg/dL
    myelin basic protein <4 ng/mL
    pressure   70 to 180 mm water
    volume   child, 60 to 100 mL
                            adult, 100 to 160 mL

feces
    coproporphyrin, 24-hr.   400 to 1200 μg/d
    fat, 72-hr. <7 g/d
    nitrogen, total ≤2 g N/d
    occult blood   negative
    protoporphyrin, 24-hr. <1500 μg/d
    urobilinogen   40 to 280 mg/d
    uroporphyrin, 24-hr.   10 to 40 μg/d

gastric acid   0 to 5 mEq/L fasting
                            10 to 60 mEq/L post stimulation

semen
    volume   2 to 4 mL
    sperm count >20 million/mL
    motility $>60\%$
    morphology $>60\%$ normal forms

sweat
    sweat chloride   normal, 0 to 35 mEq/L
                            marginal, 30 to 70 mEq/L
                            cystic fibrosis, 60 to 200 mEq/L

synovial fluid differential (%)
    polymorphonuclear cells   0 to 25
    monocytes   0 to 71
    lymphocytes   0 to 78
    clasmatocytes   0 to 26
    unclassified   0 to 21
    synovial cells   0 to 12

Table of Muscles

muscle	musculus (pl. musculi)
abdominal muscles	musculi abdominis
abdominal external oblique muscle	musculus obliquus externus abdominis
abdominal internal oblique muscle	musculus obliquus internus abdominis
abductor digiti minimi muscle of foot (abductor muscle of little toe)	musculus abductor digiti minimi pedis
abductor digiti minimi muscle of hand (abductor muscle of little finger)	musculus abductor digiti minimi manus
abductor hallucis muscle (great toe)	musculus abductor hallucis
abductor pollicis brevis muscle (abductor muscle of thumb, short)	musculus abductor pollicis brevis
abductor pollicis longus muscle (abductor muscle of thumb, long)	musculus abductor pollicis longus
accessory flexor muscle of foot (quadratus plantae muscle)	musculus flexor accessorius
adductor muscle, short	musculus adductor brevis
adductor muscle of great toe	musculus adductor hallucis
adductor muscle, long	musculus adductor longus
adductor muscle, great	musculus adductor magnus
adductor minimus muscle (adductor muscle, smallest)	musculus adductor minimus
adductor pollicis muscle (thumb)	musculus adductor pollicis
Aeby's cutaneomucous muscle	
agonistic muscles	
Albinus' muscle	
anconeus muscle	musculus anconeus
antagonistic muscles	
anterior auricular muscle	musculus auricularis anterior
anterior cervical intertransverse muscles	musculi intertransversarii anteriores cervicis
anterior rectus muscle of head	musculus rectus capitis anterior
anterior scalene muscle	musculus scalenus anterior

muscle	musculus (pl. musculi)
anterior serratus muscle	musculus serratus anterior
anterior tibial muscle	musculus tibialis anterior
antigravity muscles	
antitragus muscle	musculus antitragicus
arrector pili muscles	musculi arrectores pilorum
(erector muscles of hairs)	
articular muscle	musculus articularis
articular muscle of elbow	musculus articularis cubiti
articular muscle of knee	musculus articularis genus
articular muscle of knee	articularis genu musculus
aryepiglottic muscle	musculus aryepiglotticus
auditory ossicles, muscles of	musculi ossiculorum auditus
axillary arch muscle	pectorodorsalis musculus
back muscles	musculi dorsi
Bell's muscle (ureteric bridge)	
biceps brachii muscle	musculus biceps brachii
(biceps muscle of arm)	
biceps femoris muscle	musculus biceps femoris
(biceps muscle of thigh)	
bipennate muscle	musculus bipennatus
Bochdalek's muscle	musculus triticeoglossus
Bovero's muscle ("sucking muscle")	musculus cutaneomucosus
Bowman's muscle (ciliary muscle)	musculus ciliaris
brachial muscle (brachialis)	musculus brachialis
brachiocephalic muscle	musculus brachiocephalicus
brachioradial muscle (brachioradialis)	musculus brachioradialis
Braune's muscle	musculus puborectalis
broadest muscle of back	musculus latissimus dorsi
bronchoesophageal muscle	musculus bronchoesophageus
Brücke's muscle (Crampton's muscle)	
buccinator muscle	musculus buccinator
buccopharyngeal muscles	musculi pars buccopharyngea
(also, constrictor muscles	
of pharynx, superior)	
bulbocavernous muscle	musculus bulbospongiosus
canine muscle	musculus levator anguli oris
cardiac muscle	
Casser's perforated muscle	musculus coracobrachialis
(casserian muscle)	(ligamentum mallei anterius)

muscle	musculus (pl. musculi)
ceratocricoid muscle	musculus ceratocricoideus
cervical iliocostal muscle	musculus iliocostalis cervicis
cervical interspinal muscles	musculi interspinalis cervicis
cervical longissimus muscle (neck)	musculus longissimus cervicis
cervical muscles	musculi colli
cervical rotator muscles	musculi rotatores cervicis
Chassaignac's axillary muscle	
chin muscle	musculus mentalis
chondroglossus muscle	musculus chondroglossus
chondropharyngeal muscles	musculi pars chondropharyngea
(constrictor muscle of pharynx, middle)	(constrictor pharyngis medius)
ciliary muscle	muscularis ciliaris
coccygeal (coccygeus) muscle(s)	musculus coccygeus, musculi coccygei
Coiter's muscle	musculus corrugator supercilii
compressor muscle of naris	
congenerous muscles	
constrictor muscle of pharynx, inferior	musculus constrictor pharyngis inferior
constrictor muscle of pharynx, middle	musculus constrictor pharyngis medius
constrictor muscle of pharynx, superior	musculus constrictor pharyngis superior
coracobrachial muscle (coracobrachialis)	musculus coracobrachialis
corrugator muscle	corrugator supercilii musculus
corrugator cutis muscle of anus	musculus corrugator cutis ani
corrugator supercilii muscle	musculus corrugator supercilii
Crampton's muscle (Bruecke's muscle)	
cremaster muscle (Riolan's muscle)	musculus cremaster
cricoarytenoid muscle, lateral	musculus crico-arytenoideus lateralis
cricoarytenoid muscle, posterior	musculus crico-arytenoideus posterior
cricopharyngeal muscle	musculus cricopharyngeus
cricothyroid muscle	musculus cricothyroideus
cruciate muscle	musculus cruciatus
cutaneomucous muscle	musculus cutaneomucosus
(the "sucking muscle," also called	
Aeby's muscle, Bovero's muscle,	
Klein's muscle, Krause's muscle,	
mucocutaneous muscle)	
cutaneous muscle	musculus cutaneus
dartos muscle of scrotum	musculus tunica dartos
deep muscles of back (true back muscles)	musculi dorsi
deep flexor muscle of fingers	musculus flexor digitorum profundus

muscle	musculus (pl. musculi)
deep transverse perineal msucle	musculus transversus perinei profundus
deltoid muscle	musculus deltoideus
depressor muscle of angle of mouth	musculus depressor anguli oris
depressor muscle of epiglottis	musculus thyroepiglottic
depressor muscle of eyebrow	musculus depressor supercilii
depressor muscle of lower lip	musculus depressor labii inferioris
depressor muscle of septum of nose	musculus depressor septi
depressor superciliary muscle	musculus depressor supercilii
detrusor muscle of urinary bladder	musculus detrusor urinae (musculus detrusor vesicae)
diaphragm, diaphragmatic muscle	diaphragma
digastric muscle	musculus digastricus
dilator muscle	musculus dilatator
dilator muscle of ileocecal sphincter	musculus dilator pylori ilealis
dilator muscle of pupil	musculus dilator pupillae
dilator muscle of pylorus	musculus dilator pylori gastro-duodenalis
dorsal interosseous muscles of foot	musculi interossei dorsalis pedis
dorsal interosseous muscles of hand	musculi interossei dorsalis manus
dorsal muscles (muscles of back)	musculi dorsi
dorsal sacrococcygeal muscle	musculus sacrococcygeus dorsalis
Dupré's muscle	musculus articularis genu
Duverney's muscle	musculus orbicularis oculi
elevator muscle of anus	musculus levator ani
elevator muscle of prostate	musculus levator prostatae
elevator muscles of rib	musculi levatores costarum
elevator muscle of scapula	musculus levator scapulae
elevator muscle of soft palate	musculus levator veli palatini
elevator muscle of upper eyelid	musculus levator palpebrae superioris
elevator muscle of upper lip	musculus levator labii superioris
elevator muscle of upper lip and wing of nose	musculus levator labii superioris alaeque nasi
emergency muscles	
epicranial muscle	musculus epicranius
epimeric muscle	
epitrochleoanconeus muscle	musculus epitrochleoanconaeus
erector muscles of hairs (arrector pili)	musculi arrectores pilorum
erector muscle of penis	musculus ischiocavernosus
erector muscle of spine	musculus erector spinae

muscle	musculus (pl. musculi)
eustachian muscle	musculus tensor tympani
expression, muscles of	musculi faciales
extensor muscle of fingers	musculus extensor digitorum
extensor muscle of great toe, long	musculus extensor hallucis longus
extensor muscle of great toe, short	musculus extensor hallucis brevis
extensor muscle of hand, short (Pozzi's muscle)	musculus extensor digitorum brevis manus
extensor muscle of index finger	musculus extensor indicis
extensor muscle of little finger	musculus extensor digiti minimi
extensor muscle of thumb, long	musculus extensor pollicis longus
extensor muscle of thumb, short	musculus extensor pollicis brevis
extensor muscle of toes, long	musculus extensor digitorum longus
extensor muscle of toes, short	musculus extensor digitorum brevis
extensor muscle of wrist, radial, long	musculus extensor carpi radialis longus
extensor muscle of wrist, radial, short	musculus extensor carpi radialis brevis
extensor muscle of wrist, ulnar	musculus extensor carpi ulnaris
external intercostal muscles	musculi intercostales externi
external oblique muscle	musculus obliquus externus abdominis
external obturator muscle	musculus obturator externus
external pterygoid muscle	lateral pterygoid musculus
external sphincter muscle of anus	
extraocular muscles	musculi bulbi
extrinsic muscles	
eyeball muscles (extraocular muscles)	
facial and masticatory muscles	musculi faciales et masticatores
facial expression, muscles of	musculi faciales
facial muscles	musculi faciales
fast muscle (white muscle)	
fauces (the throat), muscles of	musculi palati et faucium
femoral muscle	musculus vastus intermedius
fibular muscle, long	musculus peroneus longus
fibular muscle, short	musculus peroneus brevis
fibular muscle, third	musculus peroneus tertius
fixation muscles, fixator muscles	
fixator muscle of base of stapes	musculus fixator baseos stapedis
flexor muscle of fingers, deep	musculus flexor digitorum profundus
flexor muscle of fingers, superficial	musculus flexor digitorum superficialis
flexor muscle of great toe, long	musculus flexor hallucis longus
flexor muscle of great toe, short	musculus flexor hallucis brevis

muscle	musculus (pl. musculi)
flexor muscle of little finger, short	musculus flexor digiti minimi brevis manus
flexor muscle of little toe, short	musculus flexor digiti minimi brevis pedis
flexor muscle of thumb, short	musculus flexor pollicis brevis
flexor muscle of thumb, long	musculus flexor pollicis longus
flexor muscle of toes, short	musculus flexor digitorum brevis
flexor muscle of toes, long	musculus flexor digitorum longus
flexor muscle of wrist, radial	musculus flexor carpi radialis
flexor muscle of wrist, ulnar	musculus flexor carpi ulnaris
Folius' muscle	ligamentum mallei laterale
fusiform muscle (spindle-shaped muscle)	musculus fusiformis
Gantzer's muscle	
gastrocnemius muscle	musculus gastrocnemius
Gavard's muscle	
gemellus muscle, inferior	musculus gemellus inferior
gemellus muscle, superior	musculus gemellus superior
genioglossal muscle	musculus genioglossus
geniohyoid muscle	musculus geniohyoideus
glossopalatine muscle (palatoglossus)	musculus palatoglossus
glossopharyngeal muscle	pars glossopharyngea musculi constrictoris pharyngis superioris
gluteal muscle, greatest	musculus gluteus maximus
gluteal muscle, least	musculus gluteus minimus
gluteal muscle, middle	musculus gluteus medius
gracilis muscle	musculus gracilis
great adductor muscle	musculus adductor magnus
greater pectoral muscle	musculus pectoralis major
greater posterior rectus muscle of head	musculus rectus capitis posterior major
greater psoas muscle	musculus psoas major
greater rhomboid muscle	musculus rhomboideus major
greater zygomatic muscle	musculus zygomaticus major
Guthrie's muscle	sphincter urethrae
hamstring muscles	
head, muscles of	musculi capitis
Hilton's muscle	musculus aryepiglotticus
Horner's muscle	musculus orbicularis oculi
Houston's muscle	compressor venae dorsalis penis
hyoglossal (hyoglossus) muscle	musculus hyoglossus

muscle	musculus (pl. musculi)
iliac muscle	musculus iliacus
iliacus minor muscle	musculus iliacus minor
iliococcygeal muscle	musculus iliococcygeus
iliocostal muscle	musculus iliocostalis
iliocostal muscle of neck	musculus iliocostalis cervicis
iliocostal muscle of loins	musculus iliocostalis lumborum
iliocostal muscle of thorax	musculus iliocostalis thoracis
iliopsoas muscle	musculus iliopsoas
incisive muscles of inferior lip	musculi incisivi labii inferioris
incisive muscles of lower lip	musculi incisivi labii inferioris
incisive muscles of superior lip	musculi incisivi labii superioris
incisive muscles of upper lip	musculi incisivi labii superioris
index extensor muscle	musculus extensor indicis
inferior constrictor muscle of pharynx	musculus constrictor pharyngis inferior
inferior gemellus muscle	musculus gemellus inferior
inferior longitudinal muscle of tongue	musculus longitudinalis inferior
inferior oblique muscle	musculus obliquus inferior
inferior oblique muscle of head	musculus obliquus capitis inferior
inferior posterior serratus muscle	serratus posterior inferior musculus
inferior rectus muscle	musculus rectus inferior
inferior tarsal muscle	musculus tarsalis inferior
infrahyoid muscles	musculi infrahyoidei
infraspinous muscle	musculus infraspinatus
innermost intercostal muscle	musculus intercostalis intimus
inspiratory muscles	
intercostal muscles	musculi intercostales
interfoveolar muscle	ligamentum interfoveolare
intermediate great muscle	musculus vastus intermedius
internal intercostal muscle	musculus intercostalis internus
internal oblique muscle	musculus obliquus internus abdominis
internal obturator muscle	musculus obturator internus
internal pterygoid muscle	musculus pterygoideus medialis
interosseous muscles	musculi interossei
interspinal muscles	musculi interspinales
intertransverse muscles	musculi intertransversarii
intra-auricular muscles	
intraocular muscles	
intrinsic muscles	
intrinsic muscles of foot	

muscle	musculus (pl. musculi)
involuntary muscles	
iridic muscles	
ischiocavernous muscle	musculus ischiocavernosus
Jarjavay's muscle	
Jung's pyramidal auricular muscle	
Klein's cutaneomucous muscle	
Kohlrausch's muscle	
Koyter's muscle	musculus corrugator supercilii
Krause's cutaneomucous muscle	musculus cutaneomucosus
Landstrom's muscle (umlaut o)	
Langer's axillary arch muscle	
larynx, muscles of	musculi laryngis
lateral cricoarytenoid muscle	musculus cricoarytenoideus lateralis
lateral great muscle	musculus vastus lateralis
lateral lumbar intertransversarii muscles	musculi intertransversarii laterales lumborum
lateral pterygoid muscle	musculus pterygoideus lateralis
lateral rectus muscle	musculus rectus lateralis
lateral rectus muscle of the head	musculus rectus capitis lateralis
lateral vastus muscle	musculus vastus lateralis
latissimus dorsi muscle	musculus latissimus dorsi
lesser rhomboid muscle	musculus rhomboid minor
lesser zygomatic muscle	musculus zygomaticus minor
levator ani muscle	musculus levator ani
levator muscles (see *elevator muscles*)	
lingual muscles	musculi linguae
long abductor muscle of thumb	musculus abductor pollicis longus
long adductor muscle	musculus adductor longus
long extensor muscle of great toe	musculus extensor hallucis longus
long extensor muscle of thumb	musculus extensor pollicis longus
long extensor muscle of toes	musculus extensor digitorum longus
long fibular muscle	musculus peroneus longus
long flexor muscle of great toe	musculus flexor hallucis longus
long flexor muscle of thumb	musculus flexor pollicis longus
long flexor muscle of toes	musculus flexor digitorum longus
long muscle of head	musculus longus capitis
longissimus muscle	musculus longissimus
longissimus muscle of back (thorax)	musculus longissimus thoracis
longissimus muscle of head	musculus longissimus capitis

muscle	musculus (pl. musculi)
longissimus muscle of neck	musculus longissimus cervicis
longitudinal muscle of tongue, inferior	musculus longitudinalis inferior linguae
longitudinal muscle of tongue, superior	musculus longitudinalis superior linguae
long muscle of head	musculus longus capitis
long muscle of neck	musculus longus colli
long palmar muscle	musculus palmaris longus
long peroneal muscle	musculus peroneus longus
long radial extensor muscle of wrist	musculus extensor carpi radialis longus
lumbar iliocostal muscle	musculus interspinalis lumborum
lumbar interspinal muscles	musculus interspinalis lumborum
lumbar quadrate muscle	musculus quadratus lumborum
lumbar rotator muscles	musculi rotatores lumborum
lumbrical muscles of foot	musculi lumbricales pedis
lumbrical muscles of hand	musculi lumbricales manus
Marcacci's muscle	
masseter muscle	musculus masseter
medial great muscle	musculus vastus medialis
medial lumbar intertransverse muscles	musculi intertransversarii mediales lumborum
medial pterygoid muscle	musculus pterygoideus medialis
medial rectus muscle	musculus rectus medialis
medial vastus muscle	musculus vastus medialis
mentalis muscle	musculus mentalis
Merkel's muscle	musculus ceratocricoideus
mesothenar muscle	musculus adductor pollicis
middle constrictor muscle of pharynx	musculus constrictor pharyngis medius
middle scalene muscle	musculus scalenus medius
mucocutaneous muscle	
Mueller's muscle	musculus orbitalis
multifidus muscles (intermediate layer of transversospinalis muscles)	musculi multifidi
multipennate muscle	musculus multipennatus
mylohyoid muscle	musculus mylohyoideus
nasal muscle	musculus nasalis
neck, muscles of	musculi colli
nonstriated muscle (smooth muscle)	
notch of helix, muscles of	musculus incisurae helicis
oblique arytenoid muscle	musculus arytenoideus obliquus
oblique auricular muscle	musculus obliquus auriculae

muscle	musculus (pl. musculi)
oblique muscle of abdomen, external	musculus obliquus externus abdominis
oblique muscle of abdomen, internal	musculus obliquus internus abdominis
oblique muscle of head, inferior	musculus obliquus capitis inferior
oblique muscle of head, superior	musculus obliquus capitis superior
obturator muscle, external	musculus obturator externus
obturator muscle, internal	musculus obturator internus
occipitofrontal muscle	musculus occipitofrontalis
Ochsner's muscles	
ocular muscles	musculi bulbi
Oddi's muscle (sphincter)	
Oehl's muscles	
omohyoid muscle	musculus omohyoideus
opposing muscle of little finger	musculus opponens digiti minimi
opposing muscle of thumb	musculus opponens pollicis
orbicular muscle	musculus orbicularis
orbicular muscle of eye	musculus orbicularis oculi
orbicular muscle of mouth	musculus orbicularis oris
orbital muscle	musculus orbitalis
organic muscle (visceral musscle)	
palate and fauces, muscles	musculi palati et faucium
palatine muscles	musculi palati
palatoglossus muscle	musculus palatoglossus
palatopharyngeal muscle	musculus palatopharyngeus
palmar interosseous muscle	musculus interosseus palmaris
palmar muscle, short	musculus palmaris brevis
palmar muscle, long	musculus palmaris longus
papillary muscle	musculus papillaris
pectinate muscles	musculi pectinati
pectineal muscle	musculus pectineus
pectoral muscle, greater	musculus pectoralis major
pectoral muscle, smaller	musculus pectoralis minor
pectorodorsalis muscle (axillary arch)	
penniform muscle	musculus unipennatus
perineal muscles	musculi perinei
peroneal muscle, long	musculus fibularis longus
peroneal muscle, short	musculus fibularis brevis
peroneal muscle, third	musculus fibularis tertius
pharyngopalatine muscle	musculus palatopharyngeus
Phillips' muscle	

muscle	musculus (pl. musculi)
piriform muscle	musculus piriformis
plantar interosseous muscle	musculus interosseus plantaris
plantar muscle	musculus plantaris
plantar quadrate muscle	musculus quadratus plantae
platysma muscle	musculus platysma
pleuroesophageal muscle	musculus pleuroesophageus
popliteal muscle	musculus popliteus
posterior auricular muscle	musculus retrahens aurem
posterior cervical intertransverse muscles	musculi intertransversarii posteriores cervicis
posterior cricoarytenoid muscle	musculus cricoarytenoideus posterior
posterior scalene muscle	musculus scalenus posterior
posterior tibial muscle	musculus tibialis posterior
Pozzi's muscle (extensor digitorum brevis muscle of hand)	musculus extensor digitorum brevis manus
procerus muscle	musculus procerus
pronator muscle, quadrate	musculus pronator quadratus
pronator muscle, round	musculus pronator teres
psoas muscle, greater	musculus psoas major
psoas muscle, smaller	musculus psoas minor
pterygoid muscle	musculus pterygoideus
pubococcygeal muscle	musculus pubococcygeus
puboprostatic muscle	musculus puboprostaticus
puborectal muscle (Braune's muscle)	musculus puborectalis
pubovaginal muscle	musculus pubovaginalis
pubovesical muscle	musculus pubovesicalis
pyloric sphincter muscle	musculus sphincter pyloricus
pyramidal auricular muscle (Jung's m.)	musculus pyramidalis auriculae
quadrate (four-sided) muscle	musculus quadratus
quadrate muscle of loins	musculus quadratus lumborum
quadrate muscle of lower lip	musculus depressor labii inferioris
quadrate muscle of sole	musculus quadratus plantae
quadrate muscle of thigh	musculus quadratus femoris
quadrate muscle of upper lip	musculus quadratus labii superioris
radial flexor muscle of wrist	musculus flexor carpi radialis
rectococcygeus muscle	musculus rectococcygeus
rectourethral muscle	musculus recto-urethralis
rectouterine muscle	musculus recto-uterinus
rectovesical muscle	musculus rectovesicalis

muscle	musculus (pl. musculi)
rectus abdominis muscle (rectus muscle of abdomen)	musculus rectus abdominis
rectus muscle of head, anterior	musculus rectus capitis anterior
rectus muscle of head, lateral	musculus rectus capitis lateralis
rectus muscle of head, greater posterior	musculus rectus capitis posterior major
rectus muscle of head, smaller posterior	musculus rectus capitis posterior minor
rectus femoris muscle (rectus muscle of thigh)	musculus rectus femoris
red muscle (slow muscle)	
Reisseisen's muscles	
rhomboid muscle, greater	musculus rhomboideus major
rhomboid muscle, lesser	musculus rhomboideus minor
ribbon muscles	musculi infrahyoidei
rider's muscles (adductor muscles of thigh)	
Riolan's muscle (cremaster muscle)	musculus cremaster
risorius muscle (Albinus' muscle, Santorini's muscle)	musculus risorius
rotator muscles	musculi rotatores
rotator muscles of neck	musculi rotatores cervicis
rotator muscles of back	musculi rotatores lumborum
rotator muscles of thorax	musculi rotatores thoracis
Rouget's muscle	
round pronator muscle	musculus pronator teres
Ruysch's muscle	
sacrococcygeal muscle	musculus sacrococcygeus
salpingopharyngeal muscle	musculus salpingopharyngeus
Santorini's muscle	musculus risorius
sartorius muscle (tailor's muscle)	musculus sartorius
scalene muscle, anterior	musculus scalenus anterior
scalene muscle, middle	musculus scalenus medius
scalene muscle, posterior	musculus scalenus posterior
scalene muscle, smallest (Albinus' m., Sibson's m.)	musculus scalenus minimus
scalp muscle (epicranius muscle)	
Sebileau's muscle	
second tibial muscle	musculus tibialis secundus
semimembranous muscle	musculus semimembranosus
semispinal muscle	musculus semispinalis
semispinal muscle of head	musculus semispinalis capitis

muscle	musculus (pl. musculi)
semispinal muscle of neck	musculus semispinalis cervicis
semispinal muscle of thorax	musculus semispinalis thoracis
semitendinous muscle	musculus semitendinosus
serratus anterior muscle	musculus serratus anterior
serratus posterior inferior muscle	musculus serratus posterior inferior
serratus posterior superior muscle	musculus serratus posterior superior
shawl muscle (trapezius muscle)	
short adductor muscle	musculus adductor brevis
short extensor musscle of great toe	musculus extensor hallucis brevis
short extensor muscle of thumb	musculus extensor pollicis brevis
short extensor muscle of toes	musculus extensor digitorum brevis
short fibular muscle	musculus peroneus brevis
short flexor muscle of great toe	musculus flexor hallucis brevis
short flexor muscle of little finger	musculus flexor digiti minimi brevis
short flexor muscle of little toe	musculus flexor digiti minimi brevis
short flexor muscle of thumb	musculus flexor pollicis brevis
short flexor muscle of toes	musculus flexor digitorum brevis
short palmar muscle	musculus palmaris brevis
short peroneal muscle	musculus peroneus brevis
short radial extensor muscle of wrist	musculus extensor carpi radialis brevis
Sibson's muscle	musculus scalenus minimus
skeletal muscles	musculi skeleti
slow muscle (red muscle)	
smaller muscle of helix	musculus helicis minor
smaller pectoral muscle	musculus pectoralis minor
smaller posterior rectus muscle of head	musculus rectus capitis posterior minor
smaller psoas muscle	musculus psoas minor
smallest scalene muscle	musculus scalenus minimus
smooth muscle (unstriated, unstriped, visceral)	
Soemmerring's muscle (levator muscle of thyroid gland)	
soleus muscle	musculus soleus
somatic muscles	musculi skeleti
sphincter muscle of anus	musculus sphincter ani
sphincter muscle of bile duct	musculus sphincter ductus choledochi
sphincter muscle of hepatopancreatic ampulla	musculus sphincter ampullae hepatopancreaticae
sphincter muscle of pupil	musculus sphincter pupillae

muscle	musculus (pl. musculi)
sphincter muscle of pylorus	musculus sphincter pyloricus
sphincter muscle of urethra	musculus sphincter urethrae
sphincter muscle of urinary bladder	musculus sphincter vesicae urinariae
spinal muscle	musculus spinalis
spinal muscle of head	musculus spinalis capitis
spinal muscle of neck	musculus spinalis cervicis
spinal muscle of thorax	musculus spinalis thoracis
spindle-shaped muscle	musculus fisiform
splenius muscle of head	musculus splenius capitis
splenius muscle of neck	musculus splenius cervicis
stapedius muscle	musculus stapedius
sternal muscle	musculus sternalis
sternochondroscapular muscle	musculus sternochondroscapularis
sternoclavicular muscle	musculus sternoclavicularis
sternocleidomastoid muscle	musculus sternocleidomastoideus
sternocostal muscle	musculus transversus thoracis
sternohyoid muscle	musculus sternohyoideus
sternomastoid muscle (sternocleidomastoid)	
sternothyroid muscle	musculus sternothyroideus
strap muscles	
striated muscle	
styloauricular muscle	musculus styloauricularis
styloglossus muscle	musculus styloglossus
stylohyoid muscle	musculus stylohyoideus
stylopharyngeal muscle	musculus stylopharyngeus
subanconeus muscle	musculus articularis cubiti
subclavian muscle	musculus subclavius
subcostal muscle	musculus subcostalis
subcrural muscle	musculus articularis genu
suboccipital muscles	musculi suboccipitales
subquadricipital muscle	musculus articularis genu
subscapular muscle	musculus subscapularis
subvertebral muscles	musculi hypaxial
superficial back muscles	
superficial flexor muscle of fingers	musculus flexor digitorum superficialis
superficial lingual muscle (of tongue)	
superficial transverse perineal muscle (Theile's muscle)	musculus transversus perinei superficialis
superior auricular muscle	musculus auricularis superior

muscle	musculus (pl. musculi)
superior constrictor muscle of pharynx	musculus constrictor pharyngis superior
superior gemellus muscle	musculus gemellus superior
superior longitudinal muscle of tongue	musculus longitudinalis superior
superior oblique muscle	musculus obliquus superior
superior oblique muscle of head	musculus obliquus capitis superior
superior posterior serratus muscle	musculus serratus posterior superior
superior rectus muscle	musculus rectus superior
superior tarsal muscle	musculus tarsalis superior
(Mueller's muscle)	
supinator muscle	musculus supinator
supraclavicular muscle	musculus supraclavicularis
suprahyoid muscles	musculi suprahyoidei
supraspinalis muscle	musculus supraspinalis
supraspinous muscle	musculus supraspinatus
suspensory muscle of duodenum	musculus suspensorius duodeni
(Treitz' ligament)	
synergic or synergistic muscles	
tailor's muscle (sartorius muscle)	
temporal muscle	musculus temporalis
temporoparietal muscle	musculus temporoparietalis
tensor muscle of fascia lata	musculus tensor fasciae latae
tensor muscle of soft palate	musculus tensor veli palati
tensor tarsi muscle	musculus orbicularis oculi
tensor muscle of tympanic membrane	musculus tensor tympani
(Toynbee's muscle)	
teres major muscle	musculus teres major
teres minor muscle	musculus teres minor
Theile's muscle (superficial transverse perineal muscle)	
third peroneal muscle	musculus peroneus tertius
thoracic interspinal muscle	musculi thoracic interspinalis
thoracic intertransverse muscles	musculi intertransversarii thoracis
thoracic longissimus muscle	musculus longissimus thoracis
thoracic rotator muscles	musculi rotatores thoracis
thorax, muscles of	musculi thoracis
thyroarytenoid muscle	musculus thyroarytenoideus
thyroepiglottic muscle	musculus thyroepiglotticus
(depressor muscle of epiglottis)	
thyrohyoid muscle	musculus thyrohyoideus

muscle	musculus (pl. musculi)
tibial muscle, anterior	musculus tibialis anterior
tibial muscle, posterior	musculus tibialis posterior
Tod's muscle (oblique auricular muscle)	
tongue, muscles of	musculi linguae
Toynbee's muscle	musculus tensor tympani
tracheal muscle	musculus trachealis
tracheloclavicular muscle	musculus tracheloclavicularis
trachelomastoid muscle	musculus longissimus capitis
tragicus muscle	musculus tragicus
(Valsalva's muscle)	
transverse arytenoid muscle	musculus arytenoideus transversus
transverse muscle of abdomen	musculus transversus abdominis
transverse muscle of auricle	musculus transversus auriculae
transverse muscle of chin	musculus transversus menti
transverse muscle of nape	musculus transversus nuchae
transverse muscle of neck	musculus transversus nuchae
transverse muscle of thorax	musculus transversus thoracis
transverse muscle of tongue	musculus transversus linguae
transversospinal muscle	musculus transversospinalis
trapezius muscle	musculus trapezius
Treitz' muscle (suspensory muscle of duodenum)	
triangular muscle	musculus triangularis
triceps muscle of arm	musculus triceps brachii
triceps muscle of hip	musculus triceps coxae
triceps muscle of calf	musculus triceps surae
trigonal muscle	
true (deep) muscles of back	musculi dorsi
two-bellied muscle (digastric muscle)	musculus digastricus
ulnar extensor muscle of wrist	musculus extensor carpi ulnaris
ulnar flexor muscle of wrist	musculus flexor carpi ulnaris
unipennate muscle	musculus unipennatus
unstriated muscle, unstriped muscle (smooth muscle)	
urogenital diaphragm, muscles of	musculi diaphragmatis urogenitalis
uvula, muscle of	musculus uvulae
Valsalva's muscle	
vastus intermedius muscle (intermediate great muscle)	musculus vastus intermedius

muscle	musculus (pl. musculi)
vastus lateralis muscle (lateral great muscle)	musculus vastus lateralis
vastus medialis muscle (medial great muscle)	musculus vastus medialis
ventral sacrococcygeal muscle	musculus sacrococcygeus ventralis
vertical muscle of tongue	musculus verticalis linguae
visceral muscle (smooth)	
vocal muscle	musculus vocalis
voluntary muscle	
white muscle (fast muscle)	
Wilson's muscle (urethral sphincter)	musculus sphincter urethrae
wrinkler muscle of eyebrow	musculus corrugator supercilii
yoked muscles	
zygomatic muscle, greater	musculus zygomaticus major
zygomatic muscle, lesser	musculus zygomaticus minor

Table of Nerves

nerve	nervus (pl. nervi)
abdominopelvic splanchnic nerves	
abducent nerve	nervus abducens
accelerator nerves	
accessory nerve	nervus accessorius
accessory nerve, vagal	ramus internus nervi accessorii
accessory phrenic nerves	nervi phrenici accessorii
acoustic nerve	
afferent nerve (centripetal; esodic)	
alveolar nerve, inferior	nervus alveolaris inferior
alveolar nerves, superior	nervi alveolares superiores
ampullar nerve, anterior	nervus ampullaris anterior
ampullar nerve, inferior	nervus ampullaris inferior
ampullar nerve, lateral	nervus ampullaris lateralis
ampullar nerve, superior	nervus ampullaris superior
anal nerves, inferior	nervi rectales inferiores
Andersch's nerve (tympanic)	
anococcygeal nerves	nervi anococcygei
anterior ampullar nerve	nervus ampullaris anterior
anterior antebrachial nerve (anterior interosseous nerve)	
anterior auricular nerves	nervi auriculares anteriores
anterior crural nerve (femoral nerve)	
anterior cutaneous nerves of abdomen (thoracoabdominal nerves)	
anterior ethmoidal nerve	nervus ethmoidalis anterior
anterior femoral cutaneous nerves	rami cutanei anteriores nervi femoralis
anterior interosseous nerve	nervus interosseous anterior
anterior labial nerves	nervi labiales anteriores
anterior scrotal nerves	nervi scrotales anteriores
anterior supraclavicular nerve (medial supraclavicular nerve)	
anterior tibial nerve (deep peroneal nerve)	

nerve	nervus (pl. nervi)
aortic nerve (Cyon's nerve, depressor nerve of Ludwig, Ludwig's nerve)	
Arnold's nerve	ramus auricularis nervi vagi
articular nerve	nervus articularis
auditory nerve (cochlear)	nervus vestibulocochlearis
augmentor nerves (cervical splanchnic nerves)	
auricular nerves, anterior	nervi auriculares anteriores
auricular nerve, great	nervus auricularis magnus
auricular nerve, internal	ramus posterior nervi auricularis magni
auricular nerve, posterior	nervus auricularis posterior
auricular nerve of vagus nerve	ramus auricularis nervi vagi
auriculotemporal nerve	nervus auriculotemporalis
autonomic nerve	nervus autonomicus
axillary nerve	nervus axillaris
baroreceptor nerve (pressoreceptor nerve)	
Bell's long thoracic nerve	nervus thoracicus longus
Bock's nerve	ramus pharyngeus ganglii pterygopalatini
buccal nerve	nervus buccalis
buccinator nerve (buccal nerve)	
cardiac nerve, cervical, inferior	nervus cardiacus cervicalis inferior
cardiac nerve, cervical, middle	nervus cardiacus cervicalis medius
cardiac nerve, cervical, superior	nervus cardiacus cervicalis superior
cardiac nerve, inferior	nervus cardiacus cervicalis inferior
cardiac nerve, middle	nervus cardiacus cervicalis medius
cardiac nerve, superior	nervus cardiacus cervicalis superior
cardiac nerves, supreme	rami cardiaci cervicales superiores nervi vagi
cardiac nerves, thoracic	rami cardiaci thoracici
cardiopulmonary splanchnic nerves	
caroticotympanic nerve	nervus carotidotympanicus
carotid sinus nerve (Hering's sinus)	ramus sinus carotici
cavernous nerves of clitoris	nervi cavernosi clitoridis
cavernous nerves of penis	nervi cavernosi penis
celiac nerves	rami coeliaci nervi vagi
centrifugal nerve (efferent)	
centripetal nerve (afferent)	

nerve	nervus (pl. nervi)
cerebral nerves	nervi craniales
cervical nerves	nervi cervicales
cervical splanchnic nerves	
(augmentor nerves)	
chorda tympani nerve	chorda tympani
ciliary nerves	nervi ciliares
circumflex nerve (axillary)	nervus axillaris
cluneal nerves	rami clunium
coccygeal nerve	nervus coccygeus
cochlear nerve	nervus cochlearis
common fibular nerve (common peroneal)	
common palmar digital nerves	nervi digitales palmares communes
common peroneal nerve	nervus fibularis communis
common plantar digital nerves	nervi digitales plantares communes
cranial nerves	nervi craniales
cranial nerve, eighth (acoustic)	nervus vestibulocochlearis
cranial nerve, eleventh (accessory	nervus accessorius
cranial nerve, fifth (trigeminal)	nervus trigeminus
cranial nerves, first (olfactory)	nervi olfactorii
cranial nerve, fourth (trochlear)	nervus trochlearis
cranial nerve, ninth (glossopharyngeal)	nervus glossopharyngeus
cranial nerve, second (optic)	nervus opticus
cranial nerve, seventh (facial)	nervus facialis
cranial nerve, sixth (abducens)	nervus abducens
cranial nerve, tenth (vagal)	nervus vagus
cranial nerve, third (oculomotor)	nervus oculomotorius
cranial nerve, twelfth (hypoglossal)	nervus hypoglossus
crural interosseous nerve	nervus interosseus cruris
cubital nerve (ulnar nerve)	nervus ulnaris
cutaneous femoral nerve, lateral	nervus cutaneus femoris lateralis
cutaneous nerve	nervus cutaneus
cutaneous nerve, femoral	nervus cutaneus femoralis
cutaneous nerve of arm, lateral, inferior	nervus cutaneus brachii lateralis inferior
cutaneous nerve of calf, medial	nervus cutaneus surae medial
cutaneous nerve of foot, dorsal, lateral	nervus cutaneus dorsalis lateralis
cutaneous nerve of forearm, medial	nervus cutaneus antebrachii medialis
cutaneous nerve of neck, anterior	nervus transversus colli
cutaneous nerve of thigh, posterior	nervus cutaneus femoralis posterior
Cyon's nerve (aortic)	

nerve	nervus (pl. nervi)
dead nerve (nonvital dental pulp)	
deep fibular nerve (deep peroneal)	
deep peroneal nerve	nervus fibularis profundus
deep petrosal nerve	nervus petrosus profundus
deep temporal nerves	nervi temporales profundi
dental nerve, inferior	nervus alveolaris inferior
depressor nerve of Ludwig (aortic)	
diaphragmatic nerve	nervus phrenicus
digastric nerve	ramus digastricus nervi facialis
digital nerves, dorsal, radial	nervi digitales dorsales nervi radialis
dorsal nerve of clitoris	nervus dorsalis clitoridis
dorsal digital nerves	
dorsal digital nerves of foot	nervi digitales dorsales pedis
dorsal digital nerves of hand	
dorsal interosseous nerve (posterior interosseous)	
dorsal lateral cutaneous nerve (lateral dorsal cutaneous)	
dorsal medial cutaneous nerve (medial dorsal cutaneous n.)	
dorsal nerve of penis	nervus dorsalis penis
dorsal nerve of scapula (dorsal scapular)	
dorsal scapular nerve	nervus dorsalis scapulae
dorsal nerves of toes	
efferent nerve (centrifugal nerve)	
eighth cranial nerve (vestibulocochlear nerve)	nervus vestibulocochlearis
eleventh cranial nerve (accessory nerve)	nervus accessorius
encephalic nerves	nervi craniales
esodic nerve (afferent nerve)	
ethmoidal nerve, anterior	nervus ethmoidalis anterior
excitor nerve	
excitoreflex nerve	
exodic nerve	
external acoustic meatus, nerve of	nervus meatus acustici externi
external carotid nerves	nervi carotici externi
external respiratory nerve of Bell (long thoracis nerve)	
external saphenous nerve (sural nerve)	

nerve	nervus (pl. nervi)
external spermatic nerve (genital branch of genitofemoral nerve)	
facial nerve	nervus facialis
femoral cutaneous nerve, intermediate	
femoral nerve	nervus femoralis
fibular nerve, superficial	nervus fibularis superficialis
fifth cranial nerve (trigeminal nerve)	nervus trigeminus
first cranial nerve (olfactory nerve)	nervus olfactorius
fourth cranial nerve (trochlear nerve)	nervus trochlearis
fourth lumbar nerve	nervus furcalis
frontal nerve	nervus frontalis
furcal nerve (fourth lumbar nerve)	
fusimotor nerves	
Galen's nerve	
gangliated nerve	
gastric nerves	truncus vagalis anterior and truncus vagalis posterior
genitocrural nerve (genitofemoral nerve)	
genitofemoral nerve	nervus genitofemoralis
glossopharyngeal nerve (ninth cranial nerve)	nervus glossopharyngeus
gluteal nerve, inferior	nervus gluteus inferior
great auricular nerve	nervus auricularis magnus
greater occipital nerve	nervus occipitalis major
greater palatine nerve	nervus palatinus major
greater petrosal nerve	
greater splanchnic nerve	nervus splanchnicus major
greater superficial petrosal nerve	nervus petrosus major
great sciatic nerve	
gustatory nerves	
hemorrhoidal nerves, inferior	nervi rectales inferiores
Hering's sinus nerve (carotid sinus)	
hypogastric nerve	nervus hypogastricus
hypoglossal nerve (twelfth cranial)	nervus hypoglossus
iliohypogastric nerve	nervus iliohypogastricus
ilioinguinal nerve	nervus ilio-inguinalis
inferior alveolar nerve	nervus alveolaris inferior
inferior cervical cardiac nerve	nervus cardiacus cervicalis inferior
inferior cluneal nerves	nervi clunium inferiores

nerve	nervus (pl. nervi)
inferior dental nerve (inferior alveolar)	
inferior gluteal nerve	nervus gluteus inferior
inferior hemorrhoidal nerves	
inferior laryngeal nerve	nervus laryngeus inferior
inferior lateral brachial cutaneous nerve	nervus cutaneus brachii lateralis inferior
inferior maxillary nerve	
inferior rectal nerves	nervi rectales inferiores
inferior vesical nerves	
infraoccipital nerve	nervus suboccipitalis
infraorbital nerve	nervus infraorbitalis
infratrochlear nerve	nervus infratrochlearis
inhibitory nerve	
intercarotid nerve	
intercostal nerves	nervi intercostales
intercostobrachial nerves	nervi intercostobrachiales
intercostohumeral nerves	
intermediary nerve	nervus intermedius
intermediate nerve	nervus intermedius
intermediate dorsal cutaneous nerve	
Jacobson's nerve (tympanic)	nervus tympanicus
jugular nerve	nervus jugularis
lacrimal nerve	nervus lacrimalis
Lancisi, nerves of	
Langley's nerves (pilomotor nerves)	
Latarget's nerve (superior hypogastric plexus)	
laryngeal nerve, recurrent	nervus laryngealis recurrens
lateral ampullar nerve	nervus ampullaris lateralis
lateral antebrachial cutaneous nerve	nervus cutaneus antebrachii lateralis
lateral anterior thoracic nerve	
lateral cutaneous nerve of calf	
lateral cutaneous nerve of forearm	
lateral cutaneous nerve of thigh	
lateral dorsal cutaneous nerve	nervus cutaneus dorsalis lateralis
lateral femoral cutaneous nerve	nervus cutaneus femoris lateralis
lateral pectoral nerve	nervus pectoralis lateralis
lateral plantar nerve	nervus plantaris lateralis
lateral popliteal nerve	
lateral supraclavicular nerve	nervus supraclavicularis lateralis

nerve	nervus (pl. nervi)
lateral sural cutaneous nerve	nervus cutaneus surae lateralis
lesser internal cutaneous nerve	
lesser occipital nerve	nervus occipitalis minor
lesser palatine nerves	nervi palatini minores
lesser petrosal nerve	
lesser splanchnic nerve	nervus splanchnicus minor
lesser superficial petrosal nerve	nervus petrosus minor
levator ani, nerve to	
lingual nerve	nervus lingualis
long buccal nerve	
long ciliary nerve	nervus ciliaris longus
longitudinal nerves of Lancisi	
long saphenous nerve	
long subscapular nerve	
long thoracic nerve	nervus thoracicus longus
lower lateral cutaneous nerve of arm	
lowest splanchnic nerve	nervus splanchnicus imus
Ludwig's nerve (aortic nerve)	
lumbar nerves	nervi lumbales
lumbar splanchnic nerves	nervi splanchnici lumbales
lumboinguinal nerve	ramus femoralis nervi genitofemoralis
Luschka, nerve of	
mandibular nerve	nervus mandibularis
masseteric nerve	nervus massestericus
masticator nerve	
maxillary nerve	nervus maxillaris
medial antebrachial cutaneous nerve	nervus cutaneus antebrachii medialis
medial anterior thoracic nerve	
medial brachial cutaneous nerve	nervus cutaneus brachii medialis
medial cutaneous nerve of arm	
medial cutaneous nerve of forearm	
medial cutaneous nerve of leg	
medial dorsal cutaneous nerve	nervus cutaneus dorsalis medialis
medial pectoral nerve	nervus pectoralis medialis
medial plantar nerve	nervus plantaris medialis
medial popliteal nerve	
medial supraclavicular nerve	nervus supraclavicularis medialis
medial sural cutaneous nerve	nervus cutaneus surae medialis
median nerve	nervus medianus

nerve	nervus (pl. nervi)
meningeal nerve	ramus meningeus medius nervi maxillaris
mental nerve	nervus mentalis
middle cervical cardiac nerve	nervus cardiacus cervicalis medius
middle cluneal nerves	nervi clunium medii
middle meningeal nerve	
middle supraclavicular nerve	
mixed nerve	nervus mixtus
motor nerve	nervus motorius
motor nerve of tongue	nervus hypoglossus
musculocutaneous nerve	nervus musculocutaneus
musculocutaneous nerve of leg	nervus fibularis profundus
musculospiral nerve (radial)	nervus radialis
myelinated nerve	
mylohyoid nerve	nervus mylohyoideus
nasal nerve	
nasociliary nerve	nervus nasociliaris
nasopalatine nerve	nervus nasopalatinus
ninth cranial nerve (glossopharyngeal nerve)	nervus glossopharyngeus
obturator nerve	nervus obturatorius
oculomotor nerve	nervus oculomotorius
olfactory nerves	nervi olfactorii
ophthalmic nerve	nervus ophthalmicus
optic nerve (second cranial nerve)	nervus opticus
orbital nerve	
palatine nerve, anterior	nervus palatinus major
parasympathetic nerve	
parotid nerves	rami parotidei nervi auriculotemporalis
pathetic nerve	
pectoral nerve, lateral	nervus pectoralis lateralis
pelvic splanchnic nerves	nervi pelvici splanchnici
parasympathetic nerve	
perforating cutaneous nerve	
perineal nerves	nervi perineales
peroneal nerve, common	nervus fibularis communis
phrenic nerve	nervus phrenicus
pneumogastric nerve	nervus vagus
popliteal nerve, external	nervus fibularis communis

nerve	nervus (pl. nervi)
popliteal nerve, internal	nervus tibialis
popliteal nerve, lateral	nervus fibularis communis
popliteal nerve, medial	nervus tibialis
posterior ampullar nerve	nervus ampullaris posterior
posterior antebrachial nerve	
posterior antebrachial cutaneous nerve	nervus cutaneus antebrachii posterior
posterior auricular nerve	nervus auricularis posterior
posterior brachial cutaneous nerve	nervus cutaneus brachii posterior
posterior cutaneous nerve of arm	
posterior cutaneous nerve of forearm	
posterior cutaneous nerve of thigh	
posterior ethmoidal nerve	nervus ethmoidalis posterior
posterior femoral cutaneous nerve	nervus cutaneus femoris posterior
posterior interosseous nerve	nervus interosseus posterior
posterior labial nerves	nervi labiales posteriores
posterior scapular nerve	
posterior scrotal nerves	nervi scrotales posteriores
posterior supraclavicular nerve	
posterior thoracic nerve	
presacral nerve	plexus hypogastricus superior
pressor nerve	
pressoreceptor nerve	
proper palmar digital nerves	nervi digitales palmares proprii
proper plantar digital nerves	nervi digitales plantares proprii
pterygoid nerve	nervus pterygoideus
pterygoid canal, nerve of	nervus canalis pterygoidei
pterygopalatine nerves	nervi pterygopalatini
pudendal nerve	nervus pudendus
pudic nerve (pudendal)	nervus pudendus
quadrate muscle of thigh, nerve of	nervus musculi quadrati femoris
radial nerve	nervus radialis
recurrent nerve	nervus laryngealis recurrens
recurrent laryngeal nerve	nervus laryngeus recurrens
recurrent meningeal nerve	nervus meningeus recurrens
recurrent ophthalmic nerve	ramus tentorii nervi ophthalmici
saccular nerve	nervus saccularis
sacral nerves	nervi sacrales
sacral splanchnic nerves	nervi splanchnici sacrales
saphenous nerve	nervus saphenus

nerve	nervus (pl. nervi)
sartorius, nerve to	
Scarpa's nerve	nervus nasopalatinus
sciatic nerve	nervus ischiadicus
second cranial nerve (optic nerve)	nervus opticus
secretomotor nerve	
secretory nerve	
sensory nerve	nervus sensorius
seventh cranial nerve (facial nerve)	nervus facialis
short ciliary nerve	nervus ciliaris brevis
short saphenous nerve	nervus saphenus brevis
sinus nerve	ramus sinus carotici nervi glossopharyngei
sinus nerve of Hering	
sinuvertebral nerves	
sixth cranial nerve (abducent nerve)	nervus abducens
small deep petrosal nerve	
smallest splanchnic nerve	
small sciatic nerve	
smell, nerve of (olfactory nerve)	nervi olfactorii
somatic nerve	
space nerve	
spinal nerves	nervi spinales
spinal accessory	
splanchnic nerve	nervus splanchnicus
stapedius muscle, nerve to	nervus stapedius
statoacoustic nerve	
subclavian nerve	nervus subclavius
subcostal nerve	nervus subcostalis
sublingual nerve	nervus sublingualis
suboccipital nerve	nervus suboccipitalis
subscapular nerves	nervi subscapulares
sudomotor nerves	
superficial cervical nerve	nervus cervicalis superficialis
superficial fibular nerve	nervus fibularis superficialis
superficial peroneal nerve	nervus fibularis superficialis
superior alveolar nerves	nervi alveolares superiores
superior cervical cardiac nerve	nervus cardiacus cervicalis superior
superior cluneal nerves	nervi clunium superiores
superior dental nerves	

nerve	nervus (pl. nervi)
superior gluteal nerve	nervus gluteus superior
superior laryngeal nerve	nervus laryngeus superior
superior lateral brachial cutaneous nerve	nervus cutaneus brachii lateralis superior
superior maxillary nerve	
supraorbital nerve	nervus supraorbitalis
suprascapular nerve	nervus suprascapularis
supratrochlear nerve	nervus supratrochlearis
sural nerve	nervus suralis
sympathetic nerve	
temporomandibular nerve	
tensor tympani muscle, nerve of	nervus tensoris tympani
tensor veli palatini muscle, nerve of	nervus tensoris veli palatini
tenth cranial nerve (vagus nerve)	nervus vagus
tentorial nerve	ramus tentorii nervi ophthalmici
terminal nerves	nervi terminales
third cranial nerve (oculomotor nerve)	nervus oculomotorius
third occipital nerve	nervus occipitalis tertius
thoracic cardiac nerves	nervi cardiaci thoracici
thoracic spinal nerves	nervi thoracici
thoracic splanchnic nerve	nervus splanchnicus thoracici
thoracoabdominal nerves	nervi thoracoabdominales
thoracodorsal nerve	nervus thoracodorsalis
thyrohyoid muscle, nerve to	ramus thyrohyoideus ansae cervicalis
tibial nerve	nervus tibialis
tibial communicating nerve	
Tiedemann's nerve	
tonsillar nerves	rami tonsillares nervi glossopharyngei
transverse nerve of neck	nervus transversus colli
trifacial nerve (trigeminal nerve)	nervus trigeminus
trigeminal nerve	nervus trigeminus
trochlear nerve	nervus trochlearis
twelfth cranial nerve (hypoglossal)	nervus hypoglossus
tympanic nerve	nervus tympanicus
tympanic membrane, nerve of	
ulnar nerve	nervus ulnaris
unmyelinated nerve	
upper lateral cutaneous nerve of arm	
upper subscapular nerve	

nerve	nervus (pl. nervi)
upper thoracic splanchnic nerves	
utricular nerve	nervus utricularis
utriculoampullar nerve	nervus utriculoampullaris
vaginal nerves	nervi vaginales
vagus nerve	nervus vagus
Valentin's nerve	
vascular nerve	nervus vascularis
vasoconstrictor nerve	
vasodilator nerve	
vasomotor nerve	
vasosensory nerve	
vertebral nerve	nervus vertebralis
vestibular nerve	nervus vestibularis
vestibulocochlear nerve (eighth cranial nerve)	nervus vestibulocochlearis
vidian nerve	nervus canalis pterygoidei
visceral nerve	nervus autonomicus
volar interosseous nerve	
Willis, nerve of	nervus accessorius
Wrisberg's nerve	nervus intermedius
zygomatic nerve	nervus zygomaticus
zygomaticotemporal nerves	ramus zygomaticotemporalis nervi

Table of Veins

vein	vena (pl. venae)
accessory cephalic vein	vena cephalica accessoria
accessory hemiazygos vein	vena hemiazygos accessoria
accessory saphenous vein	vena saphena accessoria
accessory vertebral vein	vena vertebralis accessoria
accompanying vein	vena comitans
accompanying vein of hypoglossal nerve	vena comitans nervi hypoglossi
adrenal veins	venae suprarenales
afferent veins	
anastomotic vein, inferior	vena anastomotica inferior
anastomotic vein, superior	vena anastomotica superior
angular vein	vena angularis
anonymous veins	venae brachiocephalicae
antebrachial vein, median	vena intermedia antebrachii
anterior auricular vein	vena auricularis anterior
anterior cardiac veins	venae cordis anteriores
anterior cardinal veins	
anterior cerebral vein	vena cerebri anterior
anterior facial vein	
anterior intercostal veins	venae intercostales anteriores
anterior jugular vein	vena jugularis anterior
anterior labial veins	venae labiales anteriores
anterior pontomesencephalic vein	vena pontomesencephalica anterior
anterior scrotal veins	venae scrotales anteriores
anterior vein of septum pellucidum	vena septi pellucidi anterior
anterior veins of heart	venae ventriculi dextri anteriores
anterior veins of right ventricle	venae ventriculi dextri anteriores
anterior tibial veins	venae tibiales anteriores
anterior vertebral vein	vena vertebralis anterior
appendicular vein	vena appendicularis
aqueduct of cochlea, vein of	vena aqueductus cochleae
aqueduct of vestibule, vein of	vena aqueductus vestibuli

vein	vena (pl. venae)
aqueous veins	
arciform veins of kidney	
arcuate veins of kidney	venae arcuatae renis
arterial vein	vena arteriosa, truncus pulmonalis
arterial vein of Soemmering	vena portae hepatis
articular veins	venae articulares
ascending veins of Rosenthal	venae inferiores cerebri
ascending lumbar vein	vena lumbalis ascendens
atrial veins of heart, left	venae atriales sinistrae
atrial veins of heart, right	venae atriales dextrae
atrial vein, lateral	vena lateralis atrii
atrial vein, medial	vena medialis atrii
atrioventricular veins of heart	venae atrioventriculares cordis
auditory veins, internal	venae labyrinthinae
auricular veins, anterior	venae auriculares anteriores
auricular veins, posterior	vena auricularis posterior
axillary vein	vena axillaris
azygos vein	vena azygos
basal vein, Rosenthal's	vena basalis
basilic vein	vena basilica
basivertebral vein	vena basivertebralis
Baumgarten's veins	
Boyd communicating perforation veins	
brachial veins	venae brachiales
brachiocephalic veins	venae brachiocephalicae
Breschet's vein	venae diploicae
bronchial veins	venae bronchiales
Browning's vein	
bulb of penis, vein of	vena bulbi penis
Burow's vein	
canaliculus of cochlea, vein of	vena aqueductus cochleae
capillary vein	
cardiac veins	venae cordis
cardiac veins, anterior	venae ventriculi dextri anteriores
cardiac vein, great	vena cardiaca magna
cardiac vein, middle	vena cardiaca media
cardiac vein, small	vena cardiaca parva
cardiac veins, smallest	venae cardiacae minimae
cardinal veins	

vein	vena (pl. venae)
carotid vein, external	vena retromandibularis
caudate nucleus, veins of	venae nuclei caudati
cavernous veins of penis	venae cavernosae penis
central veins of liver	venae centrales hepatis
central vein of retina	vena centralis retinae
central vein of suprarenal gland	vena centralis glandulae suprarenalis
cephalic vein	vena cephalica
cerebellar veins	venae cerebelli
cerebral veins	venae cerebri
cervical vein, deep	vena cervicalis profunda
choroid vein	vena choroidea
choroid veins of eye	
ciliary veins	venae ciliares
circumflex veins	venae circumflexae
cochlear aqueduct, vein of	vena aqueductus cochleae
cochlear canaliculus, vein of	vena aqueductus cochleae
Cockett communicating perforating veins	
colic vein, left	vena colica sinistra
colic vein, middle	vena colica media
colic vein, right	vena colica dextra
common basal vein	vena basalis communis
common cardinal veins (ducts of Cuvier)	
common facial vein	vena facialis communis
common iliac vein	vena iliaca communis
communicating veins (perforating veins)	
companion vein, companion veins	vena comitans, venae comitantes
condylar emissary vein	vena emissaria condylaris
conjunctival veins	venae conjunctivales
coronary vein, left	vena coronaria sinistra
coronary vein, right	vena coronaria dextra
corpus callosum, vein of, dorsal	vena dorsalis corporis callosi
corpus callosum, vein of, posterior	vena posterior corporis callosi
corpus striatum, vein of	
costoaxillary veins	venae costoaxillares
cubital vein, median	vena intermedia cubiti
cutaneous vein	vena cutanea
cutaneous vein, ulnar	vena basilica
Cuvier's veins	
cystic vein	vena cystica

vein	vena (pl. venae)
deep cerebral veins	venae cerebri profundae
deep cervical vein	vena cervicalis profunda
deep circumflex iliac vein	vena circumflexa iliaca profunda
deep veins of clitoris	venae profundae clitoridis
deep dorsal vein of clitoris	vena dorsalis clitoridis profunda
deep dorsal vein of penis	vena dorsalis penis profunda
deep epigastric vein	
deep facial vein	vena faciei profunda
deep femoral vein	vena profunda femoris
deep lingual vein	vena profunda linguae
deep middle cerebral vein	vena cerebri media profunda
deep vein of penis	vena profunda penis
deep temporal veins	venae temporales profundae
digital veins	venae digitales
diploic vein	vena diploica
dorsal callosal vein	vena corporis callosi dorsalis
dorsal veins of clitoris	venae dorsales clitoridis
dorsal vein of corpus callosum	vena corporis callosi dorsalis
dorsal digital veins of foot	venae digitales dorsales pedis
dorsal digital veins of toes	
dorsal lingual vein	venae dorsales linguae
dorsal metacarpal veins	venae metacarpeae dorsales
dorsal metatarsal veins	venae metatarseae dorsales
dorsal veins of penis, deep	vena dorsalis profunda penis
dorsal scapular vein	vena scapularis dorsalis
dorsispinal veins	
emissary vein	vena emissaria
emulgent vein	
epigastric veins, superior	venae epigastricae superiores
episcleral veins	venae episclerales
esophageal veins	venae esophageae
ethmoidal veins	venae ethmoidales
external iliac vein	vena iliaca externa
external jugular vein	vena jugularis externa
external nasal veins	venae nasales externae
external pudendal veins	venae pudendae externae
eyelids, veins of	
facial vein	vena facialis
femoral vein	vena femoralis

vein	vena (pl. venae)
fibular veins	venae fibulares
frontal veins	venae frontales
Galen, veins of	venae internae cerebri
gastric veins	venae gastricae
gastroepiploic vein, left	vena gastro-omentalis sinistra
gastroepiploic vein, right	vena gastro-omentalis dextra
gastro-omental vein, left	vena gastro-omentalis sinistra
gastro-omental vein, right	vena gastro-omentalis dextra
genicular veins	venae geniculares
gluteal veins, inferior	venae gluteae inferiores
gluteal veins, superior	venae gluteae superiores
great cardiac vein	vena cordis magna
great cerebral vein	
great cerebral vein of Galen	vena cerebri magna
great vein of Galen	
great saphenous vein	vena saphena magna
hemiazygos vein	vena hemiazygos
hemorrhoidal veins	venae rectales
hepatic veins	venae hepaticae
hepatic portal vein	
highest intercostal vein	vena intercostalis suprema
hypogastric vein	vena iliaca interna
ileal veins	venae ileales
ileocolic vein	vena ileocolica
iliac vein, common	vena iliaca communis
iliac vein, external	vena iliaca externa
iliac vein, internal	vena iliaca interna
iliolumbar vein	vena iliolumbalis
inferior anastomotic vein	vena anastomotica inferior
inferior basal vein	vena basalis inferior
inferior cardiac vein	
inferior veins of cerebellar hemisphere	venae hemispherii cerebelli inferiores
inferior cerebral veins	venae cerebri inferiores
inferior choroid vein	vena choroidea inferior
inferior epigastric vein	vena epigastrica inferior
inferior eyelid veins	
inferior gluteal veins	venae gluteae inferiores
inferior hemorrhoidal veins	
inferior labial vein	vena labialis inferior

vein	vena (pl. venae)
inferior laryngeal vein	vena laryngea inferior
inferior mesenteric vein	vena mesenterica inferior
inferior ophthalmic vein	vena ophthalmica inferior
inferior palpebral veins	venae palpebrales inferiores
inferior phrenic vein	vena phrenica inferior
inferior rectal veins	venae rectales inferiores
inferior thalamostriate veins	venae thalamostriatae inferiores
inferior thyroid vein	vena thyroidea inferior
inferior ventricular vein	vena ventricularis inferior
inferior vein of vermis	vena vermis inferior
innominate veins	venae brachiocephalicae
innominate cardiac veins (Vieussens' veins)	
insular veins	venae insulares
intercapitular veins	venae intercapitales
intercostal veins	venae intercostales
interlobar veins of kidney	venae interlobares renis
interlobular veins of kidney	venae interlobulares renis
interlobular veins of liver	venae interlobulares hepatis
intermediate antebrachial vein	
intermediate basilic vein	vena intermedia basilica
intermediate cephalic vein	vena intermedia cephalica
intermediate colic vein	vena colica media
intermediate cubital vein	
intermediate vein of forearm	
internal auditory veins	
internal cerebral veins	venae cerebri internae
internal iliac vein	vena iliaca interna
internal jugular vein	vena jugularis interna
internal pudendal vein	vena pudenda interna
internal thoracic vein	vena thoracica interna
interosseous veins	venae interosseae
intersegmental veins	pars intersegmentalis
intervertebral vein	vena intervertebralis
intrasegmental veins	pars intrasegmentalis
jejunal and ileal veins	venae jejunales et ilei
jugular veins	venae jejunales
key vein	
kidney, veins of	venae renis
knee, veins of	venae genus

vein	vena (pl. venae)
Krukenberg's veins	venae centrales hepatis
Labbe's vein (acute e)	vena anastomotica inferior
labial veins	venae labiales
labyrinthine veins	venae labyrinthi
lacrimal vein	vena lacrimalis
large vein	vena magna
large saphenous vein	vena saphena magna
laryngeal vein, superior	vena laryngea superior
Latarget's vein	
lateral atrial vein	vena atrii lateralis
lateral circumflex femoral veins	venae circumflexae femoris laterales
lateral direct veins	venae directae laterales
lateral vein of lateral ventricle	vena atrii lateralis
lateral recess of fourth ventricle, vein of	vena recessus lateralis ventriculi quarti
lateral sacral veins	venae sacrales laterales
lateral thoracic vein	vena thoracica lateralis
left colic vein	vena colica sinistra
left coronary vein	vena coronaria sinistra
left gastric vein	vena gastrica sinistra
left gastroepiploic vein	vena gastro-omentalis sinistra
left gastro-omental vein	vena gastro-omentalis sinistra
left hepatic veins	venae hepaticae sinistrae
left inferior pulmonary vein	vena pulmonalis inferior sinistra
left ovarian vein	vena ovarica sinistra
left superior intercostal vein	vena intercostalis superior sinistra
left superior pulmonary vein	vena pulmonalis superior sinistra
left suprarenal vein	vena suprarenalis sinistra
left testicular vein	vena testicularis sinistra
left umbilical vein	vena umbilicalis sinistra
levoatrio-cardinal vein	
lingual vein	vena lingualis
long saphenous vein	vena saphena longus
long thoracic vein	vena thoracica longus
lumbar veins	venae lumbales
Marshall's oblique vein	
masseteric veins	venae massetericae
mastoid emissary vein	vena emissaria mastoidea
maxillary vein	vena maxillaris
Mayo's vein	

vein	vena (pl. venae)
medial atrial vein	vena atrii medialis
medial circumflex femoral veins	venae circumflexae femoris mediales
medial vein of lateral ventricle	vena atrii medialis
median antebrachial vein	vena intermedia antebrachii
median basilic vein	vena intermedia basilic
median cephalic vein	vena intermedia cephalica
median cubital vein	vena intermedia cubiti
median vein of forearm	vena intermedia antebrachii
median vein of neck	vena mediana colli
median sacral vein	vena sacralis mediana
mediastinal veins	venae mediastinales
median vein	vena intermedia
medulla oblongata, veins of	venae medullae oblongatae
meningeal veins	venae meningeae
mesencephalic veins	venae mesencephalicae
mesenteric vein, inferior	vena mesenterica inferior
mesenteric vein, superior	vena mesenterica superior
metacarpal veins	venae metacarpales
middle cardiac vein	vena cordis media
middle colic vein	vena colica media
middle hemorrhoidal veins	venae rectales mediae
middle hepatic veins	venae hepaticae mediae
middle meningeal veins	venae meningeae mediae
middle rectal veins	venae rectales mediae
middle temporal vein	vena temporalis media
middle thyroid vein	vena thyroidea media
musculophrenic veins	venae musculophrenicae
nasofrontal vein	vena nasofrontalis
oblique vein of left atrium	vena obliqua atrii sinistri
obturator vein	vena obturatoria
occipital vein	vena occipitalis
occipital cerebral veins	venae occipitales
occipital emissary vein	vena emissaria occipitalis
olfactory gyrus, vein of	vena gyri olfactorii
ophthalmic vein, inferior	vena ophthalmica inferior
ophthalmic vein, superior	vena ophthalmica superior
ovarian vein, left	vena ovarica sinistra
ovarian vein, right	vena ovarica dextra
palatine vein	vena palatina

vein	vena (pl. venae)
palmar digital veins	venae digitales palmares
palmar metacarpal veins	venae metacarpeae palmares
palpebral veins	venae palpebrales
pancreatic veins	venae pancreaticae
pancreaticoduodenal veins	venae pancreaticoduodenales
paraumbilical veins	venae paraumbilicales
parietal veins	venae parietales
parietal emissary vein	vena emissaria parietalis
parotid veins	venae parotidea
pectoral veins	venae pectorales
peduncular veins	venae pedunculares
perforating veins	venae perforantes
pericardiac veins	venae pericardiales
pericardiacophrenic veins	venae pericardiacophrenicae
pericardial veins	venae pericardiacae
peroneal veins	venae peroneae
petrosal vein	vena petrosa
pharyngeal veins	venae pharyngeae
phrenic veins	venae phrenicae
plantar digital veins	venae digitales plantares
plantar metatarsal veins	venae metatarseae plantares
pontine veins	venae pontis
popliteal vein	vena poplitea
portal vein	vena portae hepatis
posterior anterior jugular vein	vena jugularis posterior anterior
posterior auricular vein	vena auricularis posterior
posterior cardinal veins	
posterior facial vein	vena retromandibularis
posterior horn, vein of	vena cornus posterioris
posterior intercostal veins	venae intercostales posteriores
posterior labial veins	venae labiales posteriores
posterior vein of left ventricle	vena posterior ventriculi sinistri
posterior marginal vein	vena corporis callosi dorsalis
posterior parotid veins	venae parotideae posterioreae
posterior pericallosal vein	vena corporis callosi dorsalis
posterior scrotal veins	venae scrotales posteriores
posterior vein of left ventricle	vena ventriculi sinistri posterior
posterior vein of septum pellucidum	vena septi pellucidi posterior
posterior tibial veins	venae tibiales posteriores

vein	vena (pl. venae)
precardinal veins	
precentral cerebellar vein	vena precentralis cerebelli
prefrontal veins	venae prefrontales
prepyloric vein	vena prepylorica
pterygoid canal, vein of	vena canalis pterygoidei
pudendal veins	venae pudendae
pulmonary veins	venae pulmonales
pyloric vein	vena gastrica dextra
radial veins	venae radiales
ranine vein	vena sublingualis
rectal veins	venae rectales
renal veins	venae renales
retromandibular vein	vena retromandibularis
Retzius' veins	
right colic vein	vena colica dextra
right gastric vein	vena gastrica dextra
right gastroepiploic vein	vena gastro-omentalis dextra
right gastro-omental vein	vena gastro-omentalis dextra
right hepatic veins	venae hepaticae dextrae
right inferior pulmonary vein	vena pulmonalis inferior dextra
right ovarium vein	vena ovarica dextra
right superior intercostal vein	vena intercostalis superior dextra
right superior pulmonary vein	vena pulmonalis superior dextra
right suprarenal vein	vena suprarenalis dextra
right testicular vein	vena testicularis dextra
Rosenthal's vein	
Ruysch's veins	
sacral veins	venae sacrales
Santorini's vein	
saphenous veins	venae saphenae
Sappey's veins	venae paraumbilicales
scleral veins	venae sclerales
scrotal veins	venae scrotales
septum pellucidum, vein of, anterior	vena anterior septi pellucidi
septum pellucidum, vein of, posterior	vena posterior septi pellucidi
short gastric veins	venae gastricae breves
short saphenous vein	vena saphena breve
sigmoid veins	venae sigmoideae
small vein of heart	vena cardiaca parva

vein	vena (pl. venae)
small cardiac vein	vena cordis parva
smallest cardiac veins	venae cordis minimae
small saphenous vein	vena saphena parva
spermatic vein	vena spermatica
spinal veins	venae spinales
spiral vein of modiolus	vena spiralis modioli
splenic vein	vena splenica
stellate veins of kidney	venulae stellatae renis
Stensen's veins	venae vorticosae
sternocleidomastoid vein	vena sternocleidomastoidea
striate veins	venae thalamostriatae inferiores
stylomastoid vein	vena stylomastoidea
subclavian vein	vena subclavia
subcostal vein	vena subcostalis
subcutaneous veins of abdomen	venae subcutaneae abdominis
sublingual vein	vena sublingualis
sublobular veins	
submental vein	vena submentalis
superficial vein	vena superficialis
superficial cerebral veins	venae cerebri superficiales
superficial circumflex iliac ven	vena circumflexa iliaca superficialis
superficial dorsal veins of clitoris	venae dorsales clitoridis superficiales
superficial dorsal veins of penis	venae dorsales penis superficiales
superficial epigastric vein	vena epigastrica superficialis
superficial middle cerebral vein	vena cerebri media superficialis
superficial temporal veins	venae temporales superficiales
superior anastomotic vein	vena anastomotica superior
superior basal vein	vena basalis superior
superior veins of cerebellar hemisphere	venae hemispherii cerebelli superiores
superior cerebral veins	venae cerebri superiores
superior choroid vein	vena choroidea superior
superior epigastric veins	venae epigastricae superiores
superior eyelid, veins of	
superior gluteal veins	venae gluteae superiores
superior hemorrhoidal vein	vena rectales superior
superior intercostal vein	vena intercostalis superior
superior labial vein	vena labialis superior
superior laryngeal vein	vena laryngea superior
superior mesenteric vein	vena mesenterica superior

vein	vena (pl. venae)
superior ophthalmic vein	vena ophthalmica superior
superior palpebral veins	venae palpebrales superiores
superior phrenic veins	venae phrenicae superiores
superior rectal vein	vena rectalis superior
superior thalamostriate vein	vena thalamostriata superior
superior thyroid vein	vena thyroidea superior
superior vein of vermis	vena vermis superior
supraorbital vein	vena supraorbitalis
suprarenal veins	venae suprarenales
suprascapular vein	vena suprascapularis
supratrochlear veins	venae supratrochleares
supreme intercostal vein	vena intercostalis suprema
sural veins	venae surales
surface thalamic veins	venae directae laterales
sylvian vein, vein of sylvian fossa	vena mediae superficiales cerebri
temporal veins	venae temporales
temporomandibular joint, veins of	venae articulares temporomandibulares
temporomaxillary vein	vena temporomaxillaris
terminal vein	vena thalamostriata superior
testicular veins	venae testiculares
thalamostriate veins	venae thalamostriatae
thebesian veins	venae cordis minimae
thoracic veins	venae thoracicae
thoracoacromial vein	vena thoracoacromialis
thoracoepigastric vein	vena thoracoepigastrica
thymic veins	venae thymicae
thyroid veins	venae thyroideae
tibial veins	venae tibiales
trabecular veins	
tracheal veins	venae tracheales
transverse cervical veins	venae transversae colli
transverse facial vein	vena transversa faciei
transverse veins of neck	venae transversae cervicis
transverse vein of scapula	venae transversae scapulae
Trolard's vein	vena anastomotica superior
tympanic veins	venae tympanicae
ulnar veins	venae ulnares
umbilical vein	vena umbilicalis
uncus, vein of	vena unci

vein	vena (pl. venae)
upper limb, veins of	venae membri superioris
uterine veins	venae uterinae
varicose veins	
vena cava, inferior	vena cava inferior
vena cava, superior	vena cava superior
ventricular veins of heart	venae ventriculares cordis
vermis, inferior vein of	vena inferior vermis
vertebral vein	vena vertebralis
vertebral column, veins of	venae columnae vertebralis
vesalian vein	
Vesalius' vein	
vesical veins	venae vesicales
vestibular veins	venae vestibulares
vestibular aqueduct, vein of	vena aqueductus vestibuli
vestibular bulb, vein of	vena bulbi vestibuli
vidian veins	venae canalis pterygoidei
Vieussens' veins	venae cardiacae anteriores
vitelline vein	vena vitellina
vortex veins (vorticose veins)	venae vorticosae